# JUDGMENTS OF RESPONSIBILITY

# JUDGMENTS OF RESPONSIBILITY

## A Foundation for a Theory of Social Conduct

### BERNARD WEINER
*University of California, Los Angeles*

**THE GUILFORD PRESS**
New York   London

© 1995 The Guilford Press
A Division of Guilford Publications, Inc.
72 Spring Street, New York, NY 10012

Printed in the United States of America

This book is printed on acid-free paper.

Last digit is print number:  9   8   7   6   5   4   3   2   1

$35- MW 8-7-96 (BX)

Library of Congress Cataloging-in-Publication Data

Weiner, Bernard, 1935–
    Judgments of responsibility : a foundation for a theory of social conduct / Bernard Weiner.
        p.     cm.
    Includes bibliographical references and index.
    ISBN 0-89862-843-1.
    1. Responsibility.   2. Stigma (Social psychology)   3. Ethics.
4. Social ethics.   I. Title
BJ1451.W45   1995
153.8—dc20                                          95-119
                                                         CIP

*To Miina*

You ask what is the use of classification, arrangement, and systematization? I answer you: order and simplification are the first steps toward the mastery of a subject.

—THOMAS MANN (*The Magic Mountain*)

The core, ethical concepts in which you most passionately believe are the language in which you are writing. These concepts probably feel like givens, like things no one ever had to make up, that have been true through all cultures and for all time. Telling these truths is your job. You have nothing else to tell us. But needless to say, you can't tell them in a sentence or a paragraph; the truth doesn't come out in bumper stickers. . . . Your whole piece is the truth, not just one shining epigrammatic moment in it. There will need to be some kind of unfolding in order to contain it, and there will need to be layers. We are dealing with the ineffable here—we're out there somewhere between the known and the unknown, trying to reel in both for a closer look. That is why it may take a whole book.

—ANNE LAMOTT (*Bird by Bird*)

# Acknowledgments

I began this book when I was a Visiting Professor at the University of Washington in the Spring of 1992, and completed it about two years later in the Spring of 1994 at my home institution, the University of California, Los Angeles (UCLA). Thirty years at UCLA have provided me with invaluable help from many students, both undergraduates and graduates; postdoctoral fellows and scholars, both American and foreign-born; and granting agencies, both intramural and extramural. The book was written while I was supported by a grant from the National Science Foundation, DBS 9211982, which was awarded because of the efforts of the co-principal (in reality, principal) investigator, Sandra Graham. I was simultaneously supported by a small grant from UCLA; these yearly sums have greatly contributed to my ability to write and conduct research. Over the years, I have benefited greatly from the contributions of the "Attribution Elders," a group of former doctoral students still located in the Los Angeles area—Jim Amirkhan, Hector Betancourt, Valerie Folkes, Sandra Graham, and Steve Lopez. Sandra Graham, in particular, contributed to this book with many important suggestions. Kathleen Nelson was my wonderful assistant, and Carol Krepack and Khanh-Van Bui provided invaluable help. Jaana Juvonen, my spouse, made my life richer and enabled me to persist in this sustained masochism.

# Preface

In writing this book, I came to understand that I had spent much of my academic life trying to explain the findings of one of my early publications, namely, that lack of effort as a cause of failure gives rise to greater reprimand from ourselves than does failure caused by absence of ability. It was sobering to think that my career had been focused on an observation that might be considered trivial and that I had not deemed very important when I first recorded those findings. Nevertheless, I also came to realize that there has been a coherence and a systematic progression in my thinking, even though I was not always consciously aware of that direction. I am puzzled as to why it took me thirty years to get to this point in my understanding, when in hindsight it appears as though the process should have taken only one or two years.

I have also been surprised to find myself looking to the legal system and to theology for clues about social motivation, whereas my training as a graduate student prepared me to think of motivation as being mathematically quantifiable. But such beliefs are far behind me. I now identify myself simply as someone who arranges, classifies, and systematizes common sense. In doing so, I attempt to develop as broad and as parsimonious a conceptual system as possible to explain everyday social conduct. If what I write strikes the reader as both true and obvious, then, in a certain sense, I have succeeded. Such a response confirms the empirical validity of my conceptual system and leaves me free to go about understanding the more specific rules of the social universe.

My goal in this book has been to identify some of the rules of social motivation. The empirical facts I have used to derive these principles have come from studying people's evaluation of achievement, their reactions to people who have been stigmatized, the way they give help to others, their aggression, and the way they manage others' impressions of them by making excuses and confessing. Hence, knowledge of these rules can be of great use to individuals in a variety of disciplines, including educational psychology, personality psychology, and clinical psychology. I like to think that there is at least something in here for many psychologists and, I hope, much for those in motivation and social psychology.

This book will also be useful as a text in academic courses and seminars that deal with the subjects of attribution theory, responsibility, social motivation, and stigmatization, and as a supplementary source in courses that deal with aggression, emotion, helping behavior, impression management, motivation, and social psychology. I have written the book primarily for professionals and graduate students, but the level of writing is within easy reach of undergraduate students as well.

# Contents

# 1

---

# The Anatomy
# of Responsibility

Let him who is without sin among you cast the first stone.
—JOHN 8:7

Judge not that ye not be judged, for with what judgment ye judge ye
shall be judged.
—MATT. 7:1

Blaming is one of the more useless human responses.
—SPINOZA

In everyday life, one is constantly confronted with questions and issues
related to responsibility, blame, and punishment. One need only open the
daily paper to confirm this. In the news section or on the editorial page we
read: Who or what is responsible for the urban riots, and what should be
done to prevent such horrors? Why are there so many homeless people? Is
this their own fault? Or we read on the sports page: Who or what is
responsible for the losses of our favorite team? Do we blame the manager,
or should we be angry at the players?

At times, responsibility appears evident and we may read about the
actions that have followed this belief. For example, we learn that a gifted
athlete is "loafing," a game was lost, and that the athlete has been fined and
"benched" by the manager. Conversely, there may be positive actions
toward another because it is inferred that this person is not responsible for
some painful state. For example, a recent widower is offered sympathy,

*1*

help, and support; or people embrace a handicapped child as she un-successfully tries to complete a race in the Special Olympics.

Stimulated by these everyday occurrences, this book examines respon-sibility, blame, anger, sympathy, punishment, and other social responses, as well as their interconnections and role in guiding human conduct. For many years, issues related to these concepts and phenomena have been central in the study of philosophy, theology, and jurisprudence. This leng-thy history, as well as the prevalent usage of these terms in daily life, provides both benefits and barriers to the research psychologist. On the positive side, languages have been formulated, distinctions have been drawn, and terms have been defined. There is much to gain from the foundation provided by our rich heritage. However, few psychologists have the courage (hubris?) to tackle issues about which Aristotle has writ-ten an entire treatise; few scientists have the capability of understanding the complex and diverse pertinent knowledge generated by philosophers, the-ologians, and legal scholars; and few researchers are willing to face the difficulties created by the idiosyncratic everyday uses of the relevant con-cepts. These historical and naive encumbrances may account for the pauc-ity of psychologists presently addressing issues associated with the relations between perceived responsibility, emotional reactions, and social conduct, in spite of the manifest centrality of this subject matter in our ongoing lives.

I also fear examining the same topic as did Aristotle; I accept that even marginal mastery of the arguments and reasoning of philosophers, theo-logians, and judges is beyond my capability; and the disparities in the layperson's utilization of the concepts considered in this book indeed create difficulties for a psychological analysis. My aims, therefore, are modest, and as an experimental social psychologist I must plow a different field than that which has been harvested by the nonempirical disciplines, while at the same time it is important to recognize and incorporate what has been reaped in these other areas of study.

Two primary goals are pursued in this book. The first goal is to docu-ment the extensity of judgments of the responsibilities of others in everyday life and their emotional and behavioral consequences. In many ways we are moral vigilantes. This intention is descriptive, although I think of this as insightful description in the sense that the readers may be made aware of truths that they have not consciously recognized. To aid in this discovery, a series of experiments for you to perform are included in the book to provide experiential knowledge. It will become evident in the course of the book that judgments of responsibility and their significance are abundant when we view achievement contexts (Chapter 2); when we consider the plights of stigmatized others, including alcoholics, the obese, and the poor (Chapter 3); when we look at homosexuals and those with AIDS (Chapter 4); when we react to the depressed, the schizophrenic, and distressed spouses (Chapter 5); when we help someone in need (Chapter 6); when we examine family abuse and aggressive retaliation (Chapter 7); and when we listen to excuses, justifications, and confessions (Chapter 8). These generally are not criminal contexts, where it is known that a central issue is to determine personal (i.e., moral) culpability. Rather, many of these situations are encountered during the course of a normal day.

So prevalent is the tendency to find if others are responsible for an event or a personal difficulty that religious tenets and secular philosophers advise us to forgo such judgments, as revealed in the quotations at the beginning of the chapter ("Let him who is without sin among you cast the first stone," "Judge not that ye not be judged, for with what judgment ye judge ye shall be judged," "Blaming is one of the more useless human responses"). But this advice has not been heeded.

My second goal for this book is theoretical—namely, to extend an attributional theory of motivation that relates thoughts and emotions to behavior. Attributional approaches in motivation have been most prominent and best applied in the achievement domain, where it has been documented that perceptions of the causes of success and failure, such as ability, effort, and luck, give rise to affects including pride and guilt. These causal thoughts and feelings, in turn, guide subsequent achievement strivings (Weiner, 1985, 1986). In the present book, it is documented that causal beliefs give rise to inferences about personal responsibility, which, in turn, generate feelings of anger and sympathy. These thoughts and feelings then direct social behavior toward others. Thus, an attributional framework that includes causal perceptions, emotions, and actions is applicable to both other- and self-perception, as well as to interpersonal behaviors and achievement strivings.

The goals of description and theory building pursued in this book are guided by two metaphors pertinent to human motivation. The history of the study of motivation has been directed by metaphors, such as the person is a machine or the person is a scientist, that suggest new ways of looking at conduct and fresh research paths (see Weiner, 1991a). One metaphor adopted here is that humans are Godlike. Hence, like God, they regard themselves as having the right or legitimacy to judge others as good or bad, innocent or guilty, or responsible or not responsible for an event or a personal plight. These inferences then give rise to affective reactions that also are ascribed to God, including anger and compassion. However, as "fair" or "just" Gods, the defendants are permitted to offer excuses, justifications, or confessions for their actions. The transgressor is then "sentenced." For example, consider the situation of a husband failing to appear at a designated time to go to a movie. The waiting wife believes that the errant husband went somewhere else instead. Because of this inference of intent and responsibility, the wife is angry and upon seeing the partner refuses to speak to him. The husband then confesses to his "sin" and asks for forgiveness, promising never to do this again. The wife is merciful and withdraws the sentence!

Very closely related to this Godlike metaphor is the metaphor that life is a courtroom where interpersonal dramas are played out and where we judge one another, gather information to determine causality and responsibility, allow for self-defense, pass sentences, consider parole, and so on. As will be seen, throughout this book the language of the courtroom and associated theological tenets related to punishment and justice are brought to bear upon social interactions.

## A SHORT STORY: THE RESPONSIBILITY PROCESS

Let me now introduce a vignette that directs the reader to thinking about perceived responsibility and its linkage to motivation and conduct. Imagine that one evening you are carefully driving home when suddenly there is a bang and a crash at the rear of your car. The trunk flies open and your car is pushed forward. Given this incident, you are likely to emerge from your automobile and immediately initiate a negative exchange with the driver of the car in back of you.

I believe that the process intervening between this adverse event and the behavioral reaction is quite complex, with many component parts. The temporal sequence is not readily discernible in the situation that was described, for the reaction may have been automatic (scripted) or the process so rapid that you, as well as any observers, were unaware of the sequential components. However, it is possible to logically as well as experimentally demonstrate the psychological steps intervening between the crash (the external stimulus) and the shouting at the rear driver (the behavioral response).

The notion that a psychological reaction has multiple inputs and sequential antecedents that are only discernible with experimental procedures and/or dialectical analyses that decompose the process is not new in social psychology or motivation. For example, the influential Schachter and Singer (1962) conception of emotion postulates that the fear one experiences at the sight of a gun is generated by two elements: arousal and the perceived situational cause of that arousal. The individual who experiences the fear, as well as observers, is unaware of these multiple and sequential influences. Schachter and Singer (1962), however, crafted an experimental situation to separate the component parts. Regardless of what one believes about the success of this attempt (see Reisenzein, 1983), Schachter and Singer's analysis is valuable in pointing out that one can isolate parts of an integrated process that is outside of the conscious awareness of the involved individual.

To aid in understanding the steps proposed as intervening between the crash and the shouting, there already exists a psychological literature concerned with this process. Three psychologists have been particularly active in exploring the pertinent issues, namely, Frank Fincham (e.g., Fincham & Roberts, 1985; Fincham & Shultz, 1981), Kelly Shaver (e.g., Shaver, 1985; Shaver & Drown, 1986), and Thomas Shultz (e.g., Shultz, Schleifer, & Altman, 1981; Shultz & Wright, 1985). I will not discuss the positions of these researchers in any detail, nor will I examine the differences between their individual positions and the scheme that I propose here. Rather, taking some liberties, these authors would interpret the mechanisms and processes that intervene between the car crash and the shouting in the following way. After the outcome, the person determines what caused the event. Under some specific conditions, another person will be held responsible—that is, there is what is called an "attribution of responsibility." Being held responsible then gives rise to blame. Blame, in turn, generates retaliation and punishment.

Thus, the motivational sequence as envisioned by Fincham, Shaver, and Shultz can be depicted as:

$$\text{Outcome} \rightarrow \text{Causal determination} \rightarrow \text{Responsibility} \rightarrow \text{Blame} \rightarrow \text{Punishment}$$

This process is based on the following premises:

1. Causal ascriptions must be distinguished from judgments of responsibility.
2. Responsibility inferences must be distinguished from blame.
3. Attributions of responsibility indirectly influence punishment and other social responses through the mediating reaction of blame. Hence, responsibility attributions and their consequences are part of a sequential process with component parts.

To provide some tests of the Fincham, Shaver, and Shultz positions, let me logically alter some of the conditions in the car crash scenario and imagine how this might change the reader's reactions to this event were he or she the driver of the car. This also will provide me with an opportunity to offer theoretical changes to the prior proposals that I regard as essential. The scenarios that are introduced might be considered *Gedankenexperiments*) ("thought experiments"), which was Fritz Heider's (1958) dominant method of scientific inquiry. The conditions that I will alter or vary depend on thoughts based, in part, on the writings of Fincham, Shaver, and

Shultz, as well as on the positions of philosophers and experts in jurisprudence (e.g., Hart, 1968; Hart & Honoré, 1959; Morse, 1992). The scenarios that I will describe are designed to illuminate six distinctions, discussed in the following pages, that I regard as necessary to understand the responsibility process. These contrasts include personal versus impersonal causality, controllability versus uncontrollability, personal controllability versus responsibility, intention versus negligence, responsibility versus blame, and blame versus anger.

## Personal versus Impersonal Causality

Imagine that as you emerge from your car, shouting and ready to engage in battle with the driver of the auto in the rear, it is discovered that a rock from a nearby hill has fallen on your back bumper. Anger and confrontation now give way to a search for where the rock had come from and for other causal information pertinent to your fate. You are still feeling "bad": demoralized, knowing that the car has to be repaired yet again; depressed about the anticipated cost; frustrated because of the time delay; and so on. But the moral judgment of holding another responsible is no longer being called forth by the situation (until you begin to wonder if the rock may have been thrown or pushed by someone on the hill).

It is evident from this vignette that causal judgments need not implicate personal causality. Rain might be the cause of a ruined picnic, an economic recession can be the cause of a business failure, and a falling rock can be the cause of car damage. In these examples, a person or a group of individuals is not held accountable for the negative outcomes. It is postulated that the assignment of responsibility requires human or personal agency (although, on some occasions, other self-initiating agents, such as a cat or dog, may be held responsible for wrecking the couch, and even God can be considered responsible for moving the rock). Given the above premise, in the prior vignette about the accident it would be appropriate to state that the rock *caused* the damage to the car, but not that the rock was *responsible* for that damage (although the latter usage may be heard in daily discourse).

There are many examples in which inferences of personal causality are made, such as a picnic canceled because of poor planning, a business failure ascribed to insufficient effort or trying, and an accident caused by another driver's speeding. Judgments of responsibility *may* then be reached, depending on other information. Inferences of responsibility, therefore, require causal beliefs of human involvement, or personal causality. But not all causal beliefs implicate personal responsibility—that is, in distinction to some psychologists (e.g., Brewer, 1977), a judgment of responsibility is not to be equated with a judgment of causality.

In sum, it is contended that an assignment of responsibility has as a first step a distinction between person versus situation causality, or thoughts about what has been called the locus of causality (see Heider, 1958; Weiner, 1986). It again and again has been documented that causal location is one of the main dimensions or properties of causal thinking. Implicit in the accident vignette was that the owner of the smashed car assumed the rear driver to be causally involved (prior to finding the rock). This might have been revealed in an accusation such as, "Look what *you* have done!" It has been suggested that there is a tendency to first search for a human agent since this makes disorderly occurrences orderly and permits us to put these causes within our future control (see Gilbert, Pelham, & Krull, 1988). Indeed, a tendency to perceive dispositional causality is considered one of the fundamental tenets of attribution theory (see Ross & Nisbett, 1991).

## Controllability versus Uncontrollability

As already indicated, in the initial car crash scenario the party that was hit implicitly assumed that the rear driver was the cause of the crash. In the absence of this belief, it is contended that shouting and confrontation would not have followed. But human involvement is just the first step in this process and does not necessarily result in an assignment of personal responsibility.

To clarify why personal causality is a necessary but not a sufficient antecedent for the assignment of responsibility, let me return to the accident story and add additional information as well as a second thought experiment. Assume that the accident was indeed caused by the rear driver but that prior to the crash the rear driver had a heart attack and fainted. Quite typically, this fact would not be available to whoever was hit. If it were, however, then it is presumed that a judgment of responsibility (as opposed to a judgment of causality) would not be rendered.

In other situations, the uncontrollability of a cause—its nonamenability to volitional change or willful regulation—is known by others. For example, if failure is caused by a lack of aptitude, if obesity is caused by a thyroid problem, and if poor performance at a sport is caused by lack of physical coordination, then the cause is located within the person but cannot be controlled. Teachers are likely to be aware of the low aptitude of a student, parents are likely to be knowledgeable about the thyroid condition of their child, and peers know of the physical limitations of their teammates. In these instances, it is asserted that the person will not be judged as responsible for a negative event or a personal plight because accountability requires that the causes of these conditions can be willfully changed. Responsibility, therefore, is intimately linked with freedom and choice.

On the other hand, failure because of lack of effort, obesity because of overeating, and causing a car accident because of fast or inattentive driving all can result in an assignment of responsibility because one can try or not, overeat or not, drive fast or slowly, and so on. Responsibility thus necessitates *internal and controllable* causality. Just as locus is known to be a basic property of phenomenal causality, so is causal controllability (see Weiner, 1986).

An inability to inhibit one's actions also can result in the cause of a negative event being perceived as uncontrollable and, therefore, can result in the person not being held responsible. So-called "crimes of passion" have produced judgments of nonresponsibility because it was presumed that the vengeful individuals in such crimes could not inhibit their retaliation (*passion* has the same linguistic root as *passive*—thus, one is "overcome with passion"). However, this supposed "irresistible impulse" was often used as a false pretext for very intentional and controllable acts against women.

A conceptually similar situation occurred in the movie classic *M*, with Peter Lorre. Lorre's character pleaded for leniency even though in this movie he was a child murderer. He argued that he "must" kill and could not prevent himself. Because he was "compelled," he declared that he was less morally culpable than the typical robber, who had a free choice to engage or not to engage in antisocial conduct. In the movie, Lorre's character is apprehended, but the director does not tell the audience if he is convicted!

In sum, an assignment of responsibility requires that there be a controllable cause of a negative event. It was the Church that first demanded that "inner facts" in addition to the amount of damage ("strict liability") be considered in the assignment of responsibility and punishment. This was because ecclesiastical law was particularly concerned with culpability and sin. This religious concern and point of view was eventually incorporated into legal proceedings.

## Causal Controllability versus Responsibility

In my prior writings, I tended not to make a distinction between causal controllability and responsibility, considering them as synonyms. But now I believe that I erred in my prior conceptual analysis: Causal controllability is not to be equated with responsibility. Controllability refers to the characteristics of a cause—causes, such as the absence of effort or lack of aptitude, are or are not subject to volitional alteration. Responsibility, on the other hand, refers to a judgment made about a person—he or she "should" or "ought to have" done otherwise, such as trying harder, eating less, or paying more attention when driving. The responsibility inference process is presumed initially to focus on causal understanding and then to shift to a consideration of the person. In a manner akin to the well-known sequence going "from acts to dispositions" (Jones & Davis, 1965), here it is being suggested that thoughts progress from a causal attribution to an inference about the person. Responsibility, therefore, is not an attribution, as others including Fincham and Shaver contend, and in this book I prefer the terms *assignment, inference,* or *judgment of responsibility,* reserving *attribution* for an exclusive linkage with causality.

## Mitigating Circumstances

There is another reason to distinguish causal controllability from responsibility. Even if the cause of an adverse event is located within the person and that cause is controllable by the individual, it still is possible that a judgment of responsibility will not be rendered. This is because there may be mitigating circumstances that negate moral responsibility. *To mitigate* means "to soften or alleviate"; hence, mitigating circumstances soften, alleviate, or totally eliminate judgments of responsibility about a person.

In the accident scenario, consider yet another thought experiment. In this situation, imagine the somewhat far-fetched possibility that the driver bumped into your car because you were headed toward an embankment that could not be seen and that was the driver's only means of stopping you, thereby saving your life. Knowing this fact would immediately result in the offset of culpability.

In other situations, mitigating circumstances are somewhat easier to introduce. Consider, for example, a business failure that is due to insufficient job-related effort. Inasmuch as goal-directed effort is located within a person and is controllable, the conditions have been met to reach a verdict of strong responsibility for failure. But now imagine that the lack of job effort was due to the time spent personally caring for a sick family member. Because of this justification (the act serves a higher moral goal), adults will not hold the person responsible for the business failure (i.e., it might be said that this cause is discounted) (see Kelley, 1972). Rather, the cause of the loss is the sick person (who, in turn, also is unlikely to be held morally accountable unless the sickness could have been prevented or ended by means of willful intervention). But perhaps the most common example of a mitigating circumstance that results in the offset of responsibility because the action serves a higher goal is the police's intentionally harming a person who is about to harm others!

Mitigating circumstances do not always involve justifications, or other moral goals. Mitigators also are inferred given incapacity on the part of the wrongdoer. Inability to comprehend the "wrongness" of an act or to discriminate right from wrong (which differs from an inability to control the behavior), as might be the case with very young children, the insane, or even with persons from other cultures that maintain contrary belief systems, can reduce or totally remove judgments of responsibility (see Kleinke & Baldwin, 1993; Roberts, Golding, & Fincham, 1987). In cases of wills or contracts, infancy, insanity, etc. are called "invalidating conditions." Thus, an adult does not hold an infant responsible for wetting the bed if that child could not prevent it (causal uncontrollability) or does not yet recognize this as "wrong" (mitigating circumstances). But if that child were two or three years of age, then responsibility would be imposed. Evidence has been reported that some types of child abuse are instigated because parents consider very young children responsible for acts that the children may not be able to control or do not perceive as transgressions (see Chapter 7).

As might be imagined, the circumstances that absolve one from responsibility because they are considered mitigating can be a difficult judgment to make, one hotly debated in courts of law as well as by philosophers. For example, assume that a gun is raised to your head and a robber demands to be helped during a robbery. You would not be considered responsible for collecting the wallets and the rings of others. Given this situation, circumstances certainly are mitigating, and moral responsibility is negated. But what if the robber threatened, "Help me or I will shoot you next week," or "Help me or I will give you a bloody nose," or "Help me or I will hit you on the arm"? In these instances, would the circumstances terminate judgments of responsibility?

The recent controversies regarding the "battered wife syndrome" also point out some of the difficulties of determining not only what is and what is not a mitigating circumstance but also when freedom of choice—and, therefore, personal responsibility—is reduced. Some have contended that battered women who kill their mates do not have (or do not perceive) the psychological option of leaving their partner. Hence, these women, who perceive killing as the only way out of a hopeless and life-threatening situation, are not responsible for their homicidal action. A judge, then, must determine whether there was a "realistic" option to leave the abuser or whether the homicide was in fact the only psychologically realistic way to escape. Note that the women were not "compelled" to kill, nor was there duress forcing the action. Nonetheless, their past history of abuse has restricted their freedom to act and, thus, is considered a mitigating circumstance. In a manner similar to "crimes of passion," there must be a separation of an intended and cold-blooded murder from an action that "could not have been otherwise," and this often is a difficult discrimination to make.

Such uncertainty is not restricted to the criminal courts. To consider a more common occurrence, assume that you break a social engagement, stating that you have to take your aged mother shopping. Will the receiver of this information release you from responsibility for the social transgression, or might it be thought that you could have (should have) managed your time better, made a different decision, and so forth? As in legal contexts, it is difficult for the accused to prove the presence of mitigating circumstances. But the onus of proof is on the accused, or the defendant.

## Reflections and Unsettled Issues

To review the discussion thus far, I have contended that judgments of responsibility presuppose human causality. In addition, the cause must be controllable if the person is to be held responsible. Furthermore, responsibility is lessened or entirely lifted if there are mitigating circumstances. The process activated in situations that give rise to judgments of responsibility and their subsequent consequences therefore can be represented with a tree diagram that includes a series of on–off judgments (see Figure 1.1). As shown in Figure 1.1, three separate stages are hypothesized as intervening between the onset of an event and the inference that another person is held responsible for that event. In the first stage, causality is allocated to the person or to the situation. If there is situation causality, then the responsibility process stops, whereas if there is person causality, then the process continues. At the next stage in the process, given person causality, it is determined whether the cause was controllable. If there was uncontrollable causality, then again the process comes to a halt. However, if there was controllable causality, then there is still the possibility of a responsibility decision. Next, it is determined if there were mitigating circumstances. If so, then again responsibility is not inferred. However, if there were no mitigators, then, in conjunction with the prior perceptions of person causality and controllability causality, a responsibility inference is made.

Although the process that has been depicted seems quite reasonable, a number of questions remain. One issue concerns whether this process is an invariant sequence: Must individuals first seek out information about situation versus personal causality, then determine whether that cause was controllable, search for mitigating circumstances, and then decide about responsibility (with the stipulation that a negative answer at any stage terminates the process)? The answer to this is an unequivocal no: This strict processing sequence is not presumed. As already indicated, if one's car is struck in the rear by another car, it is probable that responsibility is immediately imposed, and only later might this be changed if it is learned that a rock was causal (situational causality), that the person had a heart attack prior to the accident (causal uncontrollability), or that the crash was intentional to prevent a more serious accident (mitigating circumstances). That is, as some attributionists have contended, a judgment may first be made and then later invalidated as information is received (see Krull,

1993). Furthermore, one may already be aware that the person who performed a social transgression is a child or is mentally handicapped, so that mitigating circumstances are immediately available that alter the judgment of responsibility.

Thus, what has been outlined is one particular sequence, unconstrained by time requirements or other factors that might impede search and cognitive activities and starting without any preconceptions about responsibility. Furthermore, this sequence is conscious, effortful, and guided by controlled processing. It is not known how frequently or under what conditions this process actually captures the real world of inferences of responsibility, which often may be determined by unconscious and automatic processes, as might be fostered by a particular political ideology or worldview (e.g., minority people fail because of inability, people are responsible for being poor because they do not try, and so on). What is more certain is that the main ingredients, the essential component parts that determine responsibility inferences, are captured in Figure 1.1.

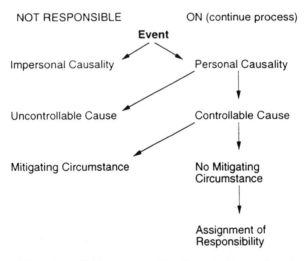

**FIGURE 1.1.** The responsibility process. The figure indicates that the responsibility process is initiated by some event. If there is a judgment of personal causality, then an inference of responsibility may be reached and the process continues. However, if there is impersonal causality, then a judgment of nonresponsibility is rendered and the process stops. The process then proceeds to determine if the cause was controllable or not, and so on. Given personal causality, a controllable cause, and no mitigating circumstances, there is an assignment of responsibility.

## Intention versus Negligence: Degrees of Responsibility

Thus far, a judgment of responsibility has been presented as an on–off decision process, which does not capture its full complexity. Personal causality, causal controllability, the presence or absence of mitigating circumstances, and the assignment of responsibility are not all-or-none inferences but vary in magnitude or degree. This has been only intimated in the discussion of mitigating circumstances, for such circumstances may not decrease responsibility beliefs to zero.

One of the major determinants of judgments of the degree of responsibility is whether a controllable act is perceived as intentionally committed or due to negligence. The differentiation between intention and negligence in the criminal domain directly relates to the distinction between murder and manslaughter or tax fraud and arithmetical error, and in more commonplace contexts the differentiation is pertinent to the difference between not appearing at a party because one did not want to go as opposed to forgetting to go, or between breaking a cup purposefully as opposed to breaking a cup through carelessness. Murder, tax fraud, failure to attend a party because of no desire to go, and purposeful breakage connote intentional actions: The person wanted to perform the socially inappropriate behavior, engaged in the conduct with foresight and knowledge of its consequences, and may even have pursued a variety of means that were responsive to "evasive" actions. As an example, if I aim my car at a person crossing the street but miss and then return to hit that individual as he runs along the sidewalk, the conclusion will be reached that the act was intentionally carried out. My conduct changed to reach my intended goal (labeled by Heider, 1958, as "equi-finality"). In a similar manner, if I say that I cannot attend a party because of a prior engagement and if the date of that party is postponed and I then indicate that I must work at that time, an inference may be made that I do not wish to be at the party (which might, in fact, be incorrect). The cause of the car's hitting the victim and the nonattendance at the party will be perceived as intentional, resulting in a judgment of high responsibility because of the presumption of a "guilty mind" (*mens rea*). It should be noted that in legal contexts the state must prove that the defendant committed the act, but the defendant must prove the "inner fact" of, for example, uncontrollability. That is, the party refuser must convince the party giver that he or she does want to go.

On the other hand, running into a pedestrian because of reckless driving, arithmetical error in a tax report, missing a party because the date was forgotten, and dropping a cup because of carelessness connote unintended actions or unintended consequences of these acts: There was no desire to have these outcomes occur, though they nonetheless did occur. There is perceived responsibility because one ought not to drive fast or make arithmetical errors, should not have forgotten the party, and should be careful when carrying a cup. A reasonable person or, as Chief Justice Holmes stated, "one of ordinary intelligence and reasonable prudence," would have foreseen the possible consequences of these maladaptive behaviors and would have prevented them from happening. Although the causes are internal and controllable, amenable to personal alteration, the individual nonetheless is not judged as harshly as when the act and the outcome were intended. Some philosophers and legal scholars have even argued that unintended acts or outcomes should not be punished inasmuch as an evil deed was not the goal of the person (i.e., there was no "guilty mind"; see review in Hart, 1968).

## CONSEQUENCES OF JUDGMENTS OF RESPONSIBILITY

I now turn from the antecedents or precursors of judgments of responsibility to their emotional and behavioral consequences. I start with a distinction between responsibility and blame because Fincham, Shaver, and Shultz suggest that responsibility judgments give rise to blame, which, in turn, influences social reactions to the person responsible. A fair amount of data have been reported in support of this position (e.g., Fincham & Shultz, 1981; Shultz, Schleifer, & Altman, 1981; Shultz & Wright, 1985).

### Responsibility versus Blame

There are compelling reasons to differentiate responsibility from blame, even though in everyday language at times these might be used interchangeably (e.g., "He is responsible for this mess," or "He is to be blamed for this mess"). The Greek conception of responsibility includes culpability and blameworthiness. But if it is stated, "She is responsible for . . . ," then this could be followed by either "our success" or "our failure." However, if it is said, "She is to be blamed for . . . ," then this can only be concluded with a negative phrase. Thus, independent of context, responsibility is affectively neutral, whereas blame conveys emotional negativity.

Another possible reason to separate responsibility from blame is that a person might be perceived as very responsible for an outcome although there could be little blame. This is because the outcome may be trivial, and outcome magnitude plausibly influences blame but not responsibility. For example, assume that one individual, with foresight and planning, murders another; a second person, with the identical foresight and planning, robs another. Both are fully responsible for their conduct. However, the murderer is likely to be blamed and punished more than the robber. In our system of justice, the harshness of the punishment relates to the amount of harm done. This is a basic principle of retribution. Or, to consider a more mundane example, imagine that a friend of yours fails to show up for a social engagement (e.g., to go to a movie). In one case, only two of you were going, while in a second situation a party of four was to meet. There may be greater blame (but not responsibility) in the former, rather than in the latter, instance because only in the two-person situation might you return home rather than go to the movie. Blame, therefore, appears to be, in part, determined by the magnitude of the consequences of an action, whereas this does not appear to be true regarding inferences of responsibility.

## Blame versus Anger

But is blame the mediator of subsequent social responses toward the transgressor, as has been contended by Fincham, Shaver, and Shultz? I would argue against this position and instead suggest that anger and sympathy mediate between perceptions of responsibility and social action. That is, a sequence of responsibility → anger and/or sympathy → social behavior, rather than responsibility → blame → social behavior is being proposed. Blame appears to be a cognition similar to responsibility, as well as an affect akin to anger. That is, it is a "blend" concept. Hence, I believe that when blame is proposed or demonstrated to mediate between responsibility and action, it is precisely because of its affective component. I therefore prefer to replace blame with the unambiguous emotion of anger (and its obverse, sympathy).

The necessary data to resolve this controversy are not available. This disagreement, therefore, may resemble a regression to an earlier, introspective Titchnerian era in psychology when one psychologist argued that green is neither yellow nor blue and another psychologist contended that green is precisely a combination of these two and is not a distinct color. In a similar manner, psychologists, in my view, have maintained that blame is distinct from responsibility (and perhaps anger), whereas I contend that blame is precisely a combination of these two (see Figure 1.2) and, therefore, does not warrant independent status when considering the sequence of cognitions and emotions that result in social action. The notion of a cognitive–affective blend also has been offered in the analysis of other psychological concepts, including anxiety. Thankfully, the main focus of this book does not require a definitive resolution of this conceptual issue. Nonetheless, a conceptual analysis of blame is of interest academically and contrasts my position with others who have conducted research in this

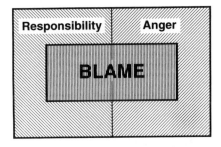

FIGURE 1.2. The association between blame, responsibility, and anger.

area. The separation or inseparation of blame from responsibility and anger is indeed a question that is amenable to empirical resolution.

## The Emotional Repercussions of Judgments of Responsibility

Imagine your feelings when an employee is not performing well because of a lack of trying, when your child is doing poorly in school because of a refusal to do homework, and when an athlete on your favorite team is "loafing." Not only are there thoughts about controllability and responsibility, but there are also feelings of anger. You are mad at the lazy employee, the rebellious child, and the lackadaisical athlete. Of course, the more you are involved with this individual or situation, the more angry you are likely to be—for most persons, there will be greater irritation with your child than with some distant athlete (see Brown & Weiner, 1984). But anger can be experienced even with minimal personal involvement. Many individuals, for example, expressed great anger at the first jurors who dismissed the charges against Rodney King and thus sparked the riots in Los Angeles, even though this decision may have had little direct effect on them. As long as a moral code has been broken and an individual is perceived as responsible for some negative action, state, or outcome, then anger may be experienced.

Now imagine your feelings about the retarded child who fails an examination in spite of putting forth great effort, or imagine your emotions about a friend who has contracted the HIV virus because of a transfusion with contaminated blood. There is more involved than dispassionate reactions to these individuals who are not responsible for their plights. Or imagine that your child performs poorly in baseball, which he or she loves, because of minimal athletic ability and coordination. Again, there is more involved than "cold" thoughts about the absence of controllability and responsibility. Compassion and sympathy are sure to be experienced, with the magnitude of these emotions likely to be dependent on how closely one is involved with the person in that situation.

Because the emotions of anger and sympathy are so closely linked with perceptions of responsibility, one cannot discuss moral accountability without also considering these feelings. I therefore turn to emotions next in this chapter. I will first contend in greater detail that anger and sympathy are generated by particular thoughts. Furthermore, it will be suggested that these emotions, rather than "cold" cognitions, determine how we react to others who have engaged in moral transgressions. One advantage of having the linkage between responsibility and action mediated by anger and sympathy rather than by blame is that this approach is able to account for positive or prosocial actions such as praising and help giving as well as negative or antisocial responses such as reprimanding and punishing.

## Anger

As already stated, anger is generated by inferences about responsibility (see Averill, 1982, 1983; Frijda, 1986; Weiner, 1986). If one is responsible for the unsuccessful attempt by another to attain a personal goal, then the person who was interfered with will experience anger. Anger is an accusation, or a value judgment, that follows from the belief that another person "could and should have done otherwise."

In one of many studies supporting this position, college students were asked to describe a recent situation in which they became angry (Weiner, Graham, & Chandler, 1982). The students most often reported that they felt anger when their boyfriend or girlfriend lied to them, when their roommates did not clean up a mess they made, or when they could not study because an inconsiderate neighbor made excessive noise. In all these situations, another person was construed as responsible for a negative state or event. That individual "should have" cleaned the room, turned down the radio volume, and so on (see Averill, 1983).

Anger can be altered if the person undergoing that feeling received information that decreased perceptions of control and, therefore, the responsibility of others. Thus, one can be "talked into" or "talked out of" anger, which further reveals the close association of this emotion to specific thoughts. If, for example, it is learned that the roommate did not clean up the room because of an electricity blackout (impersonal causality), because he became ill (lack of control), or because he had to drive a sick friend to the hospital (a mitigating justification), then anger would quite surely dissipate. As I will discuss in Chapter 8, humans have many strategies to reduce perceptions of personal responsibility and, thus, to lessen the anger of others.

Anger, then, communicates that one "should have" or "ought to have" done or not done something. The moral aspect of anger is even more evident when it is recognized that if the communicated anger is "accepted" or perceived as justified, then the recipient of this emotional message will feel guilty (see Weiner, 1986). This is because guilt follows from a self-perception of responsibility (Davitz, 1969). Guilt often is considered by psychoanalysts to be self-directed anger.

In addition to being a consequence of a thought, anger also is a stimulus for subsequent action. As I will document in the remainder of this book, anger provides a bridge between thinking and conduct. Anger directs the experiencer of this emotion to "eliminate" the wrongdoer—to go toward that person and retaliate with some form of aggressive action or to go away from that person to withhold some positive good and establish further distance (see Averill, 1983). Anger, therefore, is a "goad" or an emotion that "pushes" the person to undertake self-protective and/or retaliatory actions. In addition to this, anger has the function of "frightening" the offender by communicating that harm will be reciprocated (see Trivers, 1971). I examine these points in greater detail in subsequent chapters.

## Unsolved Issues

Associated with this conception of anger are a number of questions that are not readily resolvable. One can ask whether anger is felt if, and only if, another is held responsible. This seems contradicted by the observation that dogs and young infants give the appearance of expressing anger, although they surely do not have the cognitive capacities to make the requisite moral judgments. In addition, it appears that people are often "mad" at their nonstarting cars or flat tires (see Berkowitz, 1993, pp. 88–89). Yet, given the definitions that I have proposed in this chapter, cars and tires cannot be held responsible.

The necessity of inferences of responsibility in order for anger to be felt is a difficult issue, and a definitive answer cannot be provided. On the one hand, it could be contended that dogs, young infants, and those about to change a flat tire do not feel (are not feeling) anger. Rather, they are experiencing and expressing some other emotion, such as rage, frustration, or unhappiness. These other emotions are evoked by a threat in the environment, by pain, by the blockage of a desired goal, and so forth. Perhaps the anger reports of adults as they changed their tires would be modified if they were asked to closely consider exactly what emotion they are enduring.

A different position is to accept that anger does follow from a perception of responsibility, but this affect also may be evoked by other events or cognitions. That is, responsibility is a sufficient but not a necessary condition for evoking anger. Hence, an enemy in the visual field, pain from a diaper pin, and having a flat tire also can elicit anger.

Of these two alternatives, I am more attracted to the necessary than to the sufficient explanation (see also Roseman, Spindel, & Jose, 1990). This position is not based on definitive empirical data; rather, I consider this to be a more parsimonious path for the direction and organization of the field of emotion. The only way to settle this issue empirically is to identify the criteria that clearly differentiate affects such as anger, frustration, and unhappiness from one another. Then it can be determined which contextual and cognitive antecedents are linked with which affects. At this point in time, conclusive affective markers have not been developed (emotion researchers anxiously await the discovery of an affective X-ray). One might speculate, however, that facial expressions will differ when one is angry at another individual because of a perception of responsibility as opposed to when one is presumed angry because one's car has not started or when one experiences other types of frustration. This may, in part, be traceable to the communicative function of anger when another is the target of this emotion. If this is the case, then, indeed, one can argue that there is a difference between the emotions expressed toward a transgressing other and the emotions experienced when one's car fails to start.

Another difficult question to be raised is, If someone intentionally causes personal harm, must the wronged person feel angry? Again a definitive answer cannot be supplied, and at least two points of view are feasible. On the one hand, it could be contended that we may learn to "turn the other cheek" so that we either experience no emotion or feel some other affect, perhaps even compassion, toward the person who volitionally caused us harm. Plato accomplished this by considering all crimes against others as a disease, thus freeing criminals from responsibility and terminating anger. However, one might also accept that others are responsible and still experience no anger.

Conversely, it might be claimed that even though we express compassion following volitional harm by another, our original or initial feeling nonetheless is anger. However, this atavistic reaction, which is likely to be a product of our evolutionary heritage (see Fox, 1992; Trivers, 1971), can be masked or superseded by other learned reactions. Given this interpretation, anger must follow a perception of responsibility for a personally relevant negative event, even though it may be transient and need not be displayed or even consciously experienced.

My position on this issue—and again it is without empirical confirmation—is that one indeed can learn not to feel anger following an assignment of responsibility to another individual for a personally adverse outcome. But this is quite atypical—perhaps evident only in our most religious people.

But, in any case, why should a responsibility inference for a negative action evoke anger? What produces this linkage, or connection, between a complex moral inference and a very basic and prevalent emotion? There also are no known answers to this question. One cannot dismiss the possibility that there is a genetic or inborn association between beliefs about responsibility and anger that has aided in the preservation of the person and the social unit (see Fox, 1992). This association would have emerged with the origins of *Homo sapiens*. But, surely, socialization experiences play an important role in the identification of situations and behaviors that elicit anger as well as in the labeling of this affect. Thus, when a father says to a child, "Don't do that or I will get angry," he is conveying an association between a volitional action by the child and the feeling it will evoke in others. The child can then later generalize this sequence to other acts that involve free choice and responsibility. This position is akin to that expressed long ago by John Watson (1924), the father of behaviorism. At the present time, however, psychologists have little understanding regarding the development of any cognition–emotion linkages, including the one between responsibility beliefs and anger.

## Sympathy and the Ethos of Pathos

In contrast to the linkages between controllability, responsibility, and anger, uncontrollable causality and therefore the absence of responsibility given the personal plight of another are associated with sympathy and the related emotions of pity and compassion (these will not be differentiated in the present context). Thus, a person confined within a totalitarian state (impersonal or situational causality), athletic failure of another because of a physical handicap (internal, uncontrollable causality), or school failure because of the need to care for a sick mother (a mitigating justification) are prototypical predicaments that elicit sympathy inasmuch as the person is not perceived as responsible for his or her negative plight.

There has been relatively little research on sympathy, but some has been conducted. For example, in the Weiner et al. (1982) study previously discussed, in addition to being asked about circumstances in which they felt anger, the college student subjects also recalled instances in their lives when pity and sympathy were experienced. The most frequently reported contexts were when observing others with handicaps and when interacting with the very aged. More broadly conceived, Wispé (1991) speculated that "one will sympathize more with a brave sufferer, in a good cause, in which [the sufferer's] afflictions are beyond [his or her] control" (p. 134).

Inasmuch as sympathy and pity are evoked by uncontrollability and lack of responsibility, if these emotions are communicated to others, then the receivers of this affective message are led to believe that their negative condition is one for which responsibility cannot be assumed (see Graham, 1984, 1991). That is, their plight is not amenable to personal intervention and change. This has some positive consequences in that guilt, which is generated by self-responsibility, is not necessarily experienced and others do not necessarily get angry. However, the lack of amenability to personal intervention and change is itself aversive. Ann Sullivan, the teacher of Helen Keller, said to Ms. Keller's parents at one of their early meetings, "We do not want your pity."

As in the discussion of anger, a number of unanswered questions can be raised about this conception. It is uncertain if uncontrollability and lack of responsibility are necessary antecedents of sympathy; it is not known if, given lack of responsibility for a negative plight, sympathy must be experienced; and still uncharted is the developmental precursors of the linkage between lack of responsibility and sympathy.

For the purposes of this book, answers to the questions regarding both anger and sympathy are not essential. What is essential is the fact that perceptions of responsibility and nonresponsibility for events and states have respective linkages to the emotions of anger and sympathy. I repeatedly return to this position throughout the book.

## FROM EVENT TO ACTION: THE PSYCHOLOGICAL STEPS

I want to consider two sequences that illustrate the psychological process and the mechanisms that I propose as intervening between the onset of an event, such as a car crash, and the behavioral reactions that are exhibited, such as shouting at the rear driver. As might be anticipated from the discussion thus far, judgments of responsibility and the emotions they elicit are presumed to be the core aspects of this process.

Consider, for example, two students who are failing in school. Following failure on the examination, the teacher will search for information that will help to infer the causes that gave rise to these outcomes. In achievement contexts, two personal causes are particularly prevalent: ability and effort. Assume that, on the basis of the evidence that is available, the teacher reasons that one student failed because of lack of effort. This cause is construed as personal and controllable, inasmuch as effort can be volitionally altered. That is, the student freely chose not to try. Because the cause is personally controllable, the student may be held responsible. The teacher might then have a conference with this student to ascertain if mitigating circumstances, such as the need to be earning money at a job because of an ill mother or father, might be operating that absolve the student from responsibility, or at least lessen that judgment. If these circumstances are not present, then the student will be deemed responsible for the negative test outcome. The teacher, therefore, will be angry, and it is contended that as a result of this emotion, the teacher will impose some form of punishment. This complex sequence can be summarized as follows:

> Event (exam failure) → Causal search → Lack of effort →
> Personal and controllable cause → Responsibility
> (no mitigating circumstances) → Anger, no sympathy →
> Punishment

It is evident, therefore, that many psychological decisions and rules are presumed to intervene between something relevant that happens to the individual and the reactions that this event elicits.

Now consider a different explanation regarding the failure of the second student. This student does study hard and often seeks out help. On the basis of this information, the teacher ascribes the student's failure to low ability. Lack of ability (aptitude) is construed as uncontrollable by the student—it is an inborn characteristic not amenable to alteration through "willpower." Because this cause is uncontrollable, the student is not considered responsible for the poor outcome. As a result of this belief, the teacher feels sympathy and pity, which evokes prosocial behaviors, such as offering additional help and support. This sequence can be represented as:

> Event (exam failure) → Causal search → Lack of ability →
> Personal and uncontrollable cause → No responsibility →
> Sympathy, no anger → Help

Of course, other sequences are possible, and quite often steps are likely to be compressed, so that a judgment to punish or to help is made without a great deal of the cognitive work that might be necessary at each linkage in the hypothesized sequence. And, for example, one may help a blood relative even though that person is responsible for her plight. Nonetheless, the two postulated sequences provide the foundation for the remainder of this book, which is concerned with the emotional and behavioral consequences when another is perceived as responsible or not responsible for an action.

## GOALS AND ORGANIZATION
## OF THIS BOOK

As indicated in the very first paragraphs of this chapter, judgments of responsibility permeate our world and daily experience. My first goal in writing this book is to document the extensity of these inferences. As revealed in the introduction, the assignment of responsibility and its consequent affects and behaviors are not confined to the courtroom, for life itself is a courtroom where we all act as judges. The writing of this book was guided by the "life is a courtroom" metaphor, along with the metaphor that humans are Gods, assuming the legitimacy of acting as final judges of others.

In Chapter 2, I examine the effects of beliefs about responsibility for success and failure in achievement contexts, particularly as this inference relates to achievement evaluation. Of special importance is the distinction between lack of ability and lack of effort as causes of unsuccessful performance.

Then, in the next three chapters, I discuss the perceived causes of stigmas and the reactions that they elicit. In Chapter 3, I consider a variety of stigmas, with special attention paid to alcoholism, obesity, and poverty. In Chapter 4, I analyze reactions to homosexuals and to those who have AIDS. Then, in Chapter 5, I consider mental illness, including depression and schizophrenia.

In Chapter 6, I turn to an examination of prosocial behavior (help giving); and in Chapter 7, I examine antisocial actions, including aggression at both the individual and social level. In these chapters, the second goal of the book—namely, the construction of a theory of motivation that relates beliefs about responsibility to affective reactions and behaviors—is more fully developed. Different ways of conceptualizing the relations between thinking, feeling, and acting are outlined, and empirical evidence is presented regarding the "goodness" of the various conceptions.

In Chapter 8, I move away from the prior discussions and consider strategies or methods of impression formation and impression management that are used to decrease the extent to which others hold a person responsible. I examine denial, apology, excuses, justifications, and confession—all strategies used in everyday life to manipulate the thoughts and feelings that others have about us. This chapter documents that individuals share a naive theory about responsibility and its consequences that is quite consistent with scientific analyses. Sharing this theory allows humans to understand and regulate not only their own behavior but also the behavior of others.

In the final chapter, I address general issues within the field of motivation. This approach to social motivation is combined with the study of personal motivation, and a broader, more encompassing theory is suggested.

If the twin goals of this book—description and theory building—are attained, then the reader will be convinced of the extensity of judgments of responsibility and their centrality if everyday life. There also will be an understanding that naive psychology, the rules of the legal system, and tenets within theology have a great overlap and influence one another in mysterious ways. In addition, if my goals are met, then there will be increased recognition of the rules of human conduct, both as self-regulation and behavioral guidelines for regulating others. That is, increased practical and theoretical understanding of the laws of motivation will have been attained.

My underlying assumption in writing this book is that social judgment and social justice are among the essential human preoccupations. Hence, a general psychology cannot be constructed without incorporating principles related to causal attributions and the assignment of responsibility. Furthermore, no modern (and perhaps preliterate) society exists in which the members do not mutually understand the demands associated with moral obligation.

# 2

## Responsibility and Achievement Evaluation

*Ora est Labore* (Pray and work).
—Motto of the Benedictine monks

*Arbeit und Liebe* (Work and love).
—Freud's catalog of major life motivations

In our culture, and in other contemporary cultures, distribution of resources is *not* determined by the principle of equality, wherein all individuals receive the same amount of goods. This rule would be followed if, for example, all the sales people on a staff were paid equally, regardless of the amount of their individual sales, and perhaps if managers were paid the same as the sales staff. Instead, in America the head of a company often is paid 10 or even 20 times as much as the average worker—a far greater differential than is found in other cultures.

In a school as opposed to a work setting, a teacher may use an equality principle and base individual grading on the performance of the whole class or on the performance of groups within that class: All members of the class or the group would then receive the identical grade, determined by some imposed criteria. A few innovative classrooms that foster cooperative learning actually do use a system of equality-based grading (see Slavin, 1983). In these classes, each person's grade depends on the performance of the other students in the group. As might be intuited, such interdependence indeed increases mutual cooperation and decreases intragroup competition, so that the performance of some pupils is enhanced. But as also might be readily imagined, this grading system has the potential of arousing negative feelings in some students. In the American culture, most individuals do not prefer equality as the rule of distributive justice, as any teacher will attest. Indeed, even within cooperative groups, individual incentives often are included (see Slavin, 1983).

It is typically the case, then, that some principle of distributive justice other than equality prevails. The rule generally followed in this and most other societies as well is that successful outcomes are rewarded and unsuccessful outcomes are either unrewarded or punished for each individual. Thus, if a salesperson completes a sale, then a commission is received by that person; if there is no sale, there is no financial reward. Similarly, if a student answers all the questions correctly on a quiz, that student attains the grade of "A," whereas the student who gets few of the questions right receives a "D" or an "F."

The above appraisal reveals that a simple rule of distributive justice is being followed: Rewards are allocated according to the magnitude of the output, where output magnitude is defined as the number of test items correct for each person, the dollar value of sales for each individual, or some other indicator of output (outcome). This equity distributive rule forms the foundation of the capitalistic system: to each according to his or her performance. Indeed, the notion that outcome and reward covary is so deeply ingrained that it is difficult to conceive what American (and other cultures) would be like without it. We reason that "you get what you pay for" and "you pay for what you get," knowing there is a strong relation (although not necessarily perfect) between the quality of a good (e.g., the score on an exam) and the price (grade) that one expects to receive. This is our system of exchange. Note how closely related this is to our criminal justice system, for it is accepted that the degree of punishment for a crime should be somewhat proportional to the degree of harm done (strict liability).

Given a reward allotment determined only by outcome or performance, moral principles have no apparent role or place. But it is evident that there are moral determinants of evaluation and of the feedback given to others in achievement contexts, inasmuch as judgments concerning causal controllability and personal responsibility exert a great influence over these decisions. Consider, for example, a student who does not get many test items correct because of a mental handicap. This student does not receive the same reprimand or feedback as does the student who receives the identical low score because she did not study. In the former case, the cause (lack of aptitude) is not controllable, so that the student is not considered responsible for the poor grade. Or, if the student did not prepare for an exam because of a death in the family, then again negative sanctions would be lessened or removed entirely. There is a naive psychological belief that "my grandmother died" represents a "good" (if accepted!) excuse for missing a test. In this case, there are mitigating circumstances that decrease perceptions of responsibility and correspondent punishment. It is evident from these examples that moral precepts do affect reward and punishment in achievement settings, as in the courtroom.

There are, then, equity principles other than outcome or performance that influence the dissemination of rewards, which is consistent with the beliefs of Karl Marx. One rule considered in this chapter relates to the amount of input or the work performed, independent of its effect on output. Effort, in turn, is associated with the perception of personal responsibility inasmuch as "trying" is subject to volitional control or personal manipulation.

In this chapter, I first briefly examine what is meant by the "work ethic" and consider the salience of this value. Then an experiment is discussed that demonstrates the relative importance placed on outcome, effort, and ability as determinants of achievement evaluation. As will be the case throughout the remainder of this book, the reader will have the opportunity to complete this experiment and compare personal responses with the responses of others. I will then relate the allocation of rewards and punishments in this experiment to the analysis of perceived responsibility presented in Chapter 1.

Following this discussion, I will distinguish between responsibility for the onset and for the offset (or the continuation) of achievement failure, and I examine the relative contribution of each to the appraisal of achievement. I then consider perceptions regarding the "fairness" of others in their distribution of rewards and the use of moral principles in achievement contexts. After this, an additional area of research is explored: situations in which people may prefer that others infer that they have not tried. Individuals who desire to be thought of as having high ability rather than as expending high effort for success or as putting forth little effort rather than as failing because of low ability exhibit what might be called an "anti-effort," or at least a modified-effort, causal preference. Here again, an experiment that illuminates this issue is offered for the reader to perform.

Finally, the chapter concludes with a consideration of what adolescents communicate to peers and adults regarding the causes of their success and failure. This research documents the perceptions that these adolescents have regarding the values of their peers and adults. In all of the empirical topics discussed, the key concern is the differential reactions elicited by ability and effort as the causes of success and failure.

The underlying goals of the chapter are to (1) document that judgments of responsibility extend into achievement contexts; (2) show how the process(es) outlined in Chapter 1 are applicable in achievement settings; and (3) begin to elaborate a theory of motivation in which thinking (perceptions of responsibility), emotions (anger and sympathy), and actions (interpersonal evaluation) form a unified whole that is generalizable from the courtroom to the achievement context.

## THE ETHICS OF WORK

In his classic book *The Protestant Ethic and the Spirit of Capitalism*, Max Weber (1904) called attention to the association between achievement strivings and morality. Well before Protestantism, however, a morality of duty surely was expressed and recognized (as revealed in the motto of the Benedictine monks, "Pray and work," given at the start of the chapter). After all, members of a social group were expected to contribute to the well-being of the entire society by taking part in productive activity. This might be construed as a basic ingredient of the "social contract." Failure to do this, in the absence of lack of control or mitigating circumstances, would most likely result in some form of punishment, such as expulsion from the group. Norms of duty that capture a standard of performance below which a reasonable person was not expected to fall, must have been in force throughout the development of culture (Fuller, 1969). As Figure 2.1 illustrates, such norms remain today.

However, there also appears to be a morality of aspiration that is distinct from a morality of duty (Hamilton, Blumenfeld, & Kushler, 1988). A morality of aspiration focuses on rewards for outstanding performance, or the positive consequences of exceptional output, rather than on the punishment administered for failure to live up to a minimal standard. Weber (1904) pointed out that there is a sense of satisfaction derived from doing a job particularly well and that others recognize such accomplishments. Further, ideals of asceticism, industriousness and individuality form a syndrome that Weber described as part of the so-called Protestant Ethic. These notions formed the foundation for McClelland's (1961) studies of achievement-oriented societies.

In everyday life, putting forth effort to excel is referred to as a "work ethic." It may seem that in modern society this belief is "old fashioned" or an anachronism, far from the hedonic goals expressed by some individuals of getting the maximum personal reward with the minimum of personal investment. However, beliefs that the work ethic is no longer admired conflict with the depictions of heroes and the ideals voiced in the media by those in the public eye. For example, coaches of sports teams realize that fan support is augmented when they refer to their team as having a "blue-collar" attitude or mentality, or when they describe their team as "over-achievers," thereby implying that their success is attributable to hard work

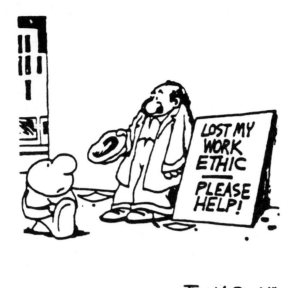

**FIGURE 2.1.** Searching for the Protestant Ethic. By Tom Wilson. Copyright 1994 by Ziggy & Friends, Inc. Reprinted by permission.

and to the overcoming of adversity through maximum exertion. (Some professional black athletes have accused the press of using this description only for white athletes and implying that African Americans are "naturally gifted" in athletic endeavors and thus do not have to work hard!) An athlete failing to exert maximum effort is not tolerated by the coach or by the public, even in those cases in which there is high output and good performance.

In one study pertinent to work values that was conducted in Australia (Feather, Volkmer, & McKee, 1991), it was found that the most successful and recognized people in that country elicited negative as well as positive feelings and attitudes. Many expressed the wish that these "tall poppies" (trees that stand above the others in the field) would be felled. However, this negative wish expressed by the Australians was directed primarily toward those individuals who were perceived as having attained their status by luck, inheritance, or by means other than hard work. Extra exertion as a cause of success is related to the belief that the rewards were earned, or "deserved," and exempts one from the "tall poppy" curse (Feather, 1992; Feather et al., 1991).

The distribution of goods and evaluation of achievement based on work input remains an accepted philosophical principle in Australia, America, and in many other cultures as well. Although Westerners tend to associate Indian philosophy with a strong belief in fate and God as determinants of outcomes and rewards, in the Indian culture the concept of Niskamakarma "teaches the individual to strive hard and do his duties sincerely to attain his goals without a concern for the reward. And therefore, higher effort on the part of the individual is worthy of reward regardless of outcome" (Eswara, 1972, p. 140). The concept of Niskamakarma is found in the Bhagavad Gita (Hindu scripture) and remains influential today.

Two equity principles of reward allocation and achievement evaluation have thus been identified: performance, or the outcome of an activity, and effort, or the input into an activity. But is one more important or significant than the other as an evaluative determinant? For example, who should receive more "goods" of these two: the pupil who does not try but performs well on an exam, or the student who tries very hard but does poorly? Or, in a school setting should the pupil who does not study and does fairly well on an exam be rewarded in the same way as the pupil who studies very hard to attain the identical outcome? Are these two students to receive the same "goods" (rewards, praise, grades, etc.)? To examine the determinants of reward allocation, or justice in achievement contexts, an experimental investigation is presented next that manipulates outcome and effort (output and input), as well as other information, so that unambiguous (unconfounded) conclusions can be reached about their relative value.

## AN EXPERIMENTAL STUDY OF THE DETERMINANTS OF ACHIEVEMENT EVALUATION

After reading the following experimental description, you are invited to complete Experiment 2.1. Fritz Heider, who was already acknowledged as the founder of attribution theory, once confided to me that prior to reading an experimental study he tried to put himself in the place of the subjects and completed the experiment himself, either actually making the judgments or thinking through what his responses might be. His approach lead me to include the key experiments in this book for the reader to carry out.

Experiment 2.1 provides information regarding performance on an exam (output), effort expenditure (input), and the level of ability of the student (along with effort, another indicator of personal causality). There are two levels of each of these three determinants of performance: (1) outcome is specified to be either a success or a failure, (2) effort expenditure is described as high or low, and (3) ability level also is designated as high or low. Then all combinations of these three sources of information

# EXPERIMENT 2.1

## Determinants of Achievement Evaluation

The following experiment includes information about eight different students. The teacher knows whether or not these students have ability, based on scores on IQ and other aptitude tests. In addition, the teacher has knowledge about how diligent the students are—if homework is handed in on time and if they study and pay attention during class. The teacher recently gave a test and the students either did well (success) or poorly (failure). Based on the information about ability, effort, and test performance, the teacher is providing feedback to each student. The feedback can be positive (with a maximum "score" of +10), or negative (with a maximum "score" of −10). You are to provide feedback to these students. Thus, for example, for Student 1, there is information that this student has high aptitude, works hard, and was successful on the test. What evaluative feedback would you give, ranging from +10 to −10?

| Student | Ability | Effort | Outcome | Evaluative feedback |
|---------|---------|--------|---------|---------------------|
| 1 | High | High | Success | _____ |
| 2 | High | High | Failure | _____ |
| 3 | High | Low | Success | _____ |
| 4 | High | Low | Failure | _____ |
| 5 | Low | High | Success | _____ |
| 6 | Low | High | Failure | _____ |
| 7 | Low | Low | Success | _____ |
| 8 | Low | Low | Failure | |

Calculations for main effects

Success (lines 1, 3, 5, 7)   =  _____
Failure (lines 2, 4, 6, 8)   =  _____
   Difference[a]   =  _____

High effort (lines 1, 2, 5, 6)   =  _____
Low effort (lines 3, 4, 7, 8)   =  _____
   Difference   =  _____

Low ability (lines 5, 6, 7, 8)   =  _____
High ability (lines 1, 2, 3, 4)   =  _____
   Difference   =  _____

[a]The reader is reminded that subtracting a negative number is equivalent to adding a positive number (forgive me for this gentle reminder).

31

are represented in eight students, so that eight different combinations of information, or eight different kinds of student situations, are depicted (2 levels of outcome × 2 levels of effort × 2 levels of ability). For example, one student is described as high in ability, low in effort, and a success (Student 3); another is characterized as high in ability, low in effort, and a failure on the exam (Student 4); and so on—so that all eight combinations of information are represented.

The effects of these three variables, representing performance outcome and two possible causes of that outcome, on achievement evaluation can then be determined. Achievement evaluation is defined in Experiment 2.1 as the feedback that a teacher gives to each student. That feedback can vary from maximum reward (arbitrarily set as +10) to maximum punishment (−10).

The reader can now take the role of the teacher and dispense rewards and punishments in these eight conditions. This might prove difficult, and you may wish to give more than one kind of feedback. However, this is not permitted here (just as it often is not possible in actual life situations, where there must be a promotion or a firing, a bonus or a cut in salary, and so on).

## The Experimental Findings

Figure 2.2 depicts the results of a variant of the experiment shown in Experiment 2.1. The variation is rather minor: There are five types of outcomes (excellent outcome, fair outcome, borderline result, moderate failure, and clear failure) rather than the two (success and failure) that were given in the experiment that you completed.

Examination of Figure 2.1 first reveals that outcome is a very important determinant of reward and punishment: Overall, good outcomes tend to be rewarded (Students 1, 3, 5, and 7) whereas poor outcomes tend to be punished (Students 2, 4, 6, and 8). As previously indicated, one equity solution guiding the distribution of reward is relative performance, or how well one has done (e.g., the number of questions correct on an exam, the number of sales made, etc.). You can determine this in your data by noting if the sum of the appraisals for Students 1, 3, 5, and 7 exceeds that for Students 2, 4, 6, and 8. Because of the factorial design, the pupils between these two groupings differ only in their outcomes, but not in effort expenditure or level of ability.

More germane to the issues addressed in this book, it also is evident from Figure 2.1 that students described as putting forth effort (Students 1, 2, 5, and 6, represented with solid lines) are rewarded more and punished less than students who do not try hard (Students 3, 4, 7, and 8, represented in Figure 2.1 with broken lines). Hence, work input, independent of its effects on outcomes, also is an important determinant of the evaluations of

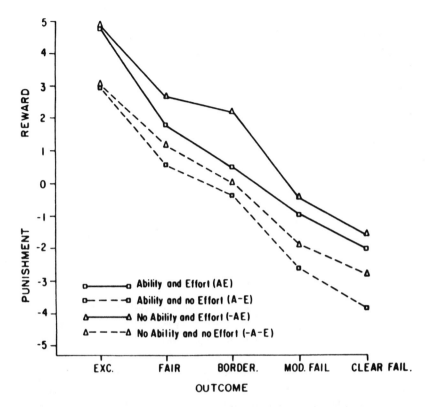

FIGURE 2.2. Achievement evaluation as a function of exam outcome, expended effort, and ability level. From Weiner and Kukla (1970, p. 3). Copyright 1970 by the American Psychological Association. Reprinted by permission of the author.

others in achievement contexts. Within each outcome, or holding outcome constant, high effort always receives a more positive evaluation than does low effort (also see Medway, 1979; Pence, Pendleton, Dobbins, & Sgro, 1982).

Finally, and perhaps what is initially most surprising, those students who are described as low in ability (Students 5, 6, 7, and 8, represented with triangles) are evaluated more positively than students characterized as high in ability (Students 1, 2, 3, and 4, represented with squares). To understand the somewhat strange finding that low ability is a "positive" characteristic in this experimental study, one has to take a closer look at the rewards and punishments given to the individual students. Figure 2.2, and quite likely your data as well, indicates that pupils who are low in ability and try hard (the top line in Figure 2.2, represented as solid with triangles), particularly given success (Student 5 in your data), are most highly rated. In our society, the handicapped person who completes a race and the marginal student who overcomes this drawback through "willpower" are most admired. This reflects the morality of aspiration. Conversely, those high in ability who do not try (represented in Figure 2.2 with broken lines and squares), particularly given failure (Student 4 in your data), are appraised most negatively. Indeed, what is more disturbing to a teacher or a coach than the "gifted" student or athlete who does not fulfill this "potential" because of lack of effort?

In life situations, ability and outcome tend to be correlated so that high ability does covary with reward. But this may be because of the performance or output equity principle, rather than because ability is in and of itself a positive determinant of achievement appraisal. I return to this issue later in the chapter when considering some of the positive consequences of having high ability, for it is obvious this is a quality that all of us desire.

## On the Historical Constraints of Psychological Laws

It was previously intimated in this chapter, as well as in Chapter 1, that moral judgments applied in the classroom or on the job are not recent additions to the culture. This is documented in Figure 2.3. The author of the work in Figure 2.3, which was published in 1642, also was concerned about students who differed in their levels of ability and effort and, as in Experiment 2.1, considered students who were high and low in ability factorially combined with high and low effort. His analyses and recommendations are quite consistent with the findings in Figure 2.2, collected about 350 years later. While some critics of social psychology have argued that our laws do not span cultures and historical contexts, these data document quite the contrary!

The reproduced original manuscript shown in Figure 2.3 is somewhat difficult to decipher, since it is written in Old English. Thus, a "translation" of this text is included below (Fuller, 1642, pp. 110–111):

> He studieth his scholars natures as carefully as their books; and ranks their dispositions into severall forms. And though it may seem difficult for him in a great school to descend to all particulars, yet experienced Schoolmasters may quickly make a Grammar of boyes natures, and reduce them all (saving some few exceptions) to these general rules.
>
> 1. Those that are ingenious and industrious. The conjunction of two such Planets in a youth presage much good unto him. To such a lad a frown may be a whipping, and a whipping death; yea where their Master whips them once, shame whips them all the week after. Such natures he useth with all gentlenesse.

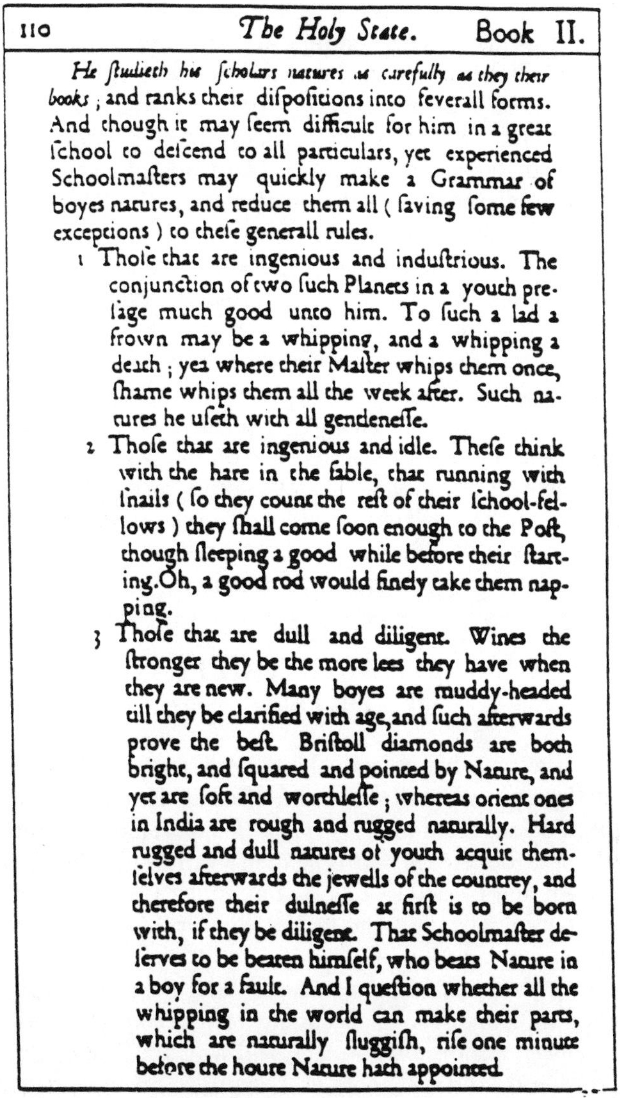

| 110 | *The Holy State.*     Book  II. |
|---|---|

He ſtudieth his ſcholars natures as carefully as they their books ; and ranks their diſpoſitions into feverall forms. And though it may ſeem difficult for him in a great ſchool to deſcend to all particulars, yet experienced Schoolmaſters may quickly make a Grammar of boyes natures, and reduce them all ( ſaving ſome few exceptions ) to theſe generall rules.

1   Thoſe that are ingenious and induſtrious. The conjunction of two ſuch Planets in a youth pre-ſage much good unto him. To ſuch a lad a frown may be a whipping, and a whipping a death ; yea where their Maſter whips them once, ſhame whips them all the week after. Such na-tures he uſeth with all gentleneſſe.

2   Thoſe that are ingenious and idle. Theſe think with the hare in the fable, that running with ſnails ( ſo they count the reſt of their ſchool-fel-lows ) they ſhall come ſoon enough to the Poſt, though ſleeping a good while before their ſtart-ing.Oh, a good rod would finely take them nap-ping.

3   Thoſe that are dull and diligent. Wines the ſtronger they be the more lees they have when they are new. Many boyes are muddy-headed till they be clarified with age, and ſuch afterwards prove the beſt. Briſtoll diamonds are both bright, and ſquared and pointed by Nature, and yet are ſoft and worthleſſe ; whereas orient ones in India are rough and rugged naturally. Hard rugged and dull natures of youth acquit them-ſelves afterwards the jewells of the countrey, and therefore their dulneſſe at firſt is to be born with, if they be diligent. That Schoolmaſter de-ſerves to be beaten himſelf, who bears Nature in a boy for a fault. And I queſtion whether all the whipping in the world can make their parts, which are naturally ſluggiſh, riſe one minute before the houre Nature hath appointed.

FIGURE 2.3. Treatment of students as a function of their levels of ability and effort. From Fuller (1642).

2.  Those that are ingenious and idle. These think with the hare in the fable, that running with snails (so they count the rest of their school-fellows) they shall come soon enough to the Post, though sleeping a good while before their starting. Oh, a good rod would finely take them napping.

3. Those that are dull and diligent. Wines the stronger they be the more lees they have when they are new. Many boyes are muddy-headed till they be clarified with age, and such afterwards prove the best. Bristoll diamonds are both bright, and squared and pointed by Nature, and yet are soft and worthless; whereas orient ones in India are rough and rugged naturally. Hard rugged and dull natures of youth acquit themselves afterwards the jewells of the countrey, and therefore their dulnesse at first is to be born with, if they be diligent. That Schoolmaster deserves to be beaten himself, who beats Nature in a boy for a fault. And I question whether all the whipping in the world can make their parts, which are naturally sluggish, rise one minute before the houre Nature hath appointed.
4. Those that are invincibly dull and negligent also. Correction may reform the latter, not amend the former. All the whetting in the world can never set a rasours edge on that which hath no steel in it. Such boys he consigneth over to other professions. Shipwrights and boatmakers will choose crooked pieces of timber, which other carpenters refuse. Those may make excellent merchants and mechanics which will not serve for Scholars.

## THEORETICAL INTERPRETATION
## OF THE FINDINGS

It is without question that individuals who fail because of a lack of effort are evaluated more negatively than those who fail because of lack of ability. This has been documented in many types of achievement situations, ranging from the classroom to the sports field; in a variety of cultures, including India and Iran; and by children as well as adults (see review in Weiner, 1986). But conceptually, how should this empirical fact be accounted for, or explained?

To answer this question, one must consider the process that, in part, includes the concepts of personal causality, causal controllability, mitigating circumstances, responsibility, anger, and sympathy. That is, there must be a progression from the phenotypical empirical relations that are

Failure → Lack of effort → High punishment

Failure → Lack of ability → Low punishment

to the genotypic, underlying, and more complex sequences that include mediating inferences about responsibility and affective reactions as depicted next:

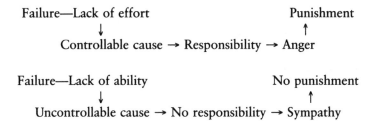

I contended in Chapter 1 that if one is to be perceived as responsible for an untoward outcome, then that event must be ascribed to a person and the cause must have been controllable by that individual. Ability as portrayed in Experiment 2.1 is not perceived as subject to volitional alteration; it is a characteristic or trait that a pupil "has." As implied in Experiment 2.1, ability is akin to an inborn aptitude, an inherited property of a person that is believed to remain constant throughout the person's life. Effort expenditure, on the other hand, can be turned "on or off." The person has control over the amount of trying.

In Experiment 2.1, ability (an uncontrollable cause) and effort (a controllable cause) were given as the determinants of exam performance. Focusing only on unsuccessful outcomes, if a person high in ability and low in effort fails, then there is no ambiguity or uncertainty about the cause of that failure. The person is held responsible because the perceived cause—namely, low effort—is considered controllable. Accordingly, without information about possible mitigators, this should produce high ratings of responsibility and anger (which, unfortunately, were not assessed in the earlier research depicted in Figure 2.2) and relatively severe punishment (which was measured).

Conversely, if a student low in ability and high in effort fails, then that student is not regarded as responsible for the outcome. The cause—lack of ability—is something that the student cannot control. Thus, there is an absence of personal responsibility (but not of personal causality, inasmuch as low ability is internal to that person). The inferred lack of responsibility theoretically elicits sympathy (which also was not measured in the prior research) and lessens negative sanctions. Again, other research has strongly supported a linkage between lack of ability and sympathy (see Weiner et al., 1982). However, it should be remembered that this causal pattern does not totally prevent some form of negative feedback, for outcome or output is another principle of appraisal that influences the allocation of rewards and punishments.

It is evident, then, that one who does not try is "immoral" but that this is not the case for a person with low ability. Achievement contexts elicit moral evaluations. One "should" put forth effort prior to an exam and is

expected to be the recipient of negative consequences (failure and reprimand) when one does not try.

## Additional Thoughts Concerning
## Why Lack of Effort Is Punished

The prior discussion considered the mechanisms or the processes that
promote the relative rewarding of effort expenditure and the punishment
that follows a lack of effort. This analysis reveals "why" high effort is
rewarded and lack of effort is punished. But another way to answer a
"why" question is to examine the function of the behavior and its
significance to the species. That is, one might ask what are the underlying
reasons why teachers, parents, and others in authority reward those who
try and reprimand the lazy?

Here some of the proposed purposes of sending a criminal to jail are
instructive. First, the student is "taught a lesson," so that lack of effort is
less likely to be a cause of failure in the future. This can be considered an
attempt to rehabilitate the student. In addition, others are informed that
this is inappropriate behavior, and a moral education is thereby provided.
This also is a utilitarian function. And additionally, one may postulate that
there is retributive justice and that society's "moral bookkeeping" is kept
in order. But why might there be "retribution" when there has been no
"harm," as would be the case given a criminal proceeding? Indeed, "strict
liability," or punishment in accord with the amount of harm done, which
is the foundation of our legal system and a basic principle for criminal
justice, seems to be totally out of place in this setting.

One may therefore have to probe still deeper and further back from
the proximal causes and seek even more distal determinants that relate to
why trying or not trying is more than a personal decision. When considering the general welfare of society, it is presumed that all must "carry their
weight." Although it could be maintained that lack of effort most harms the
individual who does not try, in that "goods" are not received by that
person, it is also the case that the entire society is adversely affected. If, for
example, a role-appropriate member of a prehistoric group does not aid in
hunting, or in the preparation of food, then that person would hamper or
tax the entire group by not contributing to the good of society. As already
revealed, a morality of duty aids in the preservation of society. The individual who does not try in school asks others to sacrifice their "personal
fitness" for his or her well-being, for it is likely to be assumed that lack of
effort at school subsequently will cause the individual to be a burden on
society. Thus, it is consistent with long-term utilitarian as well as retributive principles to punish lack of effort.

Considering the more positive side of this picture, if a student tries hard and succeeds, then rules regarding the morality of aspiration are elicited. That individual is judged as highly deserving and is especially rewarded by the society to which that person is contributing, while also serving as a role model for others to emulate.

## ONSET VERSUS OFFSET RESPONSIBILITY

Certainly the paradigm presented in Experiment 2.1 is a very simplified depiction of the complexity of the determinants of achievement evaluation and the role played by perceptions of responsibility. An additional moral-related determinant of achievement appraisal that has been experimentally studied relates to a distinction first proposed by Brickman et al. (1982) between responsibility for the onset and responsibility for the offset, or the continuation, of a problem (this is discussed in greater detail in Chapter 3). For example, one may have a heart attack because of an unknown genetic propensity (not responsible for the onset of the problem) but then not institute the necessary dietary and lifestyle changes to prevent a further attack (responsible for the continuation and the offset of the problem). The onset/offset distinction is important because it has great implications for judgments of responsibility and for emotional and behavioral responses.

Karasawa (1991) was able to separate onset and offset responsibility for a school failure and study their independent effects on evaluation. She had subjects imagine that an acquaintance enrolled in a math course and failed the midterm exam. The causes of the failure were varied so that the student was described as responsible or not responsible for the negative outcome. In one nonresponsibility condition, it was stated that the student "was sick and could not study math." In a second nonresponsibility condition, the student was described as "studying hard and doing all the homework." Hence, the inferred cause of failure was lack of ability. Finally, in the third condition the student "just did not do the reading assignments and did not do any of the homework." Hence, this student was depicted as personally responsible for the failure.

Given the discussion thus far in the book, it would be expected that the failing student in the no-effort condition would elicit greater anger, less pity, and receive more negative feedback than when described as sick or inferred to have low ability. The ratings made by the subjects, shown in Table 2.1, are entirely consistent with these expectations, with the student characterized as sick responded to somewhat more positively than the student inferred as low in ability.

Following the causal information for the onset of the problem and the ratings shown in Table 2.1, further information was communicated regard-

TABLE 2.1. Response Means after the Initial Failure Information

|           | Causal condition | | |
|-----------|------|-------------|-----------|
|           | Sick | Low ability | No effort |
| Anger     | 2.7  | 2.6         | 4.6       |
| Pity      | 6.1  | 5.2         | 3.8       |
| Criticism | 4.5  | 4.7         | 6.2       |

*Note.* Data from Karasawa (1991, p. 490).

ing the behavior of the student that related to the cause of the continuation of the problem. The vignette read:

> For the next three weeks, after having been ill (after having studied hard, after not studying), your acquaintance remained sick and could not study (studied hard, did not study or do any of the homework). The student remained behind in the classwork.

The three causes of the onset of the problem and the three causes of the continuation of the problem were factorially combined so that each subject received one of the nine possible combinations of information. For example, a subject read that the student was sick and remained sick, did not study and then became sick, studied hard and then became sick, initially was sick and then did not study, and so on. To simplify the findings, here only the sick versus no effort causal conditions will be compared, for the ratings in these two conditions following the onset information differed most from another (see Table 2.1). As shown in Table 2.2, responsibility for the continuation of the problem also influenced affective reactions and

TABLE 2.2. Response Means after the Initial Failure Information and Causes Regarding the Continuation of the Problem

|           | Onset information | | | |
|-----------|------|-----------|------|-----------|
|           | Sick | | No effort | |
|           | Offset information | | | |
|           | Sick | No effort | Sick | No effort |
| Anger     | 3.3  | 7.2       | 3.1  | 5.9       |
| Pity      | 6.5  | 2.3       | 5.4  | 3.0       |
| Criticism | 5.0  | 7.1       | 5.3  | 7.2       |

*Note.* Data from Karasawa (1991, p. 492).

criticism—and to a greater extent than did the cause of the initial failure. For example, whether the student was sick or did not try prior to the exam, he or she elicited relatively little anger when subsequently sick (ratings respectively = 3.3 and 3.1). However, following the initial exam failure, anger when the student subsequently did not try (mean of 7.2 + 5.9 = 6.5) was far greater than when the pupil was later sick (mean = 3.2).

What is of particular interest and most novel in these data is that ratings of anger are higher, and ratings of pity are lower, when a student who was initially sick subsequently did not try (anger = 7.2, pity = 2.3), as opposed to the condition in which the student never tried (anger = 5.9, pity = 3.0). Karasawa (1991) reasoned that

> no effort after recovering from the sickness did not merely mean that the target made no effort, but it also indicated that the target did not take the opportunity to better his or her condition, even though he or she had the potential for it. . . . This study suggests that there is a moral value that an individual who does not live up to his or her potential will receive negative evaluation and punishment. (p. 494)

This argument is similar to the one made regarding the negative consequences when those who have high ability fail because they did not expend effort, thereby not fulfilling their capabilities. But further, Karasawa (1991) pointed out that when conditions change from uncontrollable to controllable, persons not taking advantage of this causal change and the opportunities it provides will be severely reprimanded. One might, therefore, predict that individuals who are freed from an oppressive regime and who are then provided with chances for achievement in a democratic country but who do not put forth an effort to achieve in the new favorable circumstances will be responded to very unfavorably, while those who now work will be responded to very favorably. In accord with this line of reasoning, there are data that Conservatives respond particularly favorably toward those who have overcome prior shortcomings, such as the "recovered alcoholic" (see Skitka & Tetlock, 1993a, 1993b).

## THE PERCEIVED "FAIRNESS" OF ACHIEVEMENT EVALUATION

I have thus far been discussing the determinants of evaluation by observers. But how are these appraisals perceived? Do those who have been evaluated feel that the judgment has been fair?

Research concerned with the perception of "fairness" has found that individuals tend to think of themselves as fairer and as having more integrity than others (Liebrand, Messick, & Wolters, 1986; Messick, Bloom, Boldizar, & Samuelson, 1985; Van Lange, 1991). In one typical experimental procedure, subjects were asked to write in separate sentences as many fair and unfair behaviors as they could list. They also were instructed to begin each sentence with the personal pronoun "I" if the behavior was more applicable to themselves and with "they" if they thought the behavior was more applicable to others. It was found that subjects started more of the "fair" examples with "I" and more of the "unfair" situations with "they" (Messick et al., 1985). In a similar manner, Goethals (1986) reported that subjects rated themselves as more likely than their peers to perform a variety of moral behaviors and less likely to engage in immoral or selfish behaviors.

These self-enhancing perceptions are not recounted for all actions. For example, individuals do not report acting more intelligently than their peers (Van Lange, 1991). The difference between the self-perception of undertaking moral as opposed to intelligent behavior has been labeled the "Mohammed Ali Effect." Ali, who was known for his bravado as well as for his athletic prowess as a boxer, is quoted as saying, "I only said I was the greatest, not the smartest," after performing poorly on an exam.

As teachers, we are aware that students often feel that they have been "unfairly" graded, while we consider that our behavior was just. For example, students might believe that an essay has not been appreciated, the class curve was too low, the exam questions ambiguous, and so on. These points of student–teacher disagreement relate to the appraisal of an outcome, or the "quality" of a product. More pertinent to the present chapter and to the distinction between ability and effort is that fairness also may refer to the morality of an achievement appraisal, or a judgment as to whether a teacher gave a student credit for working hard, independent of the outcome of that effort, and took into account the extent to which the student's ability level might have been a performance impediment.

In a research investigation concerned with this issue, a colleague and I examined whether individuals perceive themselves as "fairer" evaluators of others, just as they perceive themselves as engaging in more moral behaviors (Farwell & Weiner, 1993). Fairness in this context was defined as taking into account effort and ability as determinants of performance, or considering the causal context of achievement. A fair evaluator from a moral perspective is one who would not punish failure caused by lack of ability but would punish failure caused by low effort.

In one pertinent experiment (Farwell & Weiner, 1993, p. 5), subjects responded to the following: "Pretend that you are a teacher, and one of the students fails a test because of lack of ability (effort). How would you as a teacher evaluate this student?" The subjects also were asked how a teacher would evaluate them under these two causal conditions, how they would be evaluated by someone who was not a teacher, and how the teacher would evaluate another student given this information.

As anticipated, failure ascribed to lack of effort resulted in more punishment than failure ascribed to low ability in all the conditions. More importantly, subjects perceived that they would punish another student who failed because of lack of effort more than a teacher or an unspecified person would. Conversely, the subjects believed they would punish a student less for failure caused by lack of ability than a teacher or another person would—that is, they were more "forgiving."

Figure 2.4 depicts the differences in punishment when failure is caused by effort as opposed to ability. This can be considered an index of the degree to which evaluation is guided by moral principles (perceptions of responsibility and the presence of a "guilty mind"). It is evident from Figure 2.4 that the respondents believe they are "fairer" than their teachers or another person. That is, they discriminate more clearly when it is "just" and "unjust" to reprimand another for failure, perceiving that they would punish lack of effort more than lack of ability to a greater extent than others would.

These findings suggest that even in evaluative achievement contexts, persons tend to perceive themselves as "fairer" than others, or as more

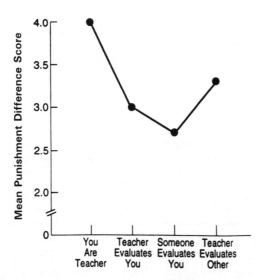

**FIGURE 2.4.** The difference in evaluative score (failure caused by lack of effort minus failure caused by lack of ability) as a function of the evaluator and the target of the evaluation. From Farwell and Weiner (1993, p. 5).

sensitive to moral rules. This also hints that individuals may view others in their achievement world as "unfair."

## WHEN WE WANT OTHERS TO THINK
## WE HAVE NOT TRIED

The findings in Figure 2.2 and Tables 2.1 and 2.2, as well as the discussion in the prior pages, leads to the conclusion that in this and most other cultures it is desirable to have others think that we are "hard workers," expending effort in school and job-related activities. After all, it is known that reward is given for "trying" and that laziness elicits punishment. And it is indeed the case that typically information is communicated that one is putting forth effort, even when this is not true. For example, a child may lock himself in his room, telling his parents that he is studying, when in fact he is calling friends; a saleswoman may state to the boss that she is leaving the office to pursue a sale, when in fact she is planning to take the afternoon off; and so forth. In research that examined what college students do to "impress" their instructors, the students reported that they worked as hard as possible or pretended to work diligently (Jagacinski & Nicholls, 1990). They did not endorse the position that they would act as if they were not trying in situations of failure in order to avoid the impression (causal ascription) that they lacked intelligence (since lack of effort rather than lack of ability would then be the apparent reason for failure). That is, the students did not indicate that they engaged in self-handicapping, or behaviors that would produce low effort and failure, as has been contended by some educational and social psychologists (see Jones & Berglas, 1978).

However, there are exceptions to the principle that we want others to think of us as making every effort to attain success. This rule may not hold in situations in which ascription of failure to low ability is particularly repugnant. In addition, groups that rebel against the dominant culture and adolescents who seek the approval of their peers may not want everyone to think they are trying hard.

### Ability and Self-Worth

High effort in achievement contexts may make it appear that one lacks ability, particularly in situations in which the outcome has been a failure. This is because ability and effort often are perceived as compensatory: If one has high ability, then hard work is unnecessary for success. Or, stated somewhat differently, if one works hard for success, then ability must be low. According to Heider (1958), the less the "can," the more the "try" is required for success.

Covington and Omelich (1979a, 1979b) have contended that high effort accompanied by low ability is a condition that is least desirous from the perspective of a failing student. These investigators ask (1979a):

> Why do others hide their effects and refuse to admit that they study hard? [This is because] there is a pervasive tendency in our society to equate the ability to achieve with human value. . . . From this self-esteem perspective, expending effort becomes a potential threat to the individual, since a combination of effort and failure invites causal ascriptions to low ability. . . . In effect, effort can become a double-edged sword for many students. On the one hand, they must exert some effort to avoid teacher punishment, but not so much as to risk public shame should they try hard and fail. (pp. 169–170)

Covington and Omelich (1979a, 1979b) contend that personal worth in our society is equated with ability level. Thus, the affect that one experiences in the face of failure depends largely on the implications that this outcome has for self-perception of ability. While the arguments of Covington and Omelich and others supporting this position (e.g., Nicholls, 1975, 1976) primarily relate self-perception to self-esteem, it also is reasonable to extend this position to social perception and the value that others place on an individual. That is, the more that others perceive a person as having high ability, the more that this person is admired, envied, accepted, and so on.

To test their self-worth theory, Covington and Omelich (1979a) asked students to imagine that they failed an exam and to indicate which of four explanations for their failure they preferred. These explanations included the four possible combinations of high and low ability with high and low effort. Hence, failure was accompanied by low ability and low effort, low ability and high effort, high ability and low effort, and high ability and high effort (where presumably some factor such as luck or circumstance caused the negative outcome). Given these alternatives, students most preferred to fail with the combination of high ability and low effort, as had been predicted by Covington and Omelich.

## Morality and Self-Evaluation

There are a number of objections one may raise about the above study, which intimates that the most "immoral" condition (high ability and low effort) is preferred as the cause of failure (see Brown & Weiner, 1984; Weiner & Brown, 1984). On the one hand, the presence of low effort may suggest that the person is uninvolved in the activity and is indifferent to the outcome. Conversely, the expenditure of effort indicates the desire to succeed. Hence, failure ascribed to a combination of high ability and low effort may be "preferred" precisely because the failure is construed as not meaningful or important.

Another possible interpretation of the Covington and Omelich results is that one may prefer failure caused by lack of effort rather than low ability because effort may be augmented, whereas ability is implied to be a more stable entity that cannot be changed. A very tasteless bumper sticker appearing in the Los Angeles area reads: "I am fat, you are ugly, I can diet." Again, this implies a particular adverse condition is preferred over another because it can be altered. There is a vast experimental literature supporting the prediction that failure ascribed to lack of effort results in lower decrements in the expectancy of future success than does failure attributed to lack of ability (see review in Weiner, 1986).

To examine the findings that expectancy of future success may have accounted for the findings reported by Covington and Omelich (1979a, 1979b), and to highlight the importance of morality in self-evaluation and presumably in the appraisal of others, Brown and Weiner (1984) conducted a series of investigations that reexamined the preference between ability versus effort as the cause of failure. One of these questionnaire studies is reproduced here (Experiment 2.2) and you are invited to respond to the questions before reading further.

In Experiment 2.2, two students as well as two older men are portrayed in the vignettes. One person within each pair was described as high in ability and low in effort; the other person in that pair was characterized as low in ability but high in effort. In addition, in one vignette the outcome was a success, while in the other it was a failure. Subjects then responded to the inquiry about which of these two individuals they would rather be.

If personal value or worth, or what others think of one, is perceived to be determined only by ability level, then in all four vignettes there should be a desire to have high ability, so that the combination of high ability and low effort would be preferred. On the other hand, if choice is only based on moral considerations, then in all four scenarios high effort and low ability should be more preferred. And finally, if there is a desire to have high ability because it is more predictive of future success than high effort is, or if there is a desire to avoid low ability because it is more predictive of future failure than lack of effort is, then one should especially prefer the high ability/low effort causal pattern when a first-year student, inasmuch as many achievement tasks lie ahead. On the other hand, future success and failure are not a consideration for the men who are reflecting on their past lives. Thus, if moral considerations influence who one "wants to be," then in these scenarios there should be a preference for the low ability/high effort causal pattern.

Brown and Weiner (1984) reported that their subjects preferred op-

## EXPERIMENT 2.2

## Achievement-Related Variables

Please select one answer in each of the following situations.

1. This is a profile of two students. Student 1 has much natural ability. This student does not study hard. During the first year of college this student maintained a B+ average. Student 2 does not have much natural ability. This student studies hard. During the first year of college this student also maintained a B+ average. Which student would you rather be? Circle one:

   a. High ability and low effort; *or*
   b. High effort and low ability.

2. This is a profile of two students. Student 1 has much natural ability. This student does not study hard. During the first year of college this student maintained a C− average. Student 2 does not have much natural ability. This student studies hard. During the first year of college this student also maintained a C− average. Which student would you rather be? Circle one:

   a. High ability and low effort; *or*
   b. High effort and low ability.

3. This is a profile of two old men. Both are reflecting upon their lives. Man 1 has much natural ability. He did not try hard. During his working life he attained moderate success. Man 2 has little natural ability. He tried very hard. He too attained moderate success. Which man would you rather be? Circle one:

   a. High ability and low effort; *or*
   b. High effort and low ability.

4. This is a profile of two old men. Both are reflecting upon their lives. Man 1 has much natural ability. He did not try hard. During his working life he attained only limited success. Man 2 has little natural ability. He tried very hard. He too attained only limited success. Which of these two men would you rather be? Circle one:

   a. High ability and low effort; *or*
   b. High effort and low ability.

tion *a* (high ability/low effort) in the student scenarios (1 and 2) but preferred option *b* (low ability/high effort) in old men scenarios (3 and 4). This documented that, when expectancy of success is ruled out as a determinant of causal preference, moral considerations affect evaluation of the self and the presumed evaluations that others would make. The reader might want to compare his or her responses with the data reported by Brown and Weiner; I expect the preferences to be the same.

## Social Approval of Adolescent Peers

Another line of research questioning the relative value of attributions to effort versus ability has examined the causes that adolescent students communicate to their peers following success and failure. Behaviors that promote social acceptance in an adolescent peer group are likely to diverge from those effortful behaviors that adults value and reward (Juvonen & Murdock, 1993). This is because adolescents may perceive diligence as a sign of competition (Slavin, 1983) or as conformity to unacceptable norms prescribed by the oppositional culture of adults. If this is the case, then adolescent students and others who oppose the dominant cultural group may convey to their peers messages about the causes of success and failure that are different from the messages given to authority figures or to others in the dominant cultural group in order to gain acceptance from everyone involved.

To test the hypothesis that adolescents use different impression management techniques when they communicate to peers as opposed to adults, Juvonen and Murdock (1993) created scenarios that depicted students as having succeeded or failed on an important exam. The predominantly middle class, white subjects were then instructed to explain to their peers, parents, and teachers why they received this grade. Specifically, the instructions stated:

> Imagine a situation in which you have done really poorly (well) on an important exam. Your parents (teachers, popular classmates) are wondering why you did so poorly (well). You need to give an explanation. You want to get along with your parents (teachers, classmates who are popular). How likely is it that you would say each of the following? (p. 1369)

Among the alternative communication options were that their failed (successful) performance was due to low (high) ability and that the performance was due to low (high) effort. The likelihood that each response would be given was rated by the subjects.

Figure 2.5 depicts the data for success (left half) and failure (right half). It is evident from Figure 2.5 that, given success, adolescents are generally less likely to endorse either internal ascription of ability or effort when they communicate to peers rather than to adult authority figures. Perhaps this reveals modesty or humbleness, but more likely it is a strategy to not be perceived as a braggart. However, they particularly are less likely to convey to their peers that they tried hard. Similarly, given failure, adolescents tell their peers that they did not try rather than say that they do not have the ability. But the subjects stated that they would communi-

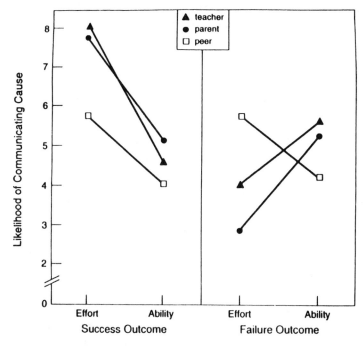

**FIGURE 2.5.** The likelihood of communicating that failure was caused by lack of effort versus lack of ability as a function of the recipient of the communication. Data from Juvonen and Murdock (1993).

cate to teachers and parents that they "cannot" rather than say that they did not try.

In sum, the data reported by Juvonen and Murdock (1993) convincingly demonstrated that adolescents (or students) prefer to tell *authority figures* (or teachers) that success was due to hard work and that failure was not due to lack of trying but was caused by lack of ability. This communication strategy is entirely consistent with the prior line of argumentation regarding the anticipated consequences of effort and ability attributions when made by authority figures. Considering only failure, the choices of communication to adults are likely to be guided by the following chains of inference or some variant that streamlines the process:

1. Adolescent fails → Adolescent communicates lack of effort → Adult ascribes the failure to low effort → Adult assumes that effort is controllable → Adult perceives the adolescent as responsible → Adult is angry → Adult will punish.

2. Adolescent fails → Adolescent communicates lack of ability → Adult ascribes the failure to low ability → Adult construes low ability as uncontrollable → Adult perceives the adolescent as not responsible → Adult feels sympathy → Adult will help and not punish.

Given these presumed chains of inferences, the adolescents (or students) will communicate low ability rather than low effort as the cause of their failure. These data, as well as the conceptual analyses, also strongly indicate that there is not a dominant desire to have others think that one has high ability.

On the other hand, adolescents prefer to communicate to popular peers, relative to adults, that success was not due to trying and that they failed precisely because they did not try. This is the opposite of what they state would be communicated to adults. Why should they do this? It seems plausible to hypothesize that this communication strategy conveys opposition to the values of adult authority figures and to the culture that adults represent. Again considering only failure, one possible interpretation of the communication to peers is captured by the following lines of reasoning:

1. Adolescent fails → Adolescent communicates lack of effort → Peer ascribes the failure to low effort → Peer assumes that effort is controllable → Peer perceives the other as intentionally violating adult rules → Peer expresses admiration → Peer accepts fellow adolescent into social network.
2. Adolescent fails → Adolescent communicates lack of ability → Peer ascribes the failure to low ability → Peer assumes that ability is uncontrollable → Peer perceives fellow adolescent as not responsible → Peer feels sympathy → Peer may help but not admit the "different" fellow adolescent into the social network.

It is evident, then, that it is not invariably the case that individuals want others to think that they are trying or that they are smart or dumb. Adolescents, and surely adults as well, are situationally discriminating and use disparate impression management strategies depending on the target of their communication and on how they want to be perceived.

## SUMMARY

It is common knowledge that legal decisions are guided by inferences about intent and the presence of a "guilty mind." It is perhaps less evident but no less important that achievement evaluation also is directed by this moral principle. In this chapter, I have documented that a distinction between failure caused by lack of ability and failure caused by lack of effort has generated a great variety of research that documents the importance of moral concerns in achievement settings.

It was first revealed that lack of effort in achievement contexts is particularly punished, whereas the expenditure of effort is especially rewarded. Paradoxically, low rather than high ability becomes a "favorable" evaluative attribute in achievement settings, inasmuch as high ability accompanied by low effort and failure is severely punished, whereas low ability accompanied by effort and success is especially rewarded. I included a book excerpt that reported the same recommendations more than 350 years ago. Furthermore, I showed that persons believe they are guided by moral considerations more than others are.

It was then argued that responsibility for the onset of a problem (failure) should be distinguished from responsibility for the continuation or the offset of that problem. When one is not responsible for an initial failure but does not work to overcome this problem when the opportunity is presented—that is, when the causes of failure change from uncontrollable to controllable—then others respond most negatively if instrumental activity is not undertaken. Thus, a student elicits very negative responses when he or she fails because of illness but then does not try when he or she is healthy.

It is not the case, however, that personal responsibility for failure is invariably avoided, compared to an ascription of failure to uncontrollable causes such as lack of ability. In situations where there will be further commerce with the task, an ascription to lack of effort may be "better" than one of low ability inasmuch as "trying" can be augmented. However, as documented in this chapter, preferences for the causes of failure when reevaluating one's life are primarily guided by moral considerations. In addition, adolescents may communicate that they are not trying in order to be popular with their peers (although they do not convey to adults that failure is due to lack of effort, but rather it is caused by inability).

The mechanisms and processes guiding these evaluation and communication decisions were outlined in Chapter 1 as well as in this chapter. I contended that effort is controllable, or subject to volitional alteration. Hence, a person who fails because of low effort is held responsible for this outcome and evokes anger. Anger, in turn, gives rise to some form of punishment. On the other hand, ability level (considering ability here as related closely to aptitude) is not construed as subject to willful change. Thus, an individual who fails because of low ability is not held responsible for that outcome, sympathy rather than anger is elicited, and punishment is withheld.

In addition to these proximal mechanisms, lack of effort may be punished because trying is instrumental to the survival of society. That is, it is functional for all persons to work and contribute to the common good; intolerance of those who do not try, then, decreases the likelihood that this behavior will continue, teaches others a moral lesson, and provides some retribution.

Just as in criminal contexts, in achievement settings the concepts of controllability, responsibility, and mitigating circumstances are central, and the affects of anger and sympathy are elicited. The linkages between causal beliefs, affects, and action lie at the heart of understanding the phenomena that have been presented. The distinction between ability and effort, is crucial to a comprehension of social responses in achievement settings.

# 3

---

# Responsibility and Stigmatization

It is a great sin to drink alcohol.
  —TOLSTOY (written at the request of the czar of
  Russia as a label to be placed on bottles of alcohol)

Does God want goodness, or the choice of goodness?
  —ANTHONY BURGESS, *A Clockwork Orange*

Just say "no."
  —REAGAN–BUSH solution to the drug problem

Thus far the responsibility process has been described, and it has been documented that responsibility judgments, which are so central in criminal contexts, also are an inherent aspect of achievement evaluation. But thoughts about responsibility are elicited by a variety of everyday behaviors that are pertinent neither to jury decisions nor to achievement-related activities. In the ensuing three chapters, evidence is provided for this assertion by considering perceptions of the stigmatized and the manner in which reactions to stigmatized persons are influenced by inferences about responsibility. I also elaborate further on the theory of motivated behavior that was incompletely presented in the initial two chapters.

First, a definition of stigma is required to identify the forthcoming topic of discussion in greater clarity. The modern usage of the term *stigma* originated with the Greek practice of branding slaves who were caught while trying to escape. The brand or mark was the letter *F*, for *fugitive*. The word for such a mark was *stigma* (from Funk, 1950). From this practice, the meaning of stigma was extended to embrace any mark or sign for perceived or inferred conditions of deviation from a norm (see Jones et al., 1984). As noted by Jones et al. (1984): "The bearer of a 'mark' . . . defines him or her as deviant, flawed, limited, spoiled, or generally undesirable" (p. 6). In a similar manner, Goffman (1963) stated that stigmas include "abominations of the body . . . blemishes of individual character inferred from a known record of, for example, mental disorder, imprisonment, addiction . . . and tribal stigma of race, nation, and religion" (p. 4). Thus, to be labeled as stigmatized, the normative deviations in physical attributes, character, behavior, and so forth must be undesirable—being different in and of itself is not stigmatizing.

In Chapter 3, I examine beliefs about responsibility and the consequences of this inference for a variety of "undesirable deviations," ranging from Alzheimer's disease to Vietnam War Syndrome. Special attention in this chapter will be devoted to the alcoholic, the obese, and the poor, marked because these characteristics define one as "deviant, flawed . . . or generally undesirable." Chapter 4 is concerned with homosexuality and acquired immuno deficiency syndrome, or what is more commonly known as AIDS. A separate chapter is devoted to AIDS because it reasonably could be described as the major stigma of this generation. Then, Chapter 5 considers a subset of stigmas in which research has examined the reactions of family members to the stigmatized and/or to one another. Included within Chapter 5 are discussions of depression, schizophrenia, and the precursor of divorce—a distressed marriage (which is not really a stigma, but nonetheless best fits here because it involves the family).

In the discussions in Chapters 3–5, I elaborate a distinction between sin (a moral transgression) and sickness (a condition of weakness). The same stigma (e.g., AIDS, cancer) may result in a person being construed as a sinner or as sick, with the applications of these labels dependent upon the perception of responsibility for the stigma. I will contend that the sin-sickness distinction in the domain of achievement is represented by the causal differentiation between lack of effort (a controllable cause of failure) and low ability (an uncontrollable cause). Indeed, the absence of effort has been conceptualized in Chapter 2 as a sin, whereas lack of ability is akin to a sickness, an "unchosen" weakness.

## AN EXPERIMENTAL DEMONSTRATION

In Chapter 2, two experiments were introduced to shed light on the ability–effort distinction and the moral connotations as well as the consequences of trying or not trying. Recall that in Experiment 2.1, evaluations were given to hypothetical students differing in exam outcome, ability, and effort. This experiment documented that output (success vs. failure) and input (trying vs. not trying) are the main determinants of evaluation, with failure associated with lack of effort and high ability evoking the greatest punishment. Then Experiment 2.2 illustrated that, when reviewing imagined life histories, individuals desire to have their capacities fulfilled through hard work, so that high effort and low ability are preferred to low effort and high ability, given that outcome is held constant and future achievements are not considered in the preference. I also am assuming (perhaps too eagerly) that these were the reports of the readers, although it must be expected that some individuals will deviate from these dominant patterns of appraisal and choice for a variety of psychologically valid and perhaps idiosyncratic reasons.

Continuing with the procedure of illuminating the main points of each chapter by providing experiential exercises, another experiment is now introduced. Again, it is in the reader's interests to undertake this experiment before reading on so that the responses to the study are not further influenced by what has been read (although some confounding already has been introduced). Let me describe the experiment first, and then the readers should indicate their responses.

In Experiment 3.1, 10 stigmas are listed. These stigmas are prevalent in our (and most other) cultures. The experiment first asks you to indicate how controllable each stigma is, that is, would it have been possible for the stigmatized person to engage in actions so as not to have this stigma? After the ratings of causal controllability, judgments regarding personal responsibility for the stigma are requested. Then you should report your emotional reactions of anger and sympathy (pity) toward the hypothetical stigmatized person. Finally, two behavioral responses are assessed: (1) The amount of personal assistance offered and (2) the amount of money allotted to each stigmatized other. Concerning monetary help, you are asked to distribute $1,000 to individuals who represent the 10 stigmas. All $1,000 may be given to one person, $100 to each one of the 10, or any other decision rule may be adopted, with the stipulation that all the money be distributed. Please complete this experiment now. However, do not yet complete the "data sheet"; this will be returned to later

## CONCEPTIONS OF ILLNESS

Prior to examining the results of Experiment 3.1, it is useful to first consider conceptions of illness that are held in everyday life and examine the manner in which illnesses are represented psychologically, or how they are construed. Understanding how illness is conceived will then provide

# EXPERIMENT 3.1
## Help to the Stigmatized

Please fill in the responses with numerical values that represent your opinions. For each question, 1 = very low (e.g., not controllable, not responsible, no anger, no sympathy, no personal aid); 7 = very high (e.g., highly controllable, etc.). For each stigma and judgment, use any number from 1 to 7. In the last column, distribute $1,000 to the 10 individuals, giving each person any amount up to $1,000 with the total not exceeding $1,000.

| Stigma | Controllability | Responsibility | Anger | Sympathy | Personal aid | Monetary award |
|---|---|---|---|---|---|---|
| AIDS | | | | | | |
| Alcoholism | | | | | | |
| Alzheimer's disease | | | | | | |
| Blindness | | | | | | |
| Cancer | | | | | | |
| Child abuser | | | | | | |
| Drug addiction | | | | | | |
| Heart attack | | | | | | |
| Obese | | | | | | |
| Paraplegia | | | | | | |

## Data Sheet for Experiment 3.1

| Stigma classification | Controllability | Responsibility | Anger | Sympathy | Personal aid | Monetary award |
|---|---|---|---|---|---|---|
| Controllable stigmas (AIDS, alcoholism, child abuser, drug addiction, obesity) | | | | | | |
| Uncontrollable stigmas (Alzheimer's, blindness, cancer, heart attack, paraplegia) | | | | | | |

some clues regarding perceptions of stigma, inasmuch as many (but not all) stigmas can be included within the category of illness. In addition, physical illness has been the subject of much thought regarding perceptions of responsibility.

Throughout history, illness has often been regarded as one form of punishment imposed for wrongdoing (see Murdock, 1980). Plagues, paralysis, and blindness are just some of the retributions imposed by divine powers on sinning others, as illustrated in the Oedipal myth. Susan Sontag (1978) points out that

> epidemic diseases were a common figure for social disorder. From pestilence (bubonic plague) came "pestilent," whose figurative meaning, according to the Oxford English Dictionary, is "injurious to religion, morals, or public peace" and "pestilential," meaning "morally baneful or pernicious." Feelings about evil are projected onto a disease. (p. 29)

If illness is conceived as a retribution, or "just deserts," then one might think that further punishment because of the illness itself is unfair and "less than human."

Rarely in modern society are illnesses thought to be imposed by powerful others seeking revenge (but see the discussion of AIDS in Chapter 4 for an exception). Nonetheless, there remain a variety of lay theories regarding the causes of sickness and differentiations of sickness according to the type of causality (see Sontag, 1978). One modern distinction that has been drawn is between a disease and an illness (see Eisenberg, 1977; Helman, 1978). A disease is something that a person or an organism "has" that is caused by a "germ." Germs are thought of as "living, invisible, malevolent entities . . . they exist only in or among people . . . the germ reveals its true personality in stages, during the course of the disease" (Helman, 1978, p. 118).

Germs originate outside of the individual. Hence, the victim of a germ-originated infection is not held responsible for its onset. Having a disease, therefore, is an acceptable reason to withdraw from work and social obligations, without any threat of punishment (considered in detail in Chapter 8). Recall from the earlier discussion that punishment for a social transgression presumes the presence of the logically prior stages in the motivational process, which include an attribution of causal controllability, inferences of personal responsibility, and feelings of anger.

In contrast to disease, "illness" is a vaguer concept as far as the origin of causality is concerned. Indeed, one can feel ill without having any identifiable disease. One common type of illness is a cold. It is a common belief that colds are brought about by something that the person has or has not done: not dressing properly, going outside with one's head still wet from a shower, walking barefoot on a cold floor. In general, not taking care of oneself and not engaging in appropriate precautions are seen as "inviting" colds. Thus, persons often are regarded as causing their own colds and are judged as responsible. Likewise, one also is responsible for the offset of a cold and getting well by means of proper behaviors (e.g., "feeding a cold").

There appear to be some cross-cultural differences in the labeling of physical problems as a disease (not controllable) as opposed to an illness (controllable). It has been suggested that in America most ill health is labeled as lifestyle induced and, therefore, as the sick person's fault. This has been called the "tyranny of the healthy over the sick." Such a belief system less characterizes the Europeans.

In sum, judgments of others are given for various physical problems. At times, the other is inferred to be responsible. These judgments, in turn, influence reactions to the sick individual.

In addition to varying on the characteristic of assigned responsibility, illnesses also differ from one another in a number of other properties. Attempts have been made to identify the properties that differentiate illnesses from one another. Table 3.1 summarizes six investigations that searched for these distinguishing characteristics. In all the studies, the dimensions were determined from ratings of illnesses on a variety of factors or from multidimensional scaling techniques. In the latter procedure, illnesses are compared in pairs and rated for similarity. Clusters then emerge that are seen in the spatial groupings of the illnesses. Identification of the basic dimensions is guided by the type of illness within each cluster.

In the first study listed in Table 3.1, conducted by Kerrick (1969), two factors, or properties, of illness were isolated: how severe and how avoidable the illness was. Examination of Table 3.1 confirms that three of the other investigations also found that illnesses are differentiated in everyday life on the basis of their severity. Kerrick's second dimension, the extent to which the illness was avoidable, is quite closely related to the familiar concepts of controllability and responsibility, which were identified as dimensions of illness by Turk, Rudy, and Salovey (1986) and by Long (1990). According to the Kerrick (1969) classification, illnesses therefore are perceived as severe and avoidable (controllable), mild and controllable, severe and uncontrollable, and mild and uncontrollable.

A number of other possible dimensions of illness also are reported in Table 3.1. These range widely, including whether the illness is treated by heat or cold, is mainly found in children or adults, is viral or nonviral, and so on. Many factors could account for the disparities between the results in the research investigations, including the illnesses that were rated, the

**TABLE 3.1.** Summary of Studies of Illness Dimensions

| Investigation(s) | Subjects | Methods | Dimensions |
|---|---|---|---|
| Kerrick (1969) | Mexican American and Anglo American teenagers | Ratings of disease | Mild/severe<br>Avoidable/unavoidable |
| D'Andrade et al. (1972) | American and Mexican adults | Ratings of disease | Contagious/noncontagious<br>Severe/not severe<br>Hot/cold treatment<br>Childhood/adult |
| Schmelkin et al. (1988) | Medical students | Ratings of diseases on disease characteristics | Psychological/physical |
| Turk et al. (1986) | Undergraduate students, nurses, and diabetics | Ratings of illness perceptions | Severe<br>Personally responsible<br>Controllable<br>Changeable |
| Bishop (1987) | Adults | Ratings of symptoms of diseases | Viral/nonviral<br>Upper body/lower body<br>Physical/psychological<br>Disruptive/nondisruptive |
| Long (1990) | Adults, nurses | Similarity ratings | Disabling<br>Controllable<br>Morally repugnant |

59

kinds of ratings made, and so on. And one can intuit still a wider array of dimensions along which physical illnesses might vary. According to Crandall and Moriarity (in press):

> Some illnesses have a distinctly moral component (e.g., syphilis), others are morally benign. . . . Some are closely related to ethnicity (e.g., testicular cancer), others are related to age (e.g., osteoporosis), social class (e.g., pneumonia) or physiological development (e.g., facial acne).

Given the empirical findings reported in Table 3.1, what is most acceptable at this point in time is that the main dimensions of illness were identified in the original study by Kerrick (1969), namely, severity (which relates to the illness itself) and personal responsibility/controllability (which relates to the cause of the outcome). Note that these two characteristics closely correspond to the determinants of evaluation in achievement contexts, that is, output (magnitude of success and failure) and input (cause of the outcome, or effort expenditure).

The two dimensions of outcome magnitude (illness severity) and responsibility for the illness are most predictive of social rejection of the ill. Crandall and Moriarity (in press) had their subjects rate 66 illnesses on 13 underlying characteristics. The dimensions were described with the following scale anchors: severe–mild, visible–concealable, highly contagious–not contagious, common–rare, treatable–not treatable, acute–chronic, a function of age–not related to age, one sex gets it–both sexes get it, caught by behavior–unaffected by behavior, avoidable–unavoidable, ethnic related–unrelated to ethnicity, hereditary–not hereditary, and sexually transmitted–not sexually transmitted. In addition to these ratings, the subjects revealed to what extent they would reject people with these sicknesses.

It was found that an illness would lead to the most rejection if it was severe, contagious, avoidable, caused by behavior, and sexually transmitted. Whether an illness is perceived as avoidable, caused by behavior, and sexually transmitted (and perhaps even contagious, as Crandall and Moriarity suggest), relates to personal control, that is, the extent to which the illness is directly or indirectly the fault of the afflicted person. Hence, the more severe the disease, and the greater the perceived controllability of the onset of the illness, the more that the individual with this problem is rejected. Again, one finds a parallel with the law: In criminal sentencing, the more severe the crime, and the greater the inferred responsibility, the greater the punishment.

The classification of illness according to the degree of personal responsibility influences not only the reactions of laypeople but also the care that practitioners, both from the medical and psychological professions, may give to their patients. In one study of psychological distress, Brewin (1984) asked medical students whether they would prescribe tranquilizing drugs to particular patients. The cause of the distress also was revealed and included 40 life events such as divorce, loss of a job, relocation, a death in the family, retirement, and so on. The respondents rated these causes on patient controllability. Brewin (1984) reported that the medical students were more willing to prescribe drugs for patients experiencing uncontrollable as opposed to controllable distressing events. This association was weakened when the severity of the event was taken into account but still had an effect in selected instances (see also Madey, DePalma, Bahrt, & Bierne, 1993). In sum, the quality of medical care may in part depend on the moral evaluation of the patient.

## CONCEPTIONS OF STIGMAS

As in the case of physical illnesses, stigmas also have been examined in order to discover their underlying properties or dimensions. And again a number of key characteristics have been proposed, including the danger posed by the person, the visibility of the stigmatizing condition, the ultimate prognosis, the aesthetic appearance of the person, the difficulty of normal social interaction with the individual, and so on (see, e.g., Jones et al., 1984; Katz et al., 1987; Siller, 1986; Tringo, 1970). Given the perspective of this book and the prior discussions, I will turn to the controllability/responsibility property and its influence on reactions to the stigmatized.

### Responsibility and Stigmatization

A great deal of research has revealed that both the stigmatized person and others search for the origin of a stigma and the possible presence of personal responsibility. As documented by Wright (1983), physically handicapped persons often ask themselves the existential attribution question, "Why me?" and frequently are confronted with the question, "How did this happen?" This search is not limited to physical abnormalities. One hears such queries as, "Why is he drinking so much?" or "What caused the nervous breakdown?" In many instances, however, the stigma itself implies a cause, thus negating the need for further information. For example, drug abuse may automatically be linked with "moral weakness," and the HIV infection associated with AIDS may be linked with promiscuous and/or aberrant sexual behavior (as will be examined in detail in the next chapter). According to the prior analysis, judged responsibility for having the stigma should guide not only affective reactions toward the stigmatized person but also as a variety of behavioral responses, including, for example, help-related actions (help might be regarded as the inverse of punishment and, therefore, should be amenable to the same analysis as was hypothesized for punishment).

In a recent investigation, I examined, along with two colleagues, the relations between stigmas, the perceived source of those stigmas, assignments of responsibility, affective reactions, and intended actions (Weiner, Perry, & Magnusson, 1988). In our investigations, 10 stigmas (AIDS, Alzheimer's disease, blindness, cancer, child abuser, drug addiction, heart disease, obesity, paraplegia, and Vietnam War Syndrome) were rated in regard to the responsibility of persons for these conditions; affective reactions of liking, anger, and pity; and help-related behaviors of charitable donations and personal assistance (unfortunately, perceptions of causal controllability were not assessed in this study). Ratings were made on nine-point scales anchored at the extremes with labels such as entirely responsible–not at all responsible or no anger–a great deal of anger. It is evident that this investigation guided the construction of Experiment 3.1, presented just a few pages ago, with some minor modifications made in the stigmas that were rated and in the exact rating scales.

The data from one study reported by Weiner et al. (1988) are given in Table 3.2. Table 3.2 shows that six of the stigmas were judged low on perceived personal responsibility (Alzheimer's disease, blindness, cancer, heart disease, paraplegia, and Vietnam War Syndrome), whereas the remaining four stigmas (AIDS, child abuser, drug addiction, and obesity) were rated high on this variable. Hence, stigmatized persons were generally not held responsible for physical problems but were judged as responsible for behavioral/mental problems. Medical doctors, therefore, treat patients generally perceived as not responsible for their problems (with some exceptions, such as AIDS), but the patients of psychologists are considered by the public as personally at fault for their plights!

Table 3.2 also shows that individuals not considered responsible for their stigmas were rated relatively high on liking, elicited pity but not anger, and generated high judgments regarding intentions to help. Conversely, persons with stigmas for which they were viewed as responsible were relatively disliked, evoked little pity and comparatively high anger, and elicited low help giving intentions.

Thus far in this book, cross-cultural comparisons have been relatively ignored. But cross-cultural data indicate the generality of the principles being proposed, and therefore, it is important to examine such data. Table 3.3 reports the findings from an exact replication of the Weiner et al. (1988) investigation that was conducted in the People's Republic of China (Lin, 1993). The subjects again were male and female college students. The general pattern of data reported by Lin (1993) is quite similar to that shown in Table 3.2. Thus, there is reason to believe that the judgments of the

**TABLE 3.2.** Mean Values on Responsibility-Related Variables

| Stigma | Responsi-bility | Blame | Liking | Pity | Anger | Assistance | Charitable donations |
|---|---|---|---|---|---|---|---|
| Alzheimer's disease | 0.8 | 0.5 | 6.5 | 7.9 | 1.4 | 8.0 | 6.9 |
| Blindness | 0.9 | 0.5 | 7.5 | 7.4 | 1.7 | 8.5 | 7.2 |
| Cancer | 1.6 | 1.3 | 7.6 | 8.0 | 1.6 | 8.4 | 8.1 |
| Heart disease | 2.5 | 1.6 | 7.5 | 7.4 | 1.6 | 8.0 | 7.5 |
| Paraplegia | 1.6 | 0.9 | 7.0 | 7.6 | 1.4 | 8.1 | 7.1 |
| Vietnam War syndrome | 1.7 | 1.5 | 5.7 | 7.1 | 2.1 | 7.0 | 6.2 |
| AIDS | 4.4 | 4.8 | 4.8 | 6.2 | 4.0 | 5.8 | 6.5 |
| Child abuser | 5.2 | 6.0 | 2.0 | 3.3 | 7.9 | 4.6 | 4.0 |
| Drug abuse | 6.5 | 6.7 | 3.0 | 4.0 | 6.4 | 5.3 | 5.0 |
| Obesity | 5.3 | 5.2 | 5.7 | 5.1 | 3.3 | 5.8 | 4.0 |

*Note.* Adapted from Weiner, Perry, and Magnusson (1988, p. 740). Copyright 1988 by the American Psychological Association. Reprinted by permission of the author.

stigmas have generality across at least two very distinct cultures and, presumably, to other cultures as well.

The data from Weiner et al. (1988) may be used to assess the temporal sequence hypothesized earlier, progressing from inferences of responsibility to affect to action. The correlations between the thinking–feeling–acting indexes in this study are shown in Table 3.4: Stigmas were treated as dichotomous variables, with a score of 1 assigned for behavioral/mental stigmas and 2 for somatic/physiological stigmas; positive affect was represented as liking + pity − anger; and helping was the combined index of personal assistance + charity intentions. Table 3.4 shows that there are significant correlations between these four indexes, in the direction intimated in the prior chapters. That is, behavioral/mental stigmas are associated with greater responsibility, less positive affect, and less help (or, conversely, somatic stimuli are related to less responsibility, more positive affect, and greater help). Further, the greater the responsibility, the less positive the affect and the lower the stated intentions to help.

Considering a proposed sequence of stigma origin → assigned responsibility → affect → action (note the absence of controllability because data were not obtained for this causal perception), Table 3.4 reveals that the

**TABLE 3.3.** Mean Values on Responsibility and Related Variables

| Stigma | Responsi-bility | Controllability-related variables | | | | | |
|---|---|---|---|---|---|---|---|
| | | Blame | Like | Pity | Anger | Assistance | Charitable donations |
| Alzheimer's disease | 3.19 | 1.69 | 4.00 | 6.83 | 2.44 | 6.83 | 6.80 |
| Blindness | 1.52 | 0.56 | 5.21 | 8.20 | 1.48 | 8.23 | 7.95 |
| Cancer | 2.19 | 0.97 | 4.76 | 7.75 | 1.55 | 7.56 | 7.69 |
| Heart disease | 2.07 | 1.03 | 5.09 | 7.15 | 1.64 | 7.71 | 6.95 |
| Paraplegia | 1.56 | 0.71 | 5.01 | 8.20 | 1.56 | 8.05 | 8.19 |
| War syndrome | 3.51 | 3.28 | 3.87 | 5.63 | 4.48 | 5.83 | 5.41 |
| Obesity | 4.60 | 3.99 | 4.07 | 4.91 | 4.04 | 5.79 | 4.12 |
| AIDS | 6.47 | 6.20 | 1.83 | 3.39 | 7.16 | 4.01 | 4.16 |
| Child abuser | 7.28 | 7.31 | 1.49 | 1.73 | 8.59 | 2.32 | 1.75 |
| Drug abuse | 6.97 | 7.00 | 1.47 | 2.80 | 7.83 | 3.44 | 2.52 |

*Note.* From Lin (1993, p. 159). Copyright 1993 by *Acta Psychologica Sinica.* Reprinted by permission.

**TABLE 3.4.** Correlations between Perceived Responsibility and Related Variables

| | Stigma source[a] | Perceived responsibility[b] | Positive affect | Help |
|---|---|---|---|---|
| Stigma source | | .59[c] | .50 | .38 |
| Perceived responsibility | | | .66 | .38 |
| Positive affect | | | | .65 |
| Help | | | | |

*Note.* Data from Weiner, Perry, and Magnusson (1988).
[a]Physically based stigmas = 2; mental/behavioral stigmas = 1.
[b]High values indicate lack of perceived responsibility.
[c]For all correlations, $p < .01$.

greater the number of steps between the variables in this postulated sequence, the lower their correlation. Specifically, when there is just one step in the path (as represented by stigma source to perceived responsibility, responsibility to affect, and affect to help), then the absolute average correlation between the two variables is $r = .63$; when the path involves two steps (stigma source to affect, perceived responsibility to help), then the average $r = .44$; and when there are three steps between the variables in the proposed path, which occurs only in the association between stigma source and help, then the correlation between the two variables is $r = .38$. This suggests that as the motivational sequence progresses, direct predictive power from the originating variable (in this case, stigma source) to the predicted variable (in this instance, help giving) is lost because of the intervention of mediating variables. For this investigation, help was strongly associated with affect but not with stigma source or inferred responsibility. The proposed affective mediator, therefore, is the proximal determinant of judgments to act.

In sum, reactions to the stigmatized are, in part, based on moral evaluations. Stigmatized persons considered responsible for their marks are construed as moral failures, which generates morality-related negative affects and, in turn, uncooperative behaviors. On the other hand, stigmatized individuals not assigned responsibility for their marks elicit altruism-generating affects as well as prosocial intentions.

## Returning to Experiment 3.1: Reacting to the Stigmatized

With these data in mind, let us now return to Experiment 3.1 to determine the correspondence between the reactions of the reader and the data in Table 3.2. To facilitate this comparison, the "data sheet" section should now be completed. There the reader is asked to combine some of his or her data. This procedure is based on the a priori belief (guided by earlier experimental findings) that 5 of the stigmas (AIDS, alcoholism, child abuser, drug addiction, and obesity) will be construed as high in controllability because they involve behavioral/mental "aberrations." On the other hand, the remaining 5 stigmas (Alzheimer's disease, blindness, cancer, heart attack, and paraplegia) are more likely to elicit perceptions of uncontrollability because of their apparent somatic origin. Of course, for any reader there might be some reversal in scores (e.g., one may conceive a heart attack is caused by smoking and alcoholism is a genetic problem). For ease of analysis, however, this possibility is ignored here. The reader, therefore, should combine his or her responses to the 5 stigmas in each category (labeled "controllable" and "uncontrollable") and calculate the mean, or average, of each set of five responses, across all six dependent variables.

If these data replicate those reported by Weiner et al. (1988), then the 5 behavioral/mental stigmas will elicit greater perceptions of controllability and responsibility, more anger, less sympathy, and relatively low values for personal aid and dollar awards. Conversely, the somatic stigmas should elicit perceptions of less controllability and responsibility, lower anger, more sympathy, and greater judgments of helping. Correlations cannot be calculated across subjects unless the readers share their ratings, in which case Table 3.3 also could be examined for replicability. (It is possible for correlations to be determined within each person, and these data may be further "purified" by combining the five stigmas rated most controllable and the five most uncontrollable rather than the a priori lists that were given).

I do believe that the judgments for the individual stigmas as shown in Table 3.2 and the data from Experiment 3.1 will be quite similar. I hope this proves to be true; if so, then I can feel quite good about the reliability of the data, a problem often encountered in studies of psychological phenomena.

## Manipulating Perceptions of Stigmas

Although it is evident that some stigmas are judged as more controllable than others—and, thus, persons are inferred to be more responsible for some stigmas than for others, there is not any direct evidence in the research presented thus far that stigma controllability and inferences of responsibility *give rise to* or cause anger, sympathy, and certain behaviors. Rather, the prior research only documented that these variables go together, or are correlated. It may be, for example, that one believes people are responsible for becoming HIV positive and is angry at them but that anger is caused by negative attitudes toward gay men and drug users and is not due to inferences about personal responsibility for getting the AIDS virus.

To examine whether controllability and responsibility actually elicit specific affects and, in turn, behaviors, Weiner et al. (1988) conducted an investigation in which the causes of stigmas were manipulated to be controllable or uncontrollable. For example, heart disease was described as caused by an unhealthy life style (controllable) or by a genetic deficit (uncontrollable); cancer was characterized as caused by smoking (controllable) or by unknowingly living in a toxic area (uncontrollable); and paraplegia was described as caused by reckless driving (controllable) or by being hit by a reckless driver (uncontrollable by the victim). Then perceptions of responsibility, the affects of pity and anger, and behavioral intentions were assessed and compared in these two opposing conditions, as well as in a third condition in which no information regarding stigma controllability was provided.

Figure 3.1 depicts just the pity and anger judgments in the three conditions that varied the information about the cause of the stigma. As anticipated, new information about the cause of the stigma altered the affective reactions. Uncontrollability increased pity and decreased anger, particularly when the stigma would ordinarily be construed as controllable, whereas controllability increased anger and decreased pity, especially given

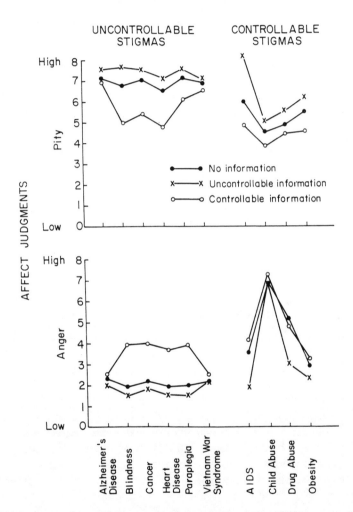

**FIGURE 3.1.** Ratings of pity (top half) and anger (bottom half) given controllable, uncontrollable, and no information for 10 stigmas. Left portion depicts stigmas normally perceived as uncontrollable; right portion depicts stigmas normally perceived as controllable. From Weiner, Perry, and Magnusson (1988, p. 745). Copyright 1988 by the American Psychological Association. Reprinted by permission of the author.

those stigmas that typically are considered uncontrollable. Thus, for example, when AIDS was depicted as onset uncontrollable (because of HIV infection through a blood transfusion), it elicited more pity and less anger than when described as controllable (because of sexual behavior) or when only the AIDS label was provided.

However, not all stigmas are amenable to such alterations. For example, it is not readily possible to convince others that one is responsible for Alzheimer's disease. There is sufficient media coverage for the public to realize that the causes and symptoms of this illness are not amenable to volitional alteration. In addition, it is very difficult to persuade others that one is not responsible for child abuse. Even information that the abuser also was abused as a child and is undergoing terrible stress does not greatly mitigate inferences of responsibility. Image reparation is very difficult in this case for it is immoral to abuse a child, regardless of the personal history of the abuser.

In sum, these data inform us that:

1. Perceptions of controllability and uncontrollability give rise to beliefs about responsibility and the affects of pity and anger.
2. These perceptions often, but not always, are subject to modification, which provides hope that entrenched beliefs and affective and behavioral reactions may be altered with appropriate educational and informational intervention techniques. This is elaborated later in this chapter.

## On Blaming the Victim

The pattern of data may make it appear that we unfairly "blame the victim"—that is, we fault those like alcoholics, the obese, the poor, and so on when they are "innocent." This is a compelling hypothesis that has attracted much attention among psychologists and laypersons. Psychologists find it appealing because it points out an "evil" aspect of human behavior that is not readily apparent; laypeople find it appealing because it points out an aspect of human nature that indeed agrees with their common sense! The data reviewed in this chapter seemingly substantiate the tendency to judge victims as responsible for their problems.

On the other hand, the empirical evidence reported in this chapter can be interpreted quite differently. Those with Alzheimer's disease, the blind, paraplegics, and so on, are surely victims. Yet the data in Table 3.2 and most likely your own reports in Experiment 3.1 reveal that individuals with these stigmas are not blamed, or held responsible, for their plights.

Thus, the general presumption that we blame victims is surely incorrect, and psychologists were premature to adopt this accusation. Do we blame the starving children in Africa? Do we even entertain the idea that they "deserve it?" The very writing of this is appalling. The correct psychological principle is not that we blame victims, but rather that we judge them. Some are then found responsible while others are not. Those with behavioral/mental stigmas tend to be blamed, and those with somatic stigmas tend not to be blamed. But for both classes of stigmas the judgments are alterable as new information about the victim is obtained.

The presumption that we blame the victim perhaps can be substantiated in instances in which there are both controllable and uncontrollable determinants of a stigma (e.g., a person with cancer who unknowingly lived in a toxic area and was a heavy smoker as well). If the smoking information is weighted more heavily than geographical knowledge in the judgment of responsibility, then perhaps it could be concluded that we blame the victim. But blameworthiness—that is, responsibility and linked anger—that is directed toward the stigmatized depends on their blameworthiness! One is not blamed for obesity because of a thyroid problem but is blamed for obesity because of overeating; when both of these determinants have contributed to the stigma, blame surely will fall between these extremes.

It is indeed the case that individuals have antiobesity attitudes, derogatory opinions and stereotypes about homosexuals, and a number of negative beliefs about those who are different. And there is a propensity for some labels, such as obesity, to elicit responsibility judgments in the absence of further causal evidence. But these judgments are modifiable when appropriate information and education are provided. That is, the inference, at least in part, is traceable to cognitive rather than to the implicit motivational factors that are conveyed with the connotation of victim blame. Like other inferences, judgments of responsibility are not necessarily veridical, and at times there could be too little as well as too much blame.

In the following sections of this chapter, I further discuss themes regarding inferences of responsibility, modification of causal beliefs, affective responses, and individual differences in reactions to the stigmatized, as I examine in greater detail the diverse stigmas of alcoholism, obesity, and poverty.

## ALCOHOLISM

Experiment 3.1, in contrast to the research by Weiner et al. (1988), included alcoholism among the rated stigmas. Given the prior discussion, it might be anticipated that alcoholics will be considered responsible for their stigma, with excessive drinking perceived as a behavioral/mental disorder that is under the volitional control of the "sinner." In support of this hypothesis, a survey at Kent State University asked approximately 700 students to what extent persons were responsible for their alcoholism (as well as homosexuality, mental illness, and obesity—four behavioral/mental stigmas). The types of items (answered from "strongly agree" to "strongly disagree") were: "An alcoholic is responsible for his or her condition" and "Alcoholism is nearly always the result of forces within the person's control."

The mean judgments of responsibility for the stigmas were as follows: mental illness, $M = 2.7$; homosexuality, $M = 5.7$; obesity, $M = 5.8$; and alcoholism, $M = 6.4$ (where 1 = not responsible and 9 = totally responsible). Thus, among these behavioral/mental stigmas, the alcoholic was the most morally condemned (although even for this group the mean judgments were far from the end point on the scale). In a similar manner, a sample of adults consisting of alcoholic caregivers, mental health professionals, educators, and judges blamed alcoholics almost twice as much as the mentally ill for their stigmas, with judges regarding the alcoholic as particularly blameworthy (Rivers, Sarata, Dill, & Anagnostopulous, 1990). Further, as Humphreys and Rappaport (1993) note:

> The most famous American[s] . . . who used an internal defect model of substance abuse were probably the advocates of prohibition, such as the Women's Christian Temperance Union. [They] . . . said that substance abuse was due to moral and spiritual weakness and a lack of willpower. At its ugliest, this model has carried with it the claim that such moral weaknesses are due to the inferiority of other races, as when the Irish Catholics were characterized as morally weak alcoholics in the 1800s, . . . when hatred of Chinese immigrants fueled the anti-opium campaign of the 1870s . . . , and when Mexican immigrants were linked with marijuana use in the 1930s. (p. 896)

However, in contrast to the cited research and opinions of some, other investigators have reported that alcoholics are perceived as having a disease. That is, in accordance with most professionals in the field, alcoholism is thought to be determined more by biological processes than by "evil" intention (see Blum, Roman, & Bennett, 1989; Titus & Thompson, 1991).

And to make matters even more muddy and complex, still other researchers report that the main perceived causes of alcoholism are neither poor morals nor genetic and biological givens. In an investigation by Furnham and Lowick (1984), 265 subjects were given a list of 30 possible explanations for excessive drinking. The most important cause was represented by the item, "They have found that alcohol helps them to reduce their anxiety." This was followed in importance by the following items:

"They find drink the only way to cope with frequent depressions," "Drinking helps them to cope with boredom in their lives," and "They suffer from considerable stress at work." Thus, immediate situational factors were perceived as causing excessive drinking, while personality and moral factors and biological and genetic deficits were among the least endorsed causes.

It is difficult (if not impossible) to reconcile the research contradictions regarding the perceived causes of drinking. However, the empirical disparities may depend upon whether an overall "responsibility" rating is made or whether lists of specific causes are considered (but see Beckman, 1979).

In addition to methodological factors, theoretical analyses also help to illuminate the reasons for the disparities in the research studies. Brickman et al. (1982) have written:

> The question of moral responsibility can be conceptualized as involving two separate issues—blame and control. We assign blame to people when we hold them responsible for having created problems. We assign control to people when we hold them responsible for influencing or changing event. . . . Responsibility for the origin of a problem, generally responsibility for a past event, clearly involves the question of deservingness and blame. Responsibility for the solution of a problem, generally responsibility for future events, clearly involves an assessment of who might be able to control events. (p. 369)

Thus, according to Brickman et al. (1982), one can be perceived as responsible for the onset and/or the offset of a problem or for neither the initiating cause nor the continuation of the stigma. Recall in Chapter 2 that I reviewed a study by Karasawa (1991) in which lack of effort or sickness caused initial failure and/or the continuation of that failure.

Figure 3.2 summarizes the Brickman et al. (1982) analysis of responsibility. As indicated, responsibility for both the onset and the continuation of a problem corresponds to what Brickman et al. (1982) label a moral problem. Conversely, one can be seen as responsible for neither the onset nor the offset of a problem. This is labeled a medical model: One has a disease. Recall that moral and medical models were the two opposing inferences often reported in prior stigma research.

Of special interest in the Brickman et al. (1982) typology are circumstances in which there is a difference between the determinants of the onset and the determinants of the offset of a problem, or stigma. Consider first the situation in which people are responsible for causing their problem but are not considered accountable for the solution. This has been labeled the "enlightenment model." People who accept this scheme must take a ne-

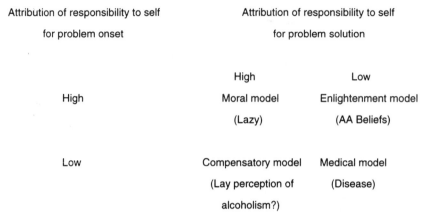

FIGURE 3.2. Models of responsibility as a function of attributions for both the onset and the offset of the problem. Adapted from Brickman et al. (1982, p. 370). Copyright 1982 by the American Psychological Association. Adapted by permission.

gative view of themselves and must accept submission to others in order to get better. As noted by Brickman et al. (1982):

> Alcoholics Anonymous (AA), one of the most successful examples of an enlightenment model organization, explicitly requires new recruits both to take responsibility for their past history of drinking (rather than blaming it on a spouse, a job, or other stressful circumstances) and to admit that it is beyond their power to control their drinking—without the help of God and the Community. . . . All bad things are blamed on the residue of the old life and good things credited to the experience of the new. (p. 374)

Finally, Brickman et al. (1982) identify what they call a "compensatory" model, wherein persons are not considered responsible for the onset of their problem but they are responsible for its offset. Thus, the onset of excessive drinking is thought of as initially beyond a person's control (because of stress, a negative life event, etc.); but once the person is drinking too much, he or she must cope with the problem and assume personal responsibility for its offset.

The compensatory model seems to best capture the naive perceptions of alcoholism. When a list of causes of alcoholism is presented, such as job stress, the implication is that one is judging responsibility for the onset of drinking. Given this methodology, alcoholics tend not to be faulted. On the other hand, when general responsibility judgments are made, individuals may be considering the offset or the continuation of the condition. In that context, which was represented in Experiment 3.1, alcoholics are held responsible. Hence, in opposition to the assumptions of AA, the common belief may be that alcoholics are not to be faulted for the onset of their problem but are responsible for its continuation.

## Alcoholism as a Perceived Cause of Criminal Behavior

The evidence is quite unequivocal linking alcoholism and crime. Robbery, wife beating, rape, and homicide are all exacerbated by drinking behavior (see Aarons et al., 1977). This is acknowledged by the lay public; surveys have repeatedly found that alcohol is believed to be a major factor in crimes of violence (see, e.g., Kidder & Cohn, 1979). Indeed, the temperance movement in the 18th and 19th centuries was both a product of this belief and in addition helped to shape this opinion (Critchlow, 1986).

A question with practical as well as theoretical significance is whether beliefs about the effect of drinking on behavior influence judgments of responsibility and punishments for crimes committed when drunk. In the first chapter, I noted that mitigating circumstances can reduce judgments of personal responsibility for a social transgression. Among the main categories of mitigators is limited capacity, or the lack of ability to distinguish right from wrong. Hence, children, the insane, the mentally retarded, and even "brainwashed" cult members are assigned lessened responsibility for an untoward act. Excessive alcoholic consumption is known to give rise to cognitive deficits, confusion, and thought disorder. These side effects should then function to reduce perceptions of responsibility and, in turn, decrease anger, increase sympathy, and reduce punishments toward wrongdoers who committed crimes while under the influence of alcohol. Summarizing the pertinent contributions of MacAndrew and Edgerton (1969) regarding this viewpoint, Critchlow (1986) writes:

> [They] have suggested that drinking provides a "time out" from usual social rules; due to alcohol's reputation as a disinhibitor, the drink rather than the drinker is blamed for untoward behavior. The major thesis of the MacAndrew and Edgerton book, that drunk people display disinhibited behavior because they can get away with it, rests on the assumption that intoxicated people are attributed less responsibility for their actions than sober people. (p. 761)

Critchlow (1986) goes on to state:

> Culturally bound beliefs about alcohol's effects provide the underlying rationale for the excuse function of drinking, in that it is the supposed powers of alcohol that lead to lessened responsibility for the

drinker. . . . In our current era of problem amplification, if greater powers are attributed to alcohol, drinking is more likely to serve as an excuse for antisocial behavior. We thus are left with a view of alcohol as a substance that is malign but that enables a number of transgressions to be partially condoned. (p. 761)

On the other hand, there is much evidence in everyday life that individuals want to increase (rather than decrease) the punishment of those committing crimes when under the influence of alcohol. Few citizen groups are more visible and powerful today than Mothers Against Drunk Drivers (MADD), which has lobbied effectively for more severe punishments against individuals who have accidents while driving when drunk.

Thus, two opposing tendencies appear to be elicited if a crime or social transgression is committed when the violator is drunk. On the one hand, being intoxicated while committing a crime may be considered a mitigating circumstance that reduces responsibility and punishment, perhaps by decreasing the inference of a "guilty mind." Conversely, persons are perceived as responsible for stopping their drinking behavior and should be aware of the dangers of, for example, driving when drunk. Some theorists have advocated that punishment for an act should be proportional to the "risks taken." This would increase perceptions of responsibility for a crime committed when intoxicated.

And what about the data? Does the research provide evidence that one or the other of these two positions—namely, that drinking decreases versus increases responsibility—is dominant? The answer is no. The data are mixed: Some researchers report that punishment is reduced when a crime, such as wife abuse, is committed while the abuser is drunk (e.g., see Richardson & Campbell, 1980). On the other hand, different researchers report an increase in responsibility and fault under these conditions (e.g., Aramburu & Leigh, 1991). Perhaps these research disparities reflect changing cultural beliefs. But today, it is likely that general statements such as "alcoholic consumption increases (decreases) responsibility and punishment" will not be substantiated. Rather, the effects of intoxication on inferences of responsibility will likely depend on the type of crime, the pattern of drinking behavior, the perceived causes of drinking, and so on. This unfortunately is not the simple rule that psychologists and other scientists prefer, but there just may not be a single principle that captures inferences about responsibility and punishment for a crime committed under the influence of alcohol.

## OBESITY

The scientific evidence indicating that obesity is in part (at times) caused by biological givens has long been established (see Chlouverakis, 1975). For example, Stunkard et al. (1986) found that measures of body fat in children are highly correlated with biological parents but not with adoptive parents. Furthermore, it is known that attempts at weight loss are generally ineffective. This is partly because energy metabolism becomes increasingly efficient when dieting, so that physiological factors make dieting both difficult and usually ineffective (Bennett & Gurin, 1982).

In spite of this evidence, which is known by some of the lay public, fatness tends to be perceived as controllable, and people are considered responsible for being overweight (men do not exercise enough; women eat too much). The constant advertising of products and programs for weight loss certainly reinforces this belief. Concerning the empirical support for the assertion that obesity is perceived as controllable, consider the study previously discussed by Weiner et al. (1988) (see Table 3.2). Table 3.2 documents that individuals are rated as highly responsible for their obesity (I suggest that the reader also examine his or her ratings in Experiment 3.1). In addition, as reported earlier regarding the survey of Kent State University students, respondents rated others as responsible for being overweight ($M = 5.8$, compared to the mental illness rating of $M = 2.7$).

Vividly capturing these data, Mackenzie (1984) stated that: "Fat people and thin people alike seem to share the notion that fatness means a loss of self-control, considered the ultimate moral failure in our culture." Furthermore, fatness is particularly construed as a woman's problem. Millman (1980) has commented:

> It is especially the case that an overweight woman is assumed to have a personal problem. She is stereotypically viewed as unfeminine ... out of control.... One of the reasons for this assumption is that despite all the gains and insights of the woman's liberation movement, women are still judged very much on the basis of physical appearance. And no matter what medical evidence we acquire to the contrary, being overweight is fundamentally viewed as an *intentional* act. In the case of women, being fat is considered such an obvious default or rebellion against being feminine that it is treated as a very significant, representative ... characteristic. (p. xi)

Obesity, then, like alcoholism, is considered a sin—a moral transgression (see Allon, 1982; Archer, 1985). It might be thought of as the morality of biology!

In a series of investigations documenting the association between perceptions of controllability, "anti-fat" attitudes (the term used by Crandall), and beliefs that obesity is a sin, Crandall (1994) first developed a measure of anti-fat attitudes. The scale consists of three components including a dislike scale, represented by such items as, "I really don't like fat people very much" and "I don't have many friends who are fat." In addition, there is a willpower scale, which includes the item, "People who weigh too much could lose at least some part of their weight through a little exercise." These two components of the anti-fat scale correlate positively, documenting the belief that weight is a function of willpower and that anti-fat attitudes are positively associated. In a cross-cultural examination of this association, Crandall and Martinez (1993) have reported that the willpower–dislike correlation is higher among Americans than Mexicans (although significant in both samples). They have suggested that the American culture, more than the Mexican, is a "culture of blame," perhaps because freedom of choice is so prevalent (see Crandall, 1994). Furthermore, in the Mexican culture a heavy body may be more positively associated with the traditional female roles of nurturance and passivity.

In an extension of these ideas to embrace political ideology, Crandall and Biernat (1990) have reported that anti-fat attitudes are related to political conservatism. Conservatives generally believe that individuals are personally responsible for their life outcomes. Crandall and Biernat (1990) therefore anticipated, and found, that conservatives also believe obesity to be controllable. Then, in a follow-up of this finding, Crandall administered his anti-fat scale (described above) to a sample of Republicans and Democrats. He found that Republicans (who were higher in conservatism than Democrats) more strongly endorsed the belief that willpower is a significant influence on weight, and they had higher anti-fat attitudes than the Democrats did.

What, then, might be some specific behavioral consequence of perceiving obesity as controllable? One might anticipate that if there are negative affects, then these will be quite pervasive inasmuch as obesity is not concealable and "engulfs the perceptual field." Furthermore, in contrast to alcoholism, obesity has a negative effect even in childhood. For example, Richardson, Hastorf, Goodman, and Dornbusch (1961) found that 10 to 11-year-olds least liked obese children. In a similar manner, obese children have been shown to be infrequently selected in sociometric studies of friendships (Staffieri, 1967). These negative appraisals continue into adulthood (see Allon, 1979; Maddox, Back, & Liederman, 1968). Among adults, the obese are less likely to be hired and do not fare well economically (see review in Crandall, 1994). Overweight women particularly receive lower wages than those who are not overweight. There is even suggestive evidence that parents, particularly if they have a conservative orientation, are less likely to send their overweight daughters to college (Crandall, in press-a, in press-b). And clinical psychologists and other mental health workers are more likely to assign negative psychological symptoms to the obese than they are to individuals of normal weight (Young & Powell, 1985).

This research, which documents an association between anti-fat attitudes and behaviors, does not however substantiate that the attitude–behavior linkage is mediated by perceptions of causal controllability and inferences of personal responsibility. In one study directly demonstrating the effect of perceptions of personal responsibility on anti-fat attitudes, Rodin, Price, Sanchez, and McElligot (1989) described two individuals applying for a job. They were identical except that one was characterized as obese because of a hormonal imbalance and the other as overweight because of overeating. In both cases, it was stated that the individual, although the best qualified job applicant, was not hired because the department head "doesn't like to be around fat people." The subjects then were asked how prejudiced this decision was. The data revealed that the department head was rated as more prejudiced in the uncontrollable than in the controllable description of obesity. That is, being rejected because one is perceived as responsible for obesity is considered relatively fair, or "deserved."

In a conceptually similar study, deJong (1980) reported data consistent with these findings. In the experiment conducted by deJong (1980), female high school students were asked to give their "first impressions" of other females based on information that included a personal photo of these females. In one condition, the picture was of an obese girl whose heaviness was described as caused by a thyroid problem. In a second condition, no cause of obesity was provided. It was found that the obese female with the thyroid problem was rated lower in self-indulgence and laziness and higher in self-discipline and liking than was the obese female who was not paired with uncontrollable causality. deJong (1980) concluded that

> the perception of responsibility does play a large role in reactions to the physical stigma of obesity. It is not the mere fact that obese people are physiologically deviant which causes them to be derogated, but that they are assumed to be responsible for their deviant status. (p. 8)

Furthermore, in the stigma study discussed earlier relating the causes of obesity to emotions and behavior, Weiner et al. (1988; see Figure 3.1) reported that when obesity is ascribed to an uncontrollable cause (a thyroid problem) as opposed to a controllable cause (overeating), then anger decreases and sympathy (pity) increases. In that study, it also was reported that significantly more help would be extended to a person with uncontrollable rather than controllable obesity.

It logically follows, then, that if perceptions of the cause of obesity could be changed from controllable to uncontrollable, then anti-fat attitudes and negative behaviors would decrease. In an investigation that included an attributional change treatment, Crandall (1994) had some subjects read a two-page report related to the genetics of obesity. The subjects were exposed to the parental correlational data and the effects of diet on metabolism that were mentioned in the prior pages. These data document the uncontrollability of obesity. Following this, his scale containing items about anti-fat attitudes and willpower was administered. Crandall (1994) found that perceptions of willpower as the cause of obesity decreased following the reading of the genetic information, as did anti-fat attitudes. Thus, information about uncontrollability and lack of responsibility can play a role in reducing negative attitudes toward the obese.

In sum, there is an abundance of data documenting the sin–sickness distinction in the perception and evaluation of obese people. The obese typically are construed as sinners, lacking willpower and the ability to control themselves. This perception is particularly true among conservatives, especially when women are considered. This causal belief generates both negative affects and aversive actions. However, the lay public also recognizes that there are uncontrollable causes that also can give rise to obesity. When these uncontrollable attributions are accepted, perceived responsibility decreases, as does general antipathy toward those who are overweight.

## POVERTY

Unlike the discussions of alcoholism and obesity, the question of causality in relation to the social stigma of poverty does not generally pit nature versus nurture, or biological destiny versus self-indulgence. Rather, causal determination involves a different (albeit related) dimension with the anchors of society versus the person, or the social system versus the individual.

Opinions differ with respect to which anchor of the this pole is the "true" cause of poverty. On the one hand, the Protestant Ethic dominates the beliefs of many Americans. Thus, it is thought that through hard work and dedication the American Dream will be fulfilled. One is therefore responsible for personal wealth and poverty. However, this ethic began to be questioned several decades ago when the welfare system was introduced and the uncontrollable forces of the economic system became apparent. In fact, the welfare system was initially developed to support widows, who were poor because of uncontrollable causes (Katz, 1986). Thus, both society and the individual are plausible causes of poverty. Let us, then, turn to the empirical literature and examine how the issue of responsibility for poverty has been studied and what has been determined.

Feagin (1972) was the first to systematically examine lay beliefs about the causes of poverty. A list of 11 causes was developed, which were categorized into three types: (1) individualistic explanations, such as laziness, which place responsibility for poverty on the poor themselves; (2) structural explanations, such as no available jobs, which hold external economic and social factors as causative; and (3) fatalistic explanations, which suggest that fate and bad luck cause poverty. A similar list and classification scheme was accepted by Feather (1974) and Furnham (1982). Table 3.5 includes the primary phenomenological causes of poverty subsumed within the specific categories of individualistic and social causes (see Zucker & Weiner, 1993).

Note that the individualistic causes are controllable by the poor (e.g., lack of effort, no attempts at self-improvement), whereas the social causes are uncontrollable by the poor (although they are considered controllable by larger social entities as, for example, the failure of industry to provide enough jobs and failure of society to provide good schools). Hence, the personal–social classification can also be considered to represent controllable versus uncontrollable attributions.

As might be anticipated, given that causality for poverty primarily is traced to individual versus social factors, political ideology will have a significant effect on causal perceptions. As Lane (1962) has pointed out: "At the roots of every ideology there are premises about the nature of causation, the agents of causation, [and] the appropriate ways of explaining complex events" (p. 318). Political ideology already has been introduced as a determinant of causal perceptions of obesity, and it was reported that conservatives think that obesity is more likely to be caused by personal indulgence than liberals do (Crandall, 1994). That being the case, then it surely is reasonable to hypothesize that ideology will play a major role in determining the perceived causes of poverty, where society is one plausible explanation. And that indeed is the case. It has been reported many times that conservatives rate individualistic causes of poverty as more important than liberals do. It also has been suggested that this ideology justifies

TABLE 3.5. Perceived Causes of Poverty

Individualistic causes
    Laziness and lack of effort
    No attempts at self-improvement
    Alcohol and drug abuse
    Lack of thrift and proper money management
Social causes
    Failure of society to provide good schools
    Failure of industry to provide enough jobs
    High taxes and no incentives
    Prejudice and discrimination
    Being taken advantage of by the rich
    Low wages in some businesses and industries

structural inequalities and the unequal distribution of rewards in society. On the other hand, liberals contend that social factors are a more important influences on poverty than conservatives do (see, e.g., Furnham, 1982; Kluegel & Smith, 1986; Skitka & Tetlock, 1992, 1993b; Williams, 1984; Zucker & Weiner, 1993). As Dionne (1991) expressed so well:

> Since the 1960s, American politics has been at war over which set of sins should preoccupy government. Conservatives preached that the good society would be created if individuals could be made virtuous. Liberals preached that the good society would create virtuous individuals.

Causal beliefs, once formed, are contended to influence the assignment of responsibility. Responsibility is then linked with affects such as sympathy and anger toward the poor, and these emotions are hypothesized to be the proximal determinants of behavioral reactions including punishment and its obverse, helping. The discussions of alcoholism and obesity indeed documented that causal perceptions of controllability do give rise to negative attitudes and correspondent behaviors. However, the thinking–feeling–acting sequence proposed in Chapters 1 and 2 and supported in Table 3.2 was not fully pursued in the examination of these stigmas. It is suitable, then, to return to this larger theoretical issue.

In one investigation that examined affective as well as behavioral reactions as a function of the perceived cause of poverty, Skitka and Tetlock (1992) presented to subjects a number of scenarios in which claimants requested help. One request was for low income housing for the poor. The reasons for the request were manipulated to be either controllable or uncontrollable by the person in need. Figure 3.3 shows the affects evoked by this request. As Figure 3.3 indicates, the positive emotions of sympathy and pity were less, and the negative emotions of disgust and distaste were greater, when the cause of the need was internal and controllable as opposed to external and/or uncontrollable. This supports the cognition–affect linkage specified by the theory that is being championed. In addition, of those needing housing for internal controllable reasons, fewer were chosen to be recipients of funds than those in need for uncontrollable reasons. These findings intimate (but certainly do not prove) that causal cognitions and emotions play a role in determining intended (and actual) action. (This study is discussed in greater detail in Chapter 6).

A more complete examination of the associations between political attitudes and behaviors, including the roles played by causal perceptions, responsibility inferences, and affective reactions, was undertaken by Zucker and Weiner (1993). We asked our respondents to rate the importance of 13 causes of poverty, most of which are listed in Table 3.5. In addition,

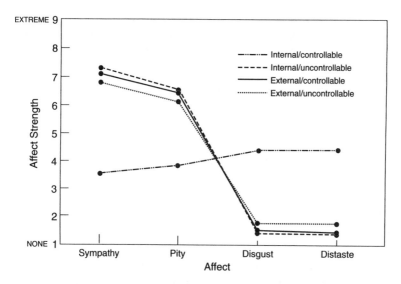

FIGURE 3.3. Affective reactions to claimants as a function of locus and control of their problem. From Skitka and Tetlock (1992, p. 507). Copyright 1992 by Academic Press. Reprinted by permission.

the subjects rated the degree to which the poor were responsible for their condition, their feelings of anger and sympathy toward the poor, and willingness to provide personal assistance to the poor. Measures of political ideology also were taken.

These data were then subject to structural equation analyses. In this statistical procedure, the associations that are reported partial out or hold constant the effects of other variables (see Chapter 6 for a fuller discussion). In addition, a temporal path is advanced that suggests (but again does not prove) a causal sequence.

The findings in this study are shown in Figure 3.4, which reveals that conservatism relates negatively ($r = -.40$) to the perception that social causes give rise to poverty and is positively related ($r = .19$) to the belief that individualistic causes generate poverty. This replicates findings reported by Crandall (1994) and others that already have been summarized. In addition, if poverty is ascribed to social causes, then the person is not held responsible ($r = -.31$); but if poverty is perceived as due to personal causes, then individuals are characterized as responsible for their plight ($r = .43$). Recall that in Chapter 1 it was contended that personal agency is a necessary condition for finding another person responsible. Responsibility, in turn, relates negatively to pity ($r = -.40$) and positively to anger ($r = .61$). That is, the more responsible the poor are for being poor, the less

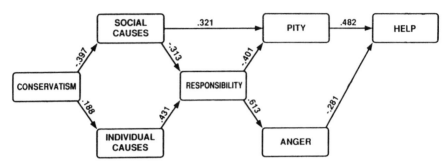

**FIGURE 3.4.** Help giving as a function of political ideology, perceptions of the causes of poverty, responsibility beliefs, and affective reactions. Adapted from Zucker and Weiner (1993, p. 937). Copyright 1993 by V. H. Winston & Sons. Adapted by permission.

are the positive affective reactions toward them and the stronger is the negative emotional response. Pity, in turn, promotes help giving ($r = .48$), whereas anger reduces help ($r = -.28$).

Note that in this analysis there is a positive advance from merely documenting a relation between political ideology and action in that there is an understanding of the psychological mechanisms that intervene to bring about this association. These mechanisms are causal beliefs, inferences of responsibility, and affects. Also worth noting in Figure 3.4 is that neither political ideology, causal beliefs, nor the assignment of responsibility are directly linked with intended behavior. Rather, these are distal causes. The proximal or immediate causes of conduct are affective reactions. That is, feelings are determined by thoughts, and then personal actions are based on those feelings rather than on the underlying cognitions.

It is now possible to return to the stigma of obesity and interpret some of the findings that were presented from the more complete theoretical perspective depicted in Figure 3.4. The same general analysis is, of course, applicable to alcoholism. For example, it was documented that people react to obesity more negatively (e.g., the person is not hired) when obesity is ascribed to overeating as opposed to a thyroid problem. Two motivational sequences are proposed to account for this finding:

1. Obesity → Thyroid problem → Uncontrollable causality → No responsibility → Pity, without anger → Relative positive reaction (hiring).
2. Obesity → Overeating → Controllable causality → Responsibility → Anger, without pity → Negative reaction (not hiring).

As already intimated, these sequences elevate the analyses beyond description in the direction of a more general theoretical understanding. I stated in Chapter 1 that this book has two primary goals. One goal is to document the extensity of everyday judgments of responsibility guided by the view of people as moral vigilantes. This chapter contributes to this aim by showing that physical illnesses, alcoholism, obesity, and poverty, as well as other stigmas, evoke thoughts about responsibility. The second goal is to develop a theoretical framework in which judgments about responsibility are embedded. It has been argued that inferences about responsibility are linked to prior beliefs concerning causal controllability and knowledge of mitigating circumstances. Further, the assignment of responsibility elicits affects and, in turn, action. Thus, responsibility is a linchpin concept, linking antecedent beliefs about causes with consequent affective and behavioral reactions. Phenomenal responsibility, therefore, lies at the very heart of psychological analyses and an understanding of everyday life.

## ON CHANGING CAUSAL BELIEFS

There is much written in the prior pages that may sadden the reader. Holding others responsible for poverty, or exhibiting anger toward the obese, does not portray a kind society. What may be especially disheartening for psychologists is that the discussion regarding stigmas has negative implications for the mental health profession regarding soliciting charitable donations, public support, and governmental funding. Mental health problems such as alcoholism and drug abuse arouse perceptions of responsibility, little sympathy, and only weak desires to help.

One course for psychologists and researchers to take is to alter perceptions of these stigmas toward uncontrollability, so that these stigmas are labeled as "diseases." It is evident that new scientific research upon which the media focuses attention, such as twin studies of the obese and the documentation that alcoholism runs in families, can help to transform public attitudes. And experimental programs, such as those undertaken in laboratory research by Crandall (1994) that provide new information about the stigmatized, can alter belief systems and, in turn, emotions and actions.

It is the case that research in mental illness has become strikingly biological in orientation. It might be maintained that merging mental/behavioral problems with biology and genetics will benefit researchers as far as ultimate funding is concerned because the needy target population no longer will be perceived as composed of sinners and those who are unworthy. But this is a complex issue, as witnessed by the recent reactions to a government-sponsored conference suggesting that violence and criminality have genetic components. Groups overrepresented in the criminal populations voiced great anger over this position!

And, to make matters even more complex, it is not entirely certain in what direction causal beliefs should be altered to benefit the stigmatized. The prior discussion clearly points to the advantages of changing causal perceptions from controllable to uncontrollable, so that affective reactions and linked behaviors will be more positive. However, this shift would not please everyone. Consider the mothers in MADD: They want to make persons more (not less) responsible for their drinking behavior and to increase the severity of punishment for accidents that take place while driving under the influence of alcohol. This position, MADD contends, is more likely to promote personal change and to aid society (see also Chapter 4).

There is no solution to the dilemma that shifting the perceptions of stigmas from controllable to uncontrollable causality is more humane as far as improving the affective reactions of others and reducing retributions are concerned, whereas controllable causality fosters the belief that one can personally do something to overcome problems. But even the argument that others are responsible for the resolution of stigmas is questionable; holding an obese individual accountable for the stigma when, in fact, the cause is uncontrollable, is inducing a false "hope" if change is not possible. Indeed, what is more demeaning than reporting for the weekly weigh-ins and seeing little change on the scale!

One very positive story regarding altered perceptions of responsibility from the self to others can be seen in the women's movement. The typical goal of most (but not all) consciousness raising for females and other disadvantaged groups is to have personal failure ascribed to factors for which others are perceived as responsible. That is, consciousness raising attempts to alter causal ascriptions so that group members no longer see themselves as personally responsible for their plights but fault others. If effective, this alters affective life from personal guilt to anger at others!

This attempt at responsibility shift is evident in the manifesto of Redstocking, an early radical feminist group that began consciousness raising. Their manifesto states: "We reject the idea that women consent to or are to be blamed for their own oppression. Women's submission is . . . the result . . . of . . . continual, daily pressure from men" (Rosenthal, 1984, p. 315). In this case, holding others responsible has aided in coping and has resulted in social and political gains.

## SUMMARY

It is evident that moral evaluation takes place in a courtroom. Rather than follow a rule of strict liability, where punishment is based solely on the magnitude of a negative outcome, intentional negative actions elicit greater sanctions than accidental negative actions. Thus, murder is punished to a greater degree than manslaughter, in good part because of the unequivocal presence of a "guilty mind" only in the former case. In a similar manner, lack of effort, as opposed to lack of ability, results in greater reprimand as a cause of failure in the classroom. This is because effort, but not ability (aptitude), is under volitional control and is freely expended or withheld. And, as documented in this chapter, behavioral/mental stigmas are judged more harshly than stigmas of somatic origin, for it is presumed that the stigmatized person is responsible for the onset and/or the continuation of the plight. Thus, one is held responsible for alcoholism and obesity, but not for Alzheimer's disease or paraplegia. Stigmas of behavioral/mental origin elicit perceptions of controllability and responsibility, negative affects, and antisocial responses, whereas uncontrollable stigmas (i.e., those of somatic origin) evoke perceptions of nonresponsibility, relatively positive affects and prosocial responses. It is hoped that this was documented in Experiment 3.1, which you completed.

I have examined three stigmas—alcoholism, obesity, and poverty—in greater detail, each emphasizing the points made above, yet having its own unique set of psychological issues. The discussion of *alcoholism* revealed that alcoholics are generally perceived as "weak individuals of flawed character." However, drinking is often perceived as caused by anxiety, depression, and stress—factors over which the alcoholic has little control. In addition, the causes of the onset of alcoholism were distinguished from the causes of its offset. Alcoholics Anonymous assumes that drinkers are responsible for the onset, but not the offset, of this condition. On the other hand, there is suggestive evidence that people perceive that alcoholics are not responsible for the onset of their drinking but are at fault for failing to bring about its offset. Similar complexity is evident in judgments of criminal responsibility for transgressions performed when drunk: At times the doer is absolved of responsibility while at other times assigned responsibility is increased.

Anti-fat attitudes are directed toward the *obese*, even by children. These attitudes are most negative toward women and are expressed particularly by conservatives. Evidence is quite clear that altering the cause of obesity from controllable (e.g., overeating) to uncontrollable (e.g., a thyroid problem) increases positive reactions.

*Poverty*, unlike the prior stigmas, does not elicit causality along a biology versus self-indulgence dimension but, rather, evokes a causal dimension with anchors of society versus the person. Conservatives locate causality within the person, and liberals see the social system as the cause of poverty. If poverty is perceived as controllable by the person (e.g., because the poverty is believed to be caused by laziness), then that person is responsible for his or her plight, anger is elicited, and help is withheld. On the other hand, if society is perceived as causal, then the poor are not considered responsible, pity is elicited, and help is provided. Studies of poverty have provided the best evidence thus far for a motivated sequence of causal controllability → inferred responsibility → affective reaction → behavioral response. The two subsets of this general rule, as previously detailed, are as follows:

1. Controllable causality → Presence of responsibility → Anger, no pity → Negative social reaction
2. Uncontrollable causality → Nonresponsibility → Pity, no anger → Positive social reaction

New information can alter which sequence is evoked by most particular stigmas, so that victim blame appears to be a cognitive, rather than (in addition to) a motivational, issue.

# 4

---

# AIDS and Stigmatization

Homosexuals have declared war on nature and now nature is
extracting an awful retribution.
   —PATRICK J. BUCHANAN (White House Communications Director
      under Ronald Reagan and former presidential aspirant)

AIDS is a largely preventable disease, and I expressed the opinion that
there is a growing public resentment about being taxed to pay for the
health care of people suffering from self-inflicted diseases.
   —ANDY ROONEY (television celebrity with the show "60 Minutes")

The story of Magic Johnson, the renowned basketball star who now carries
the HIV virus associated with AIDS (acquired immunodeficiency syndrome), recently pervaded the popular press and media, not only in the
United States but also around the world. This tragic event evokes many
emotions and public issues: sympathy for one of our most popular sports
heroes, anger at him for his behavior and toward the government for not
attacking this disease more fully, fear regarding personal infection, pity
because the virus is known to produce great suffering and eventual death,
and so on. For a psychologist, a challenging task is to step back from his
or her own feelings in order to more fully comprehend the issues, emotions, and controversies surrounding Magic Johnson. Understanding includes placing this specific event within a broader theoretical framework
that sheds light on the psychological dynamics that have been aroused. In
addition, perhaps the reactions to Magic Johnson will illuminate theoretical issues regarding AIDS stigmatization.

I begin this chapter, which focuses on the stigma of AIDS and its fusion with issues of homophobia and personal responsibility, with an analysis of the reactions to Magic Johnson. An experiment is again introduced, which in this case asks about the reader's reactions to Magic Johnson. I then examine a variety of pertinent topics including homosexuality as a stigma, homophobic influences on perceptions of those with AIDS, the historical changes in reactions to AIDS victims, and some future predictions concerning how the public and the government will view those who are HIV infected.

## MAGIC JOHNSON AND PERCEIVED RESPONSIBILITY FOR AIDS

Magic Johnson first announced that he was tested HIV-positive in a press conference held on November 7, 1991. Shortly thereafter, the popular magazine *Sports Illustrated* published a widely read article written by Johnson about his illness (November 18, 1991). This article emphasized the reasons for his contracting the virus associated with AIDS, and it documents the essential role of causal attributions. Johnson wrote: "To me, AIDS was someone else's disease. It was a disease for gays and drug users. Not for someone like me" (p. 10). He then went on to state:

> Not that being HIV-positive has been easy to accept. Not when I could easily have avoided being infected at all. All I had to do was wear condoms. I am certain that I was infected by having unprotected sex with a woman who has the virus. The problem is that I can't pinpoint the time, the place, or the woman. It's a matter of numbers. Before I was married, I truly lived the bachelor's life. I'm no Wilt Chamberlin [another basketball star known for his sexual promiscuity], but as I traveled around NBA [National Basketball Association] cities, I was never at a loss for female companionship. Even in Los Angeles, I was never far from admiring women. There are just some bachelors almost every woman in L.A. wanted to be with. ... I confess that after I arrived in L.A. in 1979, that I did my best to accommodate as many women as I could—most of them through unprotected sex. (pp. 21–22)

It is evident that Magic Johnson accepted some personal responsibility for becoming HIV-infected—he admittedly engaged in frequent casual sex. However, he did suggest that this was not entirely his fault, given that his behavior was typical in his celebrity circle (thus prompting a situational rather than a dispositional attribution; see Kelley, 1967). Concerning different impression-management strategies available to him, Magic did not call upon other causes that could have rendered him less personally responsible for his condition. He might have claimed, for example, that he contracted the HIV virus through a transfusion with contaminated blood; like many other athletes, he had operations that conceivably provided a ready excuse. Alternatively, he could have said that he was not promiscuous, but that he unluckily became infected in one of the few affairs that he had. Two other causes that may have been potentially damaging in terms of inferences of responsibility—homosexual behavior and drug use—were both explicitly denied by Mr. Johnson.

The immediate reactions to Magic Johnson's announcement were shock, overwhelming sorrow, and sympathy. A public outpouring of grief ensued. Mr. Johnson was greeted with applause on a popular talk show, and people were seen weeping and expressing genuine concern for him. Yet there soon followed other voices with a different affective tone, that of anger. An editorial from *The New York Times* stated:

> Magic Johnson is hardly a model or ideal to anyone with a sense of sexual morality. . . . Anyone with a sense of heterosexual responsibility isn't likely to get the HIV virus. . . . Magic apparently never pretended to be responsible for his sex life. . . . Earvin Johnson of the Fast Lane . . . finally got caught for speeding. (Anderson, 1991, Nov. 14, p. B-7)

In addition to professional writers commenting on the Johnson story, the newspapers began to fill with letters from readers—some voicing sympathy, others expressing anger, based on beliefs and inferences regarding personal responsibility. Here are two representative excerpts from those who held Magic Johnson responsible:

> The real tragedy is how one man's refusal to exercise discretion, self-discipline, and just plain common-sense can bring so much pain. . . . Worse has been [the press's] blatant recklessness and irresponsibility in placing this on the same level of Lou Gehrig [a baseball star] being stricken with amyotrophic lateral sclerosis [ALS]. ALS is not dictated by personal behavior; HIV/AIDS, for the most part, is. . . . Magic Johnson asks us to feel sorry for him. Believe me, I don't. (*Los Angeles Times*, Nov. 16, 1991, p. C-3)

Another person wrote:

> Johnson's flamboyant and irresponsible life-style . . . would undoubt-

edly catch up with him in the end. The misdirected national heroism showered on Johnson eclipsed the sexual irresponsibility of a man who should have known better. (*Los Angeles Times*, Nov. 16, 1991, p. C-3)

Others called for more information about causality, questioning whether Magic Johnson engaged in homosexual activity or used drugs, two causes that can be presumed to increase his level of personal responsibility. Consider this analysis of a television interview with Johnson:

Hill [the interviewer] touched on Johnson's sexuality, an issue only because of the way AIDS [i.e., the HIV virus] is transmitted. But he did not ask what is, unfortunately, a key question: Had Magic ever had a sexual encounter with a man? . . . Even after the *Sports Illustrated* story, rumors persist that Johnson is bisexual. (*Los Angeles Times*, Nov. 15, 1991, p. C-3)

Despite this general preoccupation with the cause of his illness, some contend that the assignment of responsibility is not relevant, that we should instead feel sorry for Johnson and forget about the role of causal ascriptions and responsibility in determining emotional reactions:

And now it begins. . . . Now we have to start hearing what a mistake we are making in glorifying someone so promiscuous and careless. . . . We should be expressing our outrage at this unconscionable lifestyle and how the young fool brought this thing on himself. We've got people demanding to know exactly what happened, how it happened, to whom it happened. . . . Is this really necessary? Can't we simply feel lousy about what happened? If he ever had a homosexual experience, which he denies, must we go digging and digging? . . . Magic's sick. That's all I care about. . . . Not like Lou Gehrig? No kidding. Several times, now, I have heard that Gehrig's fate was worse because his illness was something he could not have prevented. That does not make Magic's illness less relevant. . . . Can't we just feel bad? (Downey, *Los Angeles Times*, Nov. 17, 1991, p. C-1)

The issues, emotions, and controversies associated with Magic Johnson are readily amenable to the interpretation that has been proposed in the prior chapters. People are searching for why Magic Johnson is HIV-infected. He has provided an answer, which may or may not be the truth. For some, his answer appears to wholly or partially absolve him of personal responsibility; for others, he is at fault for engaging in promiscuous sexual behavior. For those in the former group, the emotion they feel toward Magic Johnson is primarily sympathy, and they grieve for him; for those in the latter group, there is less sympathy and more anger. But that is getting somewhat ahead of the story in this chapter.

## AN EXPERIMENTAL DEMONSTRATION

Prior to reading further, I would like you to complete an experiment (see Experiment 4.1) that is guided by the issues raised in the above discussion. The experimental questionnaire is composed of two sections. In Part I, you are asked to speculate about the cause of Magic Johnson's HIV-infected condition. Specifically, the questions are phrased as follows: "There are many reasons why people have gotten the AIDS virus. Why do you think that Magic Johnson got the virus? That is, what do you think caused him to get it?" Space is then provided for your free response. Next, you are asked to consider four questions (dependent variables). One question asks how responsible Magic Johnson was for contracting this illness (queries about controllability—which it has been suggested, precede decisions about responsibility—are not asked because in this impoverished context they would quite likely result in the same answers as questions about responsibility). Two queries then follow that are concerned with affects ("How much sympathy do you feel?" and "How angry are you?"). The final question examines a hypothetical behavioral intention ("Would you be willing to attend a ceremony in support of Magic Johnson?").

Part II of this questionnaire involves a manipulation of five possible causes of Magic Johnson's infection. The questionnaire begins as follows: "Now assume it is known why Magic Johnson became infected. The reason will be given and you are to answer the same questions again." Five major causes of HIV infection are provided: (1) a blood transfusion (during one of his knee operations), (2) normal (i.e., conventional) sexual behavior with a woman he knew, (3) frequent casual (promiscuous) sex with many women, (4) homosexual behavior, and (5) drug use with a contaminated needle. Each cause is given, followed by the responsibility, affect, and behavioral questions already described. Please complete this study now.

## THE EXPERIMENTAL FINDINGS REGARDING
## HIV INFECTION, RESPONSIBILITY,
## AND REACTIONS OF OTHERS

A very similar experiment to the one just completed by the reader already has been conducted (Graham, Weiner, Giuliano, & Williams, 1993). I will

# EXPERIMENT 4.1

## AIDS and Magic Johnson

Part I. As you know, Magic Johnson, the famous basketball player, recently announced that he tested positive for the AIDS virus. There are many reasons why people have gotten the AIDS virus. Why do you think Magic Johnson got the virus? That is, what do you think caused him to get it? Please write in your answer.

Circle one.

1. How much do you hold him responsible for this condition?

| 1 | 2 | 3 | 4 | 5 | 6 | 7 | 8 | 9 |

Not
at all

Entirely his
responsibility

2. How much sympathy do you have for him?

| 1 | 2 | 3 | 4 | 5 | 6 | 7 | 8 | 9 |

None
at all

As much
as possible

3. How much anger do you feel for him?

| 1 | 2 | 3 | 4 | 5 | 6 | 7 | 8 | 9 |

None
at all

As much
as possible

4. Would you be willing to attend a ceremony in support of Magic Johnson?

| 1 | 2 | 3 | 4 | 5 | 6 | 7 | 8 | 9 |

Not
at all

Definitely

Part II. Now imagine that it is known what caused Magic Johnson's condition. A number of different possibilities are given and you are asked to again answer questions about your feelings toward him.

A. He got the virus through homosexual behavior.

1. How much do you hold him responsible for this condition?

| 1 | 2 | 3 | 4 | 5 | 6 | 7 | 8 | 9 |

Not
at all

Entirely his
responsibility

2. How much sympathy do you have for him?

| 1 | 2 | 3 | 4 | 5 | 6 | 7 | 8 | 9 |

None
at all

As much
as possible

3. How much anger do you feel for him?

| 1 | 2 | 3 | 4 | 5 | 6 | 7 | 8 | 9 |
|---|---|---|---|---|---|---|---|---|

None
at all

As much
as possible

4. Would you be willing to attend a ceremony in support of Magic Johnson?

| 1 | 2 | 3 | 4 | 5 | 6 | 7 | 8 | 9 |
|---|---|---|---|---|---|---|---|---|

Not
at all

Definitely

B. He got the virus through a blood transfusion during a knee operation.

1. How much do you hold him responsible for this condition?

| 1 | 2 | 3 | 4 | 5 | 6 | 7 | 8 | 9 |
|---|---|---|---|---|---|---|---|---|

Not
at all

Entirely his
responsibility

2. How much sympathy do you have for him?

| 1 | 2 | 3 | 4 | 5 | 6 | 7 | 8 | 9 |
|---|---|---|---|---|---|---|---|---|

None
at all

As much
as possible

3. How much anger do you feel for him?

| 1 | 2 | 3 | 4 | 5 | 6 | 7 | 8 | 9 |
|---|---|---|---|---|---|---|---|---|

None
at all

As much
as possible

4. Would you be willing to attend a ceremony in support of Magic Johnson?

| 1 | 2 | 3 | 4 | 5 | 6 | 7 | 8 | 9 |
|---|---|---|---|---|---|---|---|---|

Not
at all

Definitely

C. He got the virus by using drugs with a shared needle.

1. How much do you hold him responsible for this condition?

| 1 | 2 | 3 | 4 | 5 | 6 | 7 | 8 | 9 |
|---|---|---|---|---|---|---|---|---|

Not
at all

Entirely his
responsibility

2. How much sympathy do you have for him?

| 1 | 2 | 3 | 4 | 5 | 6 | 7 | 8 | 9 |
|---|---|---|---|---|---|---|---|---|

None
at all

As much
as possible

3. How much anger do you feel for him?

| 1 | 2 | 3 | 4 | 5 | 6 | 7 | 8 | 9 |
|---|---|---|---|---|---|---|---|---|

None
at all

As much
as possible

4. Would you be willing to attend a ceremony in support of Magic Johnson?

| 1 | 2 | 3 | 4 | 5 | 6 | 7 | 8 | 9 |
|---|---|---|---|---|---|---|---|---|

Not
at all

Definitely

D. He got the virus through frequent casual sex with many women.

1. How much do you hold him responsible for this condition?

| 1 | 2 | 3 | 4 | 5 | 6 | 7 | 8 | 9 |
|---|---|---|---|---|---|---|---|---|

Not
at all

Entirely his
responsibility

2. How much sympathy do you have for him?

| 1 | 2 | 3 | 4 | 5 | 6 | 7 | 8 | 9 |
|---|---|---|---|---|---|---|---|---|

None
at all

As much
as possible

3. How much anger do you feel for him?

| 1 | 2 | 3 | 4 | 5 | 6 | 7 | 8 | 9 |
|---|---|---|---|---|---|---|---|---|

None
at all

As much
as possible

4. Would you be willing to attend a ceremony in support of Magic Johnson?

| 1 | 2 | 3 | 4 | 5 | 6 | 7 | 8 | 9 |
|---|---|---|---|---|---|---|---|---|

Not
at all

Definitely

E. He got the virus through normal sexual behavior with a woman he knew.

1. How much do you hold him responsible for this condition?

| 1 | 2 | 3 | 4 | 5 | 6 | 7 | 8 | 9 |
|---|---|---|---|---|---|---|---|---|

Not
at all

Entirely his
responsibility

2. How much sympathy do you have for him?

| 1 | 2 | 3 | 4 | 5 | 6 | 7 | 8 | 9 |
|---|---|---|---|---|---|---|---|---|

None
at all

As much
as possible

3. How much anger do you feel for him?

| 1 | 2 | 3 | 4 | 5 | 6 | 7 | 8 | 9 |
|---|---|---|---|---|---|---|---|---|

None
at all

As much
as possible

4. Would you be willing to attend a ceremony in support of Magic Johnson?

| 1 | 2 | 3 | 4 | 5 | 6 | 7 | 8 | 9 |
|---|---|---|---|---|---|---|---|---|

Not
at all

Definitely

present these data and the reader can then compare his or her responses to what already has been found. Once more, I am optimistic that the two sources will yield comparable data. Unfortunately, in the Graham et al. (1993) study a measure of intended behavior was not included, so that a full analysis of the theory that has been proposed and a complete comparison with the responses of the reader cannot be made.

In the prior experiment by Graham et al. (1993), two samples of subjects were tested, each within days of Magic Johnson's announcement. One group consisted of college students, the typical respondents in psychological experiments. The second sample was composed primarily of adults, all of African American descent. An African American sample was desired because Magic Johnson is believed to be particularly important to the Black community, which could therefore influence the assignment of responsibility and the evoked affect. In addition, it is crucial to test the generality of the findings beyond the population of American college students. The consistency between the ratings of stigmas in the People's Republic of China and America certainly increased the credulity of the arguments in the prior chapter.

Consider first the results related to the manipulation of the causes. Figure 4.1 shows the responsibility ratings as a function of the imagined cause. There is least responsibility when the HIV-infected condition was caused by a blood transfusion, which in this experiment would be considered the only uncontrollable cause of Magic Johnson's illness. The next degree of responsibility was linked with conventional sexual behavior, after which came both promiscuous sex and homosexual behavior, with most responsibility ascribed for drug use. The data from the two samples are quite consistent, with slightly higher responsibility ratings given by the adult African American sample than by the primarily white college students.

Figure 4.2 depicts the sympathy and anger ratings for the two samples as a function of the hypothetical cause of Magic Johnson's HIV infection.

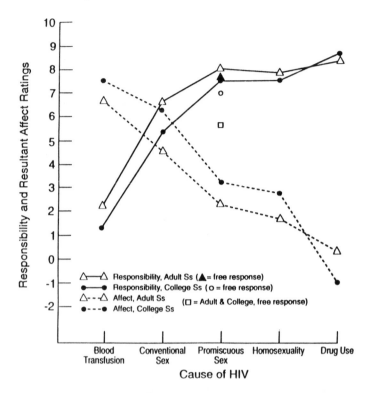

**FIGURE 4.1.** Responsibility ratings and affective reactions toward Magic Johnson as a function of the manipulated cause of his HIV infection. From Graham, Weiner, Giuliano, and Williams (1993, p. 1006). Copyright 1993 by V. H. Winston & Sons. Reprinted by permission.

Sympathy and anger are inversely related, with sympathy greatest and anger least when a blood transfusion is the cause and with anger greatest and sympathy least when drug use with a shared needle is the reason for Magic Johnson's infection. Again, trends for both samples are identical, although college students reported somewhat more sympathy than the African American adults did.

A "resultant affect" index was then created by Graham et al. (1993) by subtracting the anger ratings from the sympathy ratings. This index reflects the relative positivity of the emotional reactions toward Magic Johnson. Inspection of Figure 4.1 documents what has been contended in the prior chapters—namely, that there is an inverse relation between perceptions of responsibility for a negative action, event, or state and the

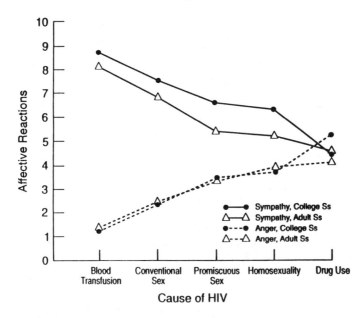

**FIGURE 4.2.** Affective reactions of anger and sympathy toward Magic Johnson as a function of the manipulated cause of his HIV infection. From Graham, Weiner, Giuliano, and Williams (1993, p. 1005). Copyright 1993 by V. H. Winston & Sons. Reprinted by permission.

positivity of reported feelings toward the responsible party. Emotional reactions were most favorable when blood transfusion was the cause of AIDS and were least favorable in the case of drug abuse.

The results of a more sophisticated procedure examining the association between responsibility inferences and affective reactions are shown in Figure 4.3. In contrast to Figures 4.1 and 4.2, in Figure 4.3 the distances between the causes on the horizontal axis are determined by their responsibility ratings. That is, rather than spacing the causes equally, as in the prior two figures, the causes are set at intervals according to their psychological meaning (i.e., their implications for perceptions of responsibility). The resultant affect ratings are again depicted for the five manipulated causes. Figure 4.3 reveals that the large increment in responsibility between blood transfusion and normal sexual behavior as the causes of HIV infection is accompanied by relatively little (but some) decrease in resultant positive affect. That is, although one is held much more responsible for contracting the virus associated with AIDS by means of normal sexual behavior rather than through a blood transfusion, there is nevertheless a great deal of

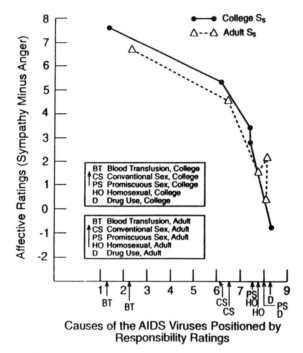

**FIGURE 4.3.** Affective ratings of sympathy minus anger toward Magic Johnson as a function of the responsibility ratings of the manipulated cause of his HIV infection. From Graham, Weiner, Giuliano, and Williams (1993, p. 1007). Copyright 1993 by V. H. Winston & Sons. Reprinted by permission.

sympathy and relatively little anger with either cause. After that, however, there is an "inflection point," or a point on the curve where change takes place; small increases in perceived responsibility are now accompanied by large decreases in relative sympathy. Thus, for example, although people report that others are almost as responsible for HIV infection from promiscuous sexual behavior as from drug use, there is much less sympathy for the drug user. The function relating responsibility to reported affect is nearly identical for both respondent populations.

The reader may now wish to examine his or her data for similar trends. Simply plot the responsibility ratings as a function of the cause of Magic Johnson's HIV infection, and then do the same for the sympathy and anger ratings. This might even be done within Figures 4.1, 4.2, and 4.3. I expect the results shown in these figures to be fully replicated.

Thus far the open-ended causal responses reported by Graham et al.

(1993) have not been discussed. This is because the responses did not yield very revealing data. Virtually all the respondents believed what Magic Johnson had communicated—namely, that his HIV infection was due to promiscuous sexual behavior. Figure 4.1 includes the responsibility and affect ratings made in response to this cause for the two subject populations; the data are located above the horizontal axis where promiscuous sex was placed as the imagined cause. Finally, consistent with the manipulation data, Graham et al. (1993) report a significant inverse correlation (average $r = -.39$) between these responsibility and affective ratings (i.e., the greater the responsibility assigned, the less positive the feelings toward Magic Johnson). Again the reader might now want to plot his or her data in the free response condition and examine the correspondence between those ratings and the responses made to the manipulated causes.

In addition, you are able to examine the relations between the judgments of responsibility, affective reactions, and the intended behavioral responses. Recall that ratings of behavioral intentions were not collected by Graham et al. (1993). According to the discussions in the prior chapters, the greater the sympathy relative to anger, the more positive (or, the less negative) will be the response tendency. Hence, it is likely that prosocial responses will be most evident in the blood transfusion condition (high sympathy, low anger) and will be least displayed when drug abuse is the cause (low sympathy, high anger).

## General Conclusions

People seek to know why events have happened. We ask: What caused the damage to the car? Why did this student fail the exam? Why is this person alcoholic, obese, or poor? Why is Magic Johnson HIV-positive? Reports in the newspaper and the other media in response to Magic Johnson's situation confirm this position. Indeed, according to attribution theorists, causal knowledge is most desired for a negative, unexpected, and important event (see Weiner, 1985), which characterizes the Magic Johnson story for many individuals.

Magic Johnson has been responsive to this informational desire and has provided a reason for his illness—promiscuous sexual behavior. The data reported by Graham et al. (1993), as well as reports in the media, confirm that this cause has been accepted by the public. However, as was documented in Chapter 3, causal inferences are amenable to alteration with the availability of new information, so it is possible that this explanation will be called into question in the future. Indeed, there has been some suspicion that Magic Johnson was not telling the truth and that his HIV infection is due to a homosexual encounter. He has denied this accusation.

It has been proposed further that there is a relation between perceptions of responsibility and emotions, with responsibility for a negative event hypothesized to be directly related to anger and inversely related to sympathy. Both the correlational data generated by the freely given cause (promiscuous sexual behavior) and the experimental data (in response to the five manipulated causes) confirm this hypothesis. Given promiscuous sexual behavior as the reported cause, the more that others ascribed personal responsibility to Magic Johnson for his behavior, the less positive were their feelings. And given a range of manipulated causes, blood transfusion generated the least amount of responsibility and the most positive resultant affect, whereas drug use evoked the greatest degree of personal accountability and the most negative affective reactions.

In sum, Magic Johnson provided a "real life" opportunity to explore the value and validity of the conceptual approach that has been championed. The results are supportive and encouraging regarding the associations between controllable causality, perceived responsibility, and emotion, with two specific patterns of connections evident:

1. Blood transfusion as the cause, low perceptions of responsibility, high sympathy, and low anger.
2. Drug use as the cause, high perceptions of responsibility, low sympathy, and high anger.

Although it has been contended that controllability, responsibility, and emotions are connected sequentially, the data presented by Graham et al. (1993) only confirm that stigma origin (which presumably relates to perceptions of control) does give rise to anticipated responsibility beliefs and affective reactions.

In addition to these empirical and theoretical contributions, the data yielded some unexpected results and avenues for further exploration. For both samples, homosexual behavior was not associated with significantly greater responsibility or less positive affect than was promiscuous heterosexuality. Thus, if Magic Johnson was not telling the truth (as a few still wonder) and truly engaged in homosexual activity, then these data suggest that a "cover-up" was not necessary as far as the affective responses of the public were concerned. However, if at a subsequent time evidence is provided that favors an explanation of homosexual activity, then there is quite likely to be very negative consequences because Johnson's prior communications were untrue (see Weiner, Graham, Peter, & Zmuidinas, 1991, and Chapter 8). In addition, the notion of an inflection point regarding the relation between inferences about responsibility and emotional reactions suggests new insights into this connection that had not previously been considered.

## REACTIONS TO OTHER PEOPLE
## WITH HIV INFECTION/AIDS

The discussion thus far in this chapter has concerned Magic Johnson, one of the best-known and best-liked American athletes. It may be that because of his status and personality, the reactions to Magic Johnson differ from those elicited by others infected with the HIV virus. He may, for example, elicit more sympathy; conversely, perhaps Magic Johnson evokes greater inferences of responsibility than others do.

An answer to the question of how the public responds to others infected with the HIV virus already has been provided. In Chapter 3, I reported an experiment by Weiner et al. (1988) that gathered ratings regarding a number of stigmas. Included within this stigmatizing list was AIDS. Both Table 3.2 (American respondents) and Table 3.3 (respondents from the People's Republic of China) reveal that AIDS evokes reactions similar to those for other mental/behavioral stigmas (child abuser, obesity, and drug abuse) because it is perceived as controllable and because comparatively high resultant negative affect as well as low helping intentions are expressed.

However, it also is evident from the discussion in the prior chapters and from Figure 3.1 that negative affects and behavioral intentions can be altered with information that HIV infection was due to a blood transfusion or other uncontrollable factors rather than sexual activity and drug use. As was the case for Magic Johnson, this dramatically reduces perceptions of responsibility assigned to other persons infected with the HIV virus and increases positive and prosocial responses (see Chapman & Levin, 1989; Levin & Chapman, 1990; Strasser & Damrosch, 1992). In sum, the reactions to Magic Johnson depicted in Figures 4.1, 4.2, and 4.3, and quite likely your responses as well, do not seem to differ from the responses to most (i.e., noncelebrity) persons infected with the HIV virus.

As already intimated, AIDS is perceived in part as a sexually transmitted disease, particularly prevalent in the gay community. Thus, attitudes toward those with AIDS must be considered in the context of general reactions toward homosexuals (see Weiner, 1993). I turn to this issue next, considering first homosexuality as a stigma and then examining the relation of homophobia to responses directed at those who are HIV-infected or have full-blown AIDS.

## HOMOSEXUALITY

A recent scientific discovery has attracted much attention among the media and lay public, as well as within the biological and genetic academic communities. It has been reported that in gay men the tiny area in the brain believed to control sexual activity is less than one-half the size found in heterosexual males and is approximately equal in size to that found in females. About the same time that this discovery was announced, it also was reported that if one identical twin is gay (identical twins share all genes), then the other twin is three times more likely to be gay than if the paired twin is fraternal (fraternal twins do not hold all genes in common). These two investigations strongly suggest that genetic makeup influences sexual orientation (there have been criticisms of both these research investigations, but this issue is too far removed from the topic of this chapter).

Of course, locating a genetic marker or sign for sexual orientation within a male or a female brain is a significant finding for genetic and biological sciences. But this has major social implications as well that relate to the main theme of this section of the book. If homosexuals are "born that way," then sexual orientation is uncontrollable. Hence, homosexuals should not be held responsible for their "sins," and their parents or caregivers need not feel "guilty" because of presumed child-rearing "errors" (which, for Freudians, includes a hostile relationship between father and son). Furthermore, if homosexuality is not a free choice, then can it be considered a sin by the Church? After all, sin as conceived within the Church has been associated with free will, just as crime as perceived by the criminal justice system requires freedom of choice (i.e., personal responsibility). It should not come as a surprise that gay groups have maintained that sexual direction is not a "choice," and thus they prefer the term "sexual orientation" to "sexual preference."

Do causal attributions for homosexuality empirically relate to attitudes toward gays? An abundance of studies have found that people who believe that homosexuality is genetically or biologically based—and, therefore, not controllable by the gay person—have less negative attitudes toward gays than those who believe that homosexuality is a learned behavior or is just preferred (see Aguero, Bloch, & Byrne, 1984; Schneider & Lewis, 1984; VanderStoep & Green, 1988). In one correlational study related to this issue, Whitley (1990) had subjects report the main cause of homosexuality and then rate that cause for controllability. The subjects also responded to scales assessing their attitudes toward gays. Whitley found that high perceived controllability was strongly associated with negative attitudes toward homosexuals. He went on to speculate:

> This relationship between perceptions of the controllability of the causes of homosexuality and antigay attitudes among heterosexuals may explain some of the success of college sexuality courses in ameliorating those attitudes (see review by Stevenson, 1988). Textbooks in this area typically present a number of biological explanations—

implying uncontrollability for sexual preference development. (Whitley, 1990, p. 375)

A 1993 survey conducted by *The New York Times* and the Columbia Broadcasting system, reproduced in Table 4.1, also revealed that those who say that homosexuality cannot be changed (and, thus, is a biological given) believe that homosexuals should have more jobs and rights, and expressed more liberal attitudes toward gays, than did individuals who endorsed the opinion that homosexuality is a free choice.

Of course, many (including myself) feel that it is irrelevant "why" persons are gay. It is argued that sexual behavior is neither a sickness nor a sin, so that causal uncontrollability and mitigating factors that reduce responsibility have no consequences. Further, the possibility that there may be a biological basis for homosexuality raises fear of biological intervention to "eliminate" this "deficit." The genetic research, therefore, raises a host of social issues that again fall beyond the scope of this chapter. What is apparent, however, is that individuals want to know "why" this stigma comes into being. The answer to this question then determines if homosexuality is perceived as a disease or a sin (or neither); and attitudes, feelings, and behaviors are in part driven by the answer to this causal question. Thus, if the cause of homosexuality is, as suggested by scientists, uncontrollable, and if this explanation becomes accepted by the general public, then science will exert a profound influence on attitudes toward homosexuality and quite likely on attitudes toward people with AIDS. One might also ask will this scientific evidence alter the stance of the Church?

## AIDS, HOMOSEXUALITY, AND HOMOPHOBIA

The quotation at the start of this chapter asserting that "homosexuals have declared war on nature and now nature is extracting an awful revenge" reflects a sentiment expressed by many in the general public. For example, in a survey by Wallack (1989), it was reported that 26% of a sample of nurses and 11% of a sample of physicians either fully agreed with or considered the following statement as possibly true: "AIDS is God's punishment to homosexuals" (see also Pryor & Reeder, 1993). This sentiment is similar to the perceived origin of plagues expressed at an earlier point in our history, as previously pointed out by Sontag (1978). Even more dramatically documenting a connection between antigay attitudes (homophobia) and AIDS is that "gay bashing" considerably increased following the onset of AIDS (as will be elaborated later in this chapter). That is, attitudes toward homosexuals have been damaged because of their association with HIV infection and AIDS.

**TABLE 4.1.** Attitudes toward Homosexuals as a Function of Beliefs about the Origin of Homosexuality

The respondents were first classified according to how they answered the following question: "Do you think being homosexual is something people choose to be, or do you think it is something they cannot change?" The general population was almost evenly split on this response.

| Total adults | | Those who say homosexuality . . . | |
|---|---|---|---|
| | | is a choice | cannot be changed |
| Jobs and Rights | | | |
| 78% | Say homosexuals should have equal rights in terms of job opportunities | 68% | 90% |
| 42 | Say it is necessary to pass laws to make sure homosexuals have equal rights | 30 | 58 |
| 11 | Object to having an airline pilot who is homosexual | 18 | 4 |
| 49 | Object to having a doctor who is homosexual | 64 | 34 |
| 55 | Object to having a homosexual as a child's elementary school teacher | 71 | 39 |
| Personal Judgments | | | |
| 46 | Say homosexual relations between consenting adults should be legal | 32 | 62 |
| 36 | Say homosexuality should be considered an acceptable alternative life style | 18 | 57 |
| 55 | Say homosexual relations between adults are morally wrong | 78 | 30 |
| 43 | Favor permitting homosexuals to serve in the military | 32 | 54 |
| 34 | Would permit their child to play at the home of a friend who lives with a homosexual parent | 21 | 50 |
| 36 | Would permit their child to watch a prime-time television situation comedy with homosexual characters in it | 27 | 46 |

*Note.* From *New York Times* (March 5, 1993, p. A14). Copyright 1993 by The New York Times Company. Reprinted by permission.

The survey data and observations of reactions to gays suggests that the negative attitudes and behaviors displayed toward individuals with AIDS may be generated by general negative reactions toward homosexuals (see St. Lawrence, Husfeldt, Kelly, Hood, & Smith, Jr., 1990). This might be represented as follows:

$$\left.\begin{array}{l}\text{Homophobia}\\ \text{1. AIDS} \rightarrow \text{Caused by}\\ \quad\text{homosexual behavior}\end{array}\right\} \rightarrow \text{Anger, no sympathy} \rightarrow \text{Antisocial conduct}$$

In addition, as already discussed, negative reactions toward persons with AIDS also may be generated by the fact that infection with the virus associated with AIDS is typically viewed as controllable:

2. AIDS → Caused by homosexual behavior → Controllable → Inference of personal responsibility → Anger, no sympathy → Antisocial conduct

The former explanation appears to be unrelated to a causal responsibility analysis, whereas the latter dynamic is consistent with a responsibility approach to social motivation (see Anderson, 1992). However, it also is possible that homophobia influences beliefs about causality (homophobia increases perceptions of personal controllability and, therefore, of assigned responsibility), so that the two approaches can be integrated in the following manner:

$$\left.\begin{array}{l}\text{Homophobia}\\ \text{3. AIDS} \rightarrow \text{Caused by}\\ \quad\text{homosexual behavior}\end{array}\right\} \rightarrow \begin{array}{l}\text{Controllable} \rightarrow \text{Responsible} \rightarrow \text{Anger,}\\ \text{no sympathy} \rightarrow \text{Antisocial conduct}\end{array}$$

The motivational process suggested in this model is consistent with the findings of Whitley (1990) that homophobics perceive homosexuality as more controllable than nonhomophobics do.

Two scientific procedures have been used to examine the effects of homophobia on reactions toward people with AIDS and to separate or distinguish between the three conceptual models outlined above to account for hostile actions against those who have AIDS. One type of study is correlational, with attitudes towards gays assessed and related to attitudes about those who have AIDS. For example, Pryor, Reeder, Vinacco, and Kott (1989) found that those holding negative attitudes toward homosexuals tended to view AIDS and, by implication, its causes, as "immoral," "disgusting," "dirty," and "God's punishment for homosexuals" (see also Bishop, Alva, Cantu, & Rittman, 1991).

However, these data do not address the question of whether antisocial feelings and conduct against those with AIDS is more traceable to perceptions of responsibility or to homophobia and whether homophobia is or is not associated with beliefs about the causal controllability of the behavior that may lead to AIDS. To answer these questions, Mallery (1991) conducted an experimental study that manipulated both the controllability of the cause of AIDS and the sexual orientation of the victim. His subjects read vignettes in which a coworker was described as becoming infected with the virus associated with AIDS. Four vignettes were created:

1. The coworker is homosexual and caught [the virus associated with] AIDS because he did not use a condom while having sex with a man he met in a gay bar.
2. The coworker is heterosexual and caught [the virus associated with] AIDS because he did not use a condom while having sex with a woman he met in a bar.
3. The coworker is homosexual and caught [the virus associated with] AIDS during a blood transfusion he received after a ski accident.
4. The coworker is heterosexual and caught [the virus associated with] AIDS during a blood transfusion he received after a ski accident.

Note that vignettes 1 and 2 differ from 3 and 4 in that infection with the HIV virus is controllable in the first and second but is uncontrollable in the third and fourth vignettes. Furthermore, in vignettes 1 and 3 the infected person is homosexual, whereas in vignettes 2 and 4 the infected person is heterosexual. Hence, the effects of controllability and the sexual orientation of the infected person (which would activate homophobic beliefs) were separated in this experimental design. In each condition, Mallery (1991) assessed the controllability of the cause of infection, the amount of pity and anger that would be experienced, the degree of personal help that would be extended, and the likelihood that someone will do harm (e.g., telling the boss that a coworker has AIDS so that the coworker might lose his or her job).

The data from this study are shown in Table 4.2. For ease of comparison, in this table the main effects of control and sexual orientation are shown. It is evident from the table that pity and, to a lesser extent, help, are greater with an uncontrollable etiology, whereas anger and, to a lesser extent, harm are augmented with a controllable etiology. This corroborates the prediction depicted in Model 2 that responsibility mediates the reactions toward those with AIDS, although the data are stronger regarding

**TABLE 4.2.** Mean Ratings on the Dependent Variables as a Function of the Controllability of HIV infection and the Sexual Orientation of the Person with AIDS

| Manipulations | Controllability | Pity | Anger | Help | Harm |
|---|---|---|---|---|---|
| Controllable | 6.13 | 4.75 | 3.79 | 5.41 | 2.21 |
| Uncontrollable | 1.63 | 6.43 | 1.38 | 5.98 | 1.87 |
| Homosexual | 4.12 | 5.26 | 2.88 | 5.42 | 2.16 |
| Heterosexual | 3.64 | 5.92 | 2.29 | 5.97 | 1.92 |

*Note.* Data from Mallery (1991).

emotional than behavioral reactions. In addition, when homosexual victims are compared to heterosexuals, slightly more pity and help are directed toward the heterosexuals, whereas there is somewhat greater anger and intended harm directed at the homosexuals. This supports the predictions in Model 1 that antisocial thoughts and acts pertaining to those with AIDS are due to homophobia. However, it is evident from Table 4.2 that the controllability manipulation has a greater effect or influence on the responsibility and the affective judgments (but not on help or harm) than does the sexual orientation of the infected individual, thereby providing more support for Model 2 than for Model 1. In addition, the data reveal that for homosexuals HIV infection, given the same manipulated reason, is perceived as more controllable than for heterosexuals. Hence, the process depicted in Model 3 also finds support (also see Collins, in press).

Mallery (1991) also administered a measure of homophobia, consisting of items such as "homosexuals do not contribute positively to society." The correlations of homophobia with the other measures already discussed (determined by summing the ratings over all four vignettes) are shown in Table 4.3, which reveals that homophobia does relate positively with perceptions of the controllability of HIV infection (which also was inferred

**TABLE 4.3.** Correlations among the Dependent Variables and Individual Differences in Homophobia

| Manipulations | Controllability | Pity | Anger | Help | Harm |
|---|---|---|---|---|---|
| Homophobia | .30 | −.24 | .21 | −.53 | .32 |
| Controllability | | −.32 | .15 | −.28 | .09 |
| Pity | | | −.30 | .43 | −.16 |
| Anger | | | | −.33 | .38 |
| Help | | | | | −.55 |

*Note*: Data from Mallery (1991). All correlations greater than $r = .16$ are significant.

from Table 4.2). In addition, the remaining affective and behavioral variables are associated in the manner specified by a causal understanding:
controllability relates negatively to pity and help, and positively with anger
and harm; pity correlates positively with help and negatively with harm,
whereas anger displays the opposite pattern of relations; and so on.

The path models presented in Chapter 3 relating, for example, causal
controllability to help for the poor, were not performed by Mallery (1991).
However, the pattern of correlations certainly is consistent with Model 3
presented above in which (1) homophobia affects beliefs about controllability as the cause of infection with the virus associated with AIDS, (2)
controllability then influences (in these data, correlates with) emotion, and
(3) emotion is associated with (and theoretically directs or guides) conduct.
In addition, Mallery (1991) documented that homophobia (as inferred
from the sexual orientation of the victim) also influences reactions to those
with AIDS, independent of causal beliefs. Two specific motivational sequences capturing reactions toward those with AIDS, therefore, are proposed. In these models, homophobia influences affect and action indirectly
through an influence on perceptions of controllability, and directly without
intervention of other beliefs.

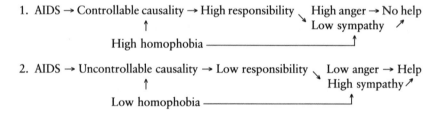

## Instrumental versus Symbolic Attitudes

Negative attitudes toward people with AIDS conceivably could be driven
by two distinct sources of attitudes, labeled instrumental and symbolic
(Herek, 1987). Instrumental attitudes are defined as serving self-interest,
such as having a negative attitude toward infected persons because of fear
of becoming personally infected. Symbolic attitudes, on the other hand, are
not clearly tied to self-interest, but rather concern more abstract values and
emotions (Kinder & Sears, 1981; Sears, 1988). Measures of symbolic
attitudes consist of items that are "almost wholly abstract, ideological, and
symbolic in nature ... with no conceivable personal relevance to the
individual, but have to do with his [or her] moral code or his [or her] sense
of how society should be organized" (Sears & Kinder, 1971, p. 66).

It has been contended by Pryor and his colleagues (Pryor et al., 1989;
Pryor, Reeder, & McManus, 1991) that individuals who have negative

attitudes toward homosexuals also have negative opinions about those with AIDS because of symbolic rather than instrumental reasons. To test this hypothesis, Pryor et al. (1989) examined the effects of persuasive messages upon attitudes toward an HIV-infected coworker. A movie stressing that one could not be infected with the HIV virus through casual work-related contact did not reduce negative attitudes toward the HIV-infected co-worker among persons who were homophobic (which they consider synonymous with symbolic-drive attitude), whereas nonhomophobics who expressed negative attitudes toward the individual were more positive in their attitudes following the education film, suggesting that their negative beliefs were instrumentally driven. Pryor et al. (1989) contend that for those who are homophobic, AIDS signals "homosexual promiscuity and moral decadence."

## COMPLEXITY OF REACTIONS TO PEOPLE WITH AIDS

The preceding discussion intimated that a wide variety of emotions and behaviors are elicited by persons who are infected with HIV or who have AIDS. Table 4.4 summarizes some of the reactions that have been observed or inferred. Table 4.4 indicates that HIV infection caused by sexual behavior is controllable and evokes anger and neglect; controllable infection traced to homosexual behavior and drug use elicits anger and moral repugnance, as well as neglect and/or aggression; regardless of onset causality, because the virus associated with AIDS is communicable, it evokes fear, which leads to neglect and/or nonaltruistic (i.e., self-interested) help; regardless of onset causality, because AIDS is terminal and offset uncontrollable, pity and altruistic concerns are aroused; and when the cause of the HIV infection is uncontrollable (e.g., obtained through a blood transfusion or transmitted from an HIV-infected parent), then pity and again altruistic help are elicited. Thus, for example, a homosexual infected with the HIV virus through homosexual behavior is expected to arouse the emotions of anger, moral repugnance, fear, and sympathy, and the behavioral tendencies to neglect, to aggress, and to provide both altruistic and nonaltruistic-instigated help. It is no wonder that, as Freud voiced, life is fraught with conflict!

Because it is known by the public that HIV infection can be controllable or uncontrollable (in contrast, say, to Alzheimer's disease), because it is unlike other stigmas in being both terminal and communicable (in contrast, say, to obesity and alcoholism), and because the fear of AIDS may interfere with or hinder normal biological urges and behaviors, AIDS has a special status as an elicitor of multiple affective reactions. Of course,

TABLE 4.4. Cognitive Antecedents, Affective Reactions, and Subsequent Behavioral Tendencies toward Persons with AIDS

| Cognitive antecedents | Causal controllability | Affective reactions | Behavioral tendencies |
|---|---|---|---|
| Sexual behavior | Controllable | Anger | Neglect |
| Homosexual behavior Drug use | Controllable | Anger, moral repugnance | Neglect, aggression |
| Communicable | Controllable or Uncontrollable | Fear | Neglect, nonaltruistic help |
| Terminal | Controllable or Uncontrollable (onset only) | Pity, sympathy | Altruistic help |
| Blood transfusion, Children of AIDS parents | Uncontrollable | Pity, sympathy | Altruistic help |

Note. Data from Weiner (1988, p. 126).

the magnitude of all the emotions depend on a number of variables, including the relationship between the HIV-infected person and the person experiencing the emotion, the stage of the illness, and so on.

## Historical Analysis of Reactions to People with AIDS

Although multiple reactions to AIDS are displayed, the feelings that have been expressed to this illness have quite likely varied in the short history (just about one decade) since AIDS was first identified (see Weiner, 1988, 1993a). When AIDS was initially reported in 1981, relatively minor organized intervention was undertaken. The slow acknowledgment of this disease has been subject to much criticism directed at the United States and other governments. One reason for the inaction was that little was known about the illness. However, even after some initial understanding was attained, there was still limited responsiveness. It is suggested that AIDS was ignored because it was perceived as only onset-controllable, so that persons contracting this disease were held personally responsible for their plight. Hence, individuals with this illness elicited anger, relatively little pity, and neglect from others. In addition, AIDS was associated with homosexuality (and shortly thereafter with drug use). Independent of the perceived controllability of HIV infection, persons with AIDS therefore elicited negative reactions. This initial stage in the historical analysis is summarized in the first rows of Table 4.5.

**TABLE 4.5.** Historical Analysis of Reactions to Persons with AIDS

---

Stage 1 (1981–1984)
   [a]AIDS—onset controllable—responsible—little pity, anger—neglect
   [b]AIDS—contracted by gay males—sexual hostility—little pity, anger—neglect

Stage 2 (1985)
   [a]AIDS—onset controllable—responsible—little pity, anger—neglect
   [b]AIDS—contracted by gay males—sexual hostility—little pity, anger—neglect
   [b]AIDS—perceptions of communicability—anger—aggression

Stage 3 (1985–1987)
   [a]AIDS—onset controllable—responsible—little pity, anger—neglect
   [b]AIDS—contracted by gay males—sexual hostility—little pity, anger—neglect
   [b]AIDS—perceptions of communicability—anger—aggression
   [b]AIDS—perceptions of communicability—fear—nonaltruistic help

Stage 4 (1987–present)
   [a]AIDS—onset controllable—responsible—little pity, anger—neglect
   [b]AIDS—contracted by gay males—sexual hostility—little pity, anger—neglect
   [b]AIDS—perceptions of communicability—anger—aggression
   [b]AIDS—perceptions of communicability—fear—nonaltruistic help
   [a]AIDS—onset uncontrollable—no responsibility—pity and sympathy, no
      anger—altruistic help
   [b]AIDS—terminal—pity—altruistic help

---

*Note.* Adapted from Weiner (1988, p. 126). Copyright 1988 by Abt. Books. Adapted by permission.
[a]Responsibility-based reactions.
[b]Nonresponsibility-based reactions.

A short time later, when AIDS began to spread and its communicability—as well as its threat to the heterosexual population—became more evident, anger toward the carriers of this disease began to flourish. As Triplet and Sugarman (1987) have summarized:

> Homosexual rights legislation that was pending in several state legislatures has been tabled in the face of acrimonious debate.... A Gallop poll has indicated that attitudes towards homosexuals have generally become more negative ... and Haitian immigrants have faced increasing discrimination in housing and employment.... Even among college students, a traditionally tolerant segment of the population, 47.8% currently approve of legislation prohibiting homosexual relations. (pp. 265–266)

Furthermore, there was an alarming growth of aggressive action that was directly traced to "retaliation" for the carrying and spreading of the

HIV virus by homosexuals. Thus, not only was AIDS perceived as some form of "revenge" from God, but having the disease promoted further human reprisal. That is, the "punishment" itself provoked additional punishment! These reactions to AIDS are shown in Stage 2 of Table 4.5.

As personal fear began to grow because of the communicability of this illness, private and governmental support soon was augmented. This is illustrated in the following report:

> In the last six months, there has been an enormous change in the responses of foundations, corporations, and the public generally," said Dr. Mathilde Krim, a research biologist who established the AIDS Medical Foundation in 1983. "I cannot pinpoint any single event or reason, but people finally have caught on that AIDS is a potential threat to everybody and has an impact on health, the economy, and our lives," said Dr. Krim, who has frequently complained about the public apathy toward the spread of the disease. (Teltsch, *New York Times*, July 28, 1987, p. 9)

Hence, the help that was provided was not altruistically motivated or generated by pity or sympathy; rather, it was driven by concerns and fear for the self. This characterizes the recent past and is shown in Stage 3 of Table 4.5. Note that in Stage 3 of the hypothesized historical sequence (which is loose regarding exact boundary dates), there are two determinants of responding that are unrelated to thoughts about responsibility (negative attitudes toward homosexuals and beliefs of communicability) and there is one responsibility-generated source that relates to perceived controllability. Two of these influences contribute to neglect and one to aggression, whereas only fear of transmission gives rise to help giving— although, as already indicated, this is help that protects the self and is unrelated to prosocial conduct as far as its motivational source is concerned.

The virus associated with AIDS continues to be viewed as contracted by gay males and drug users, and therefore remains considered as onset controllable. At the same time, however, it also is perceived as onset uncontrollable, infecting blood recipients and infants. Thus, another source of help captured in Table 4.5 that is operating at present is altruistically motivated sympathy. This emotion also is experienced because AIDS is now known to be terminal.

## The Future

It is quite likely that Stage 4 soon will give way to yet another period, for the perceived causes and course of AIDS are in flux. If the spread of AIDS among heterosexuals in America drops or is less than anticipated, if the new blood detection methods are infallible, and if there are increasing abortions by potential mothers with AIDS, then this could result in a shift in the direction from Stage 4 back to Stage 3 regarding the affective and behavioral dynamics of this disease. That is, the virus associated with AIDS will no longer be perceived as onset uncontrollable and the infection will be linked exclusively to gays and drug users. This is likely to have quite negative consequences for help giving and financial support inasmuch as the altruistic origins of help (save for the terminal nature of the illness) would decrease. This is rather dramatically revealed in the following report:

> Another federal physician put it more bluntly: "Everybody has got their own agenda, and the thing that fuels the resources for AIDS is the threat of heterosexual transmission. The people who are spending money basically don't care if a bunch of Gay men and drug users get AIDS. They really don't. So the thing that's driving the money is the fear of heterosexual transmission. And the people who run the laboratories that get the money know that." (Scheer, *Los Angeles Times*, Aug. 14, 1987, p.18)

On the other hand, if AIDS dramatically rises among the heterosexual population—which is the case, for example, in Asia—then a different array of dominant affects is likely to be displayed.

## *Assimilation and Contrast*

Another reason for affective alteration as a function of who contracts the HIV virus and for what reason is that reactions are determined by the entire social context in which AIDS is judged. For example, if the vast majority of HIV infections were due to blood transfusions with contaminated blood, then those few individuals infected because of sexual behavior would be judged especially harshly since that behavior would be contrasted with the dominant uncontrollable determinants of HIV infection. One might make the perhaps surprising prediction that if all uncontrollable causes of HIV infection are eliminated, then the persons with AIDS would be judged more (rather than less) leniently because of the lack of a contrasting causal group.

## THE DILEMMA OF AIDS EDUCATION

It is quite evident from the past discussion that HIV infection can be caused by a variety of factors. However, those most common are sexual behavior and sharing a contaminated needle for drug injection. Both these causes are controllable, and the person becoming infected for either of these two reasons is held responsible. Hence, AIDS prevention techniques focus upon "safe sex," and some drug programs are distributing free needles to potential drug users in order to keep down the incidence of HIV infection and AIDS.

Yet there is an unintended consequence of the educational programs. By teaching that persons are responsible for acquiring the HIV virus, the degree of perceived responsibility of those who are infected is raised, thereby increasing anger, decreasing sympathy, and minimizing the likelihood of providing help. Thus, the educational programs create costs as well as benefits by pitting the positive and negative consequences of holding another responsible for acquiring the virus associated with AIDS (see also Chapter 3). On the one hand, it is essential that persons assume individual responsibility for their actions. This surely promotes personal change and is the basis for many psychotherapies. However, altruistic actions from others are augmented by perceptions of uncontrollability. In this context, the dual consequences of education are more of theoretical than practical interest, for surely the educational programs create more benefit than harm.

It is, of course, theoretically possible to induce perceived controllability while increasing help giving. But this would require asking individuals to accept that the acquisition of the HIV virus is due to a personal "moral failure," while at the same time asking them to ignore this information or to forgive those who have "fallen." This is a difficult request for many.

## The Christian Dilemma

One might think that the quandary of whether to help or neglect those with AIDS would be particularly exacerbated among those holding strong religious beliefs. Homosexuality among Christians is regarded as a sin against God. To justify this position, they turn (perhaps unexpectedly) to the Old Testament Book of Leviticus (20:13), which contains the following passage: "If a man also lie with mankind, as he lieth with a woman, both of them have committed an abomination: they shall surely be put to death; their blood shall be upon them." On the other hand, religions also advocate coming to the help of those in need—being good Samaritans. Love, justice, compassion, mercy, and faith are preached. Hence, given strong prohibitions against actions that cause HIV infection, and given strong directions to help those in need, it would be expected that solicitation of funds to help people with AIDS would activate deep moral conflicts. It also is the case, however, that religiosity correlates highly with conservatism, and it is known that conservatives see persons as responsible for their HIV infections (as well as for poverty and other social problems). They also are less likely to help. So perhaps the moral dilemma characterizes only a small subset of this population.

## SUMMARY

Perhaps the most stigmatizing condition in contemporary society is AIDS. A research investigation regarding Magic Johnson, the famous basketball star, confirmed what also is known to be true for other stigmas—namely, that infection from controllable causes such as sexual behavior and drug use results in greater inferences of responsibility, more anger, and less sympathy than does infection from uncontrollable causes such as a transfusion with contaminated blood.

AIDS is a stigma that is associated with two other stigmas: homosexuality and drug use. Hence, reactions to those with AIDS are linked with general attitudes toward homosexuals. Individuals who have negative attitudes toward homosexuals not only judge those with AIDS as more responsible than persons who are not homophobic but also express greater anger and less prosocial actions toward people with AIDS than do those who have more positive opinions about homosexuality. However, information about causal controllability exerts a more powerful effect than on reactions to those with AIDS. There also is evidence that the negative attitudes of homophobics toward persons with AIDS is symbolic rather than instrumental in origin; information that could alleviate their fears about others infected with the virus does not alter their opinions and behaviors.

It is proposed that reactions to others with AIDS have varied in the short history of this illness as the cause of the infection, its communicability, and its lethal course have become known. Specifically, the theoretical perspective that has been advanced in this chapter leads to the observation that as blood transfusion became known as a cause of HIV infection, then sympathy for the infected increased; as the communicability of the HIV virus became known, then fear and anger toward those with the virus grew; and as it became evident that AIDS is terminal, pity for those with AIDS increased. It also is proposed that education about the controllability of HIV infection, while producing desirable self-protective behavior, will result in less altruistic behavior toward others who are infected because inferences of responsibility will increase. In addition, those holding strong religious beliefs may experience conflicting feelings about persons with AIDS because religious tenets to help the needy coexist with an interpretation of the Bible asserting that homosexual behavior should be condemned.

Reactions to AIDS are more complex than are responses to other stigmas because of the greater number of influencing factors. However, these reactions are amenable to the theoretical reasoning that already has been proposed. A motivational sequence of causal thinking → emotional reactivity → behavioral responses provides a conceptual framework that incorporates many of the observations. The key concepts of controllable causality and inferences about responsibility are as salient in the study of AIDS as they are when teachers react to students who are not trying as opposed to those who have low ability. The underlying distinctions that the layperson addresses is whether AIDS in a particular case is a sin or a sickness or both.

# 5

Responsibility,
Stigmatization, Mental
Illness, and the Family

Teresa of Avila (1515–1582) declared that the unwanted conduct, the
reported visions, should be treated as if they were symptoms of illness
... accounted for by natural causes.... Since the person is not the
agent of action in sickness, he or she cannot be held responsible....
Teresa effectively sidetracked the Inquisitors from their usual practice
of locating the cause of unauthorized visions in the visionary's
intentional commerce with the devil.

—SARBIN (1990)

The discussion in the prior two chapters focused on perceptions of stigmatized persons and the consequences of beliefs regarding the cause of their stigmas. The larger social system, or the social context in which the stigmatized person is included, has been neglected, although this does require attention when considering the dynamics of stigmatization. For example, it is known that the obese face great obstacles in employment. This obviously has economic consequences for their families that could promote accusations of laziness or neglect by their spouse, parents, and so on. Family conflict therefore arises, and interpersonal bonds are weakened. Clearly, then, stigmatization takes place within a social and cultural context.

In Chapter 5, I begin to modestly redress this shortcoming by considering the social context of stigmatization, particularly the role of the family unit. Three stigmas, each linked with a distinct psychological issue, are examined: (1) depression, and the consequences of conveying negative emotions to others; (2) schizophrenia, and its exacerbation by the reactions it elicits from family members (labeled "expressed emotions"); and (3) divorce, as accelerated by spousal judgments of intentionality for undesired interpersonal behaviors. I must admit that a distressed marriage certainly is not a stigma, and in today's American society neither is divorce. Hence, I have stretched the boundaries of this chapter to include a literature that deserves your attention yet has no appropriate location in the book. The decision to include the distressed marriage literature here weakens the coherence of the chapter, which starts with two mental illnesses, but I do believe that it strengthens the entire book and is meaningfully related to the discussion of depression and schizophrenia.

By including depression and schizophrenia, for the first time common categories of mental illness are introduced into the discussion of reactions to the stigmatized. As was the case with physical illnesses, implicit in the understanding of mental illness, conveyed by labels such as depression and schizophrenia, is whether the onset of the illness was controllable, and whether the mentally ill person was responsible for the illness (Schoeneman, Segerstrom, Griffin, & Gresham, 1993). Individuals generally are held responsible for anorexia and other eating disorders, for example, but are not perceived as responsible for retardation, the experience of multiple personalities, and the like. Virtually all the other stigmas that have been considered, including alcoholism, obesity, homosexuality, and AIDS, have implications for the entire family and, in turn, for the stigmatized person. Hence, rather than provide an exhaustive account of the interdependence of stigmatization and the social context, the stigmas that were selected for analysis were intended to illustrate some selected psychological topics. I also have limited my analysis, leaving sociologists and anthropologists to point out the connections between stigmatization and the larger social system and cultural factors.

## DEPRESSION

There is a huge literature documenting that causal thoughts of the depressed person play a role in bringing about or maintaining certain kinds of depression. Attributions of the causes of personal problems to unchangeable sources may give rise to hopelessness, while beliefs that the causes of difficulties are due to the self can result in low self-esteem as well as guilt and/or shame. The emotions of hopelessness, low self-esteem, guilt, and shame may bring about and/or accompany certain types of depression. Of course, maladaptive causal thinking is merely one antecedent of depression, along with stressful events such as a death in the family, hormonal imbalance, and so on.

In this book, the thoughts of the depressed person are not examined, inasmuch as I have confined my analysis to the perception of others, not the self. Rather, following the suggestion of Coyne, Kahn, and Gotlib (1987), attention will be directed to the social context in which depressive symptoms are expressed. I am particularly concerned with the manner in which others who interact with the depressed person are influenced by beliefs about the cause of the unhappiness of that individual. These causal inferences elicit particular feelings and actions that are directed toward the depressed person and may ameliorate or deepen his or her depression.

Prior to examining these and related issues, I do want to make it clear that in these few pages I am neither foolhardy nor wise enough to propose a theory of depression. My goals are much more modest: I merely want to point out that the conception guiding this book also appears amenable to the understanding of some possible dynamics associated with depression. This position is consistent with a current experimental literature based on the assumption that behavior associated with depression is interwoven with a corresponding pattern of responses from others (Coyne, 1976a, 1976b).

## Reactions to the Depressed

What, then, are the emotional reactions to the depressed? Reviews of the literature clearly reveal that depressed persons elicit rejection from others (Coates & Wortman, 1980; Coyne et al., 1987; Gurtman, 1986). Rejection is manifested in both distance from and active dislike of the depressed. Thus, people are unwilling to interact with others who are depressed. In one simple experiment documenting this aversion, subjects spoke over the phone with either a depressed or a nondepressed person. Those talking with the depressed person became more depressed and hostile and voiced rejection of the person with whom they had communicated (Coyne, 1976a). Even following an imagined interaction with someone who is depressed, subjects actively reject the possibility of future interaction (Winer, Bonner, Blaney, & Murray, 1981). In general, depressed individuals create a negative effect on others. At best, the emotional reactions they elicit are ambivalent or mixed, and at worst the affective responses are only negative, with anger being the most dominant affective component (see the reviews cited above). Marital interactions with a depressed spouse also are characterized by negative affect and tension (see Coyne et al., 1987).

In sum, a vast psychological literature documents that being depressed has a dramatic negative effect on social relationships, resulting in the absence of positive, supportive involvements with others. Some theories of depression contend that anger toward the depressed and rejection contribute to the depth and the perpetuation of the depression that is being experienced (Coyne et al., 1987). This is in part because individuals under severe stress have a special need for close, supportive relationships (see Coates & Wortman, 1980). Indeed, lack of social support has been documented to have a direct effect on depression (see Coyne et al., 1987).

But why do the depressed elicit negative responses? What are the mechanisms that intervene between the perception of the depressed other and these aversive reactions? A number of explanations have been offered, all supported by some empirical evidence. Perhaps the negativity and the sadness of the depressed person induce a bad mood in others, and this mood triggers antisocial reactions (Winer et al., 1981). Or, perhaps any individuals who reveal pain and suffering tend to be judged as poorly adjusted and, thus, unfit (Coates & Wortman, 1980). Or perhaps expressed depression evokes fears in others of personal dependence, which entails "costs" that the other does not want to bear. To prevent this possibility, the depressed individual is rejected. And yet another possible explanation—one that is consistent with the theme of this book—relates to beliefs about personal responsibility for the stigma (which, in this instance, is an emotional state) and the negative affects linked with judgments of responsibility for expressed unhappiness.

Prior to exploring this latter explanation in detail, you are once more asked to participate in an experiment (Experiment 5.1). This experiment attempts to document that the process applicable to the analysis of why depressed individuals elicit personal rejection is not unique to this abnormal state but rather can be called upon to explain reactions to normal individuals as well. I will next describe this experiment and I suggest that Experiment 5.1 be completed after reading the following brief description.

In Experiment 5.1, you are asked to assume that you or another person is feeling happy or unhappy. Then two causes of these feelings are to be considered: something unspecified about the person (e.g., the kind of person you or that other individual is, the way of viewing the world, etc.), or something unspecified about the environment (e.g., something that happened, the particular circumstances, etc.). You are asked to rate the likelihood that each of these is the cause of the two emotions for both the self and the other. Thus, eight responses are to be given in this factorial design: two emotions (happy and unhappy) × two individuals (self and other) × two causes (disposition and situation). Please do this now. It should be noted that, in distinction to the other chapters, here inferences of personal versus situational causality are assessed. Recall from Chapter 1 that personal causality is one of the necessary antecedents for an inference of responsibility, whereas situational causality results in the offset of the responsibility process. Hence, these judgments later will be interpreted in

## EXPERIMENT 5.1

# The Perceived Causes of Positive and Negative Feelings

Assume the following emotional states, experienced by you or someone else, and indicate what caused them by circling one number on the rating scale.

1. You are feeling happy. To what extent is this due to something about you (the kind of person you are, your way of viewing the world, etc.)?

| 1 | 2 | 3 | 4 | 5 | 6 | 7 | 8 | 9 |
|---|---|---|---|---|---|---|---|---|

Not at all
due to me

Entirely due
to me

2. You are feeling happy. To what extent is this due to something about the environment (something good that happened, the particular circumstances, etc.)?

| 1 | 2 | 3 | 4 | 5 | 6 | 7 | 8 | 9 |
|---|---|---|---|---|---|---|---|---|

Not at all due
to the environment

Entirely due to
the environment

3. You are feeling unhappy. To what extent is this due to something about you (the kind of person you are, your way of viewing the world, etc.)?

| 1 | 2 | 3 | 4 | 5 | 6 | 7 | 8 | 9 |
|---|---|---|---|---|---|---|---|---|

Not at all
due to me

Entirely due
to me

4. You are feeling unhappy. To what extent is this due to something about the environment (something bad that happened, the particular circumstances, etc.)?

| 1 | 2 | 3 | 4 | 5 | 6 | 7 | 8 | 9 |
|---|---|---|---|---|---|---|---|---|

Not at all
due to me

Entirely due
to me

5. Someone else is feeling happy. To what extent is this due to something about the person (the kind of person he or she is, their way of viewing the world, etc.)?

| 1 | 2 | 3 | 4 | 5 | 6 | 7 | 8 | 9 |
|---|---|---|---|---|---|---|---|---|

Not at all
due to them

Entirely due
to them

6. Someone else is feeling happy. To what extent is this due to something about the environment (something good that happened, the particular circumstances, etc.)?

| 1 | 2 | 3 | 4 | 5 | 6 | 7 | 8 | 9 |
|---|---|---|---|---|---|---|---|---|

Not at all due
to the environment

Entirely due to
the environment

7. Someone else is feeling unhappy. To what extent is this due to something about them (the kind of person he or she is, their way of viewing the world, etc.)?

| 1 | 2 | 3 | 4 | 5 | 6 | 7 | 8 | 9 |
|---|---|---|---|---|---|---|---|---|

Not at all                                        Entirely due
due to them                                        to them

8. Someone else is feeling unhappy. To what extent is this due to something about the environment (something bad that happened, the particular circumstances, etc.)?

| 1 | 2 | 3 | 4 | 5 | 6 | 7 | 8 | 9 |
|---|---|---|---|---|---|---|---|---|

Not at all                                        Entirely due
due to them                                        to them

terms of inferences of responsibility. The experiment is phrased in this manner to be consistent with prior research.

## The Perceived Causes of Emotional States

Investigations similar to Experiment 5.1 already have been reported, although they are more extensive than what has been asked of you (Karasawa, in press; Liu, Karasawa, & Weiner, 1992). In one of a series of studies by Karasawa (in press), situation and disposition causality were rated for a number of positive and negative emotions assumed to be experienced by both the self and another person. The findings, shown in Figure 5.1, reveal that for positive emotions including happiness, it is believed that the situation was causally more important in bringing forth the emotion than the person was (see left half of Figure 5.1). This is true

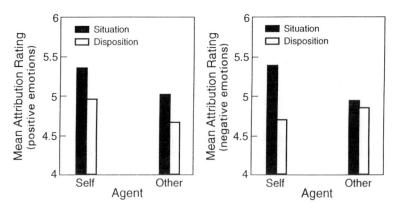

**FIGURE 5.1.** Attributional ratings to situation and disposition as a function of the valence of the emotion (positive vs. negative) and the experiencer of the emotion (self vs. other). Data from Karasawa (in press).

for judgments regarding both the self and the other. Happiness therefore is generally attributed to something that has happened, rather than to something dispositional about the person experiencing this feeling.

The pattern of data for the negative emotions, including unhappiness, is more complex (see Figure 5.1, right half). When judging why one might personally experience unhappiness, again the main attribution is to the situation—something bad has happened. However, when someone else is unhappy, then this is perceived as caused by something dispositional about that person as much as it is ascribed to the situation. Thus, only when judging the negative feelings of others is there a tendency to perceive that the person is as causally implicated as the situation.

In a second investigation exploring the reliability of these findings, Karasawa (in press) examined only negative emotions and again found the pattern of results just reported. However, in this investigation the differences between the causal judgments made about the self and those made about others were even more pronounced, with dispositional ratings exceeding those for the situation when judging the negative emotions of another.

You should now examine your data to determine if the same results are found—that is, happiness is more ascribed to the situation than to personal dispositions for both the self and the other, whereas unhappiness is thought to be caused by the situation for the self but relatively more by the person when judging the other. Hence, only given the unhappiness of the other is the individual judged to be as much of the cause as is the situation. I believe that this will be the case in your data as well.

Liu et al. (1992) then elaborated the research by Karasawa (which, although in press, was actually conducted prior to Liu et al., 1992). They provided a situational cause for an emotion and asked subjects if additional causes might have contributed to produce this feeling. For example, in vignettes it was stated that "Tom felt excited when starting a new job" or that "Tom felt angry when his roommate left a pile of dishes in the sink." The subjects rated if other factors might have contributed to these emotional responses. The additional emotional determinants to be considered were three general categories of causality: dispositional ("something about the kind of person he is also caused or contributed to this emotional reaction"), situational ("something else about the immediate situation or recent past also caused or contributed to this emotional reaction"), and current mood.

The data from one investigation reported by Liu et al. (1992) are shown in Figure 5.2, which reveals that when a positive emotion is experienced by another, all three additional potential causes of that reaction are rated as somewhat high and nearly equal (the ratings were made on 7-point scales). On the other hand, when the emotion is negative, percep-

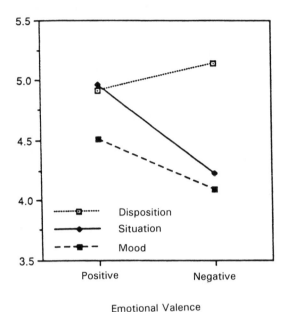

FIGURE 5.2. Mean causal ratings to disposition, situation, and mood as a function of the valence of the emotion. From Liu, Karasawa, and Weiner (1992, p. 609). Copyright 1992 by Sage Publications, Inc. Reprinted by permission.

tions of disposition as a further cause increase relative to judgments about positive emotions, whereas situation and mood causal judgments decrease.

Other research, using an entirely different methodology, supports the conclusion that depression is attributed to the depressed person. For example, Rippere (1977) examined a variety of naive beliefs about depression. Among the most endorsed items were the following:

1. If someone is feeling depressed, there's probably something he can do about it (91% agreement).
2. When a depressed person recovers, he should take most of the credit himself (93% agreement).
3. When someone is feeling depressed, he ought to try to deal with it himself rather than consult a psychiatrist (82% agreement).

Taken together, the investigations reported by Karasawa (in press), Liu et al. (1992), and Rippere (1977) document that when others express unhappiness, there is a strong tendency to judge that something about the other (i.e., his or her disposition) causes this feeling.

But what consequence might the inclination to attribute depression to the depressed person have? Karasawa (in press) reported that ascription of a negative emotional state to the person as opposed to the situation has far-reaching interpersonal ramifications. To examine the effects of causal beliefs about another's emotion, Karasawa gave subjects the following story stem:

> You recently moved into a new apartment with a new roommate . . . You planned to study together for an exam . . . but could not because of the roommate's emotional state. When your roommate came back, he/she indicated that he/she felt _____ (angry, anxious, depressed, guilty, sad, or ashamed). You asked why, and your room-mate talked about an event that happened at work

This was followed by a situational or a dispositional ascription for the feeling:

1. Indeed, what happened there was something that made people feel _____, and you understood why your roommate felt _____ because of it—others would have felt that way.
2. However, what happened there was minor, and you thought that your roommate's personality was the real reason for his/her _____.

After reading the vignettes, the subjects indicated how responsible the roommate was for having this feeling and how the subject would respond emotionally toward the roommate.

The data revealed that responsibility was perceived as greater when the other's personality disposition, rather than the situation, was the cause of the emotional state. This is consistent with the conclusion in Chapter 1 that responsibility necessitates person causality. Further, as displayed in Figure 5.3, the observer's affective reactions were markedly positive when the situation was the cause but were almost equally negative when person-ality was manipulated as causal.

Finally, in a follow-up of this research, Karasawa (in press) repeated the above scenarios but merely indicated the emotional experience of the roommate without supplying a cause. The respondents rated their percep-tions of dispositional and situational causality, as well as the roommates responsibility for the emotion, their own emotional reactions toward the roommate, and their intended behaviors of comforting (providing social support) and avoiding personal interaction with this individual (rejection).

The correlations between these ratings are shown in Table 5.1. Table 5.1 reveals a replication of what is displayed in Figure 5.3: If a negative

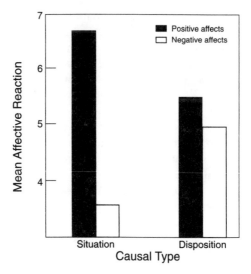

**FIGURE 5.3.** Mean positive and negative affective reactions as a function of the attribution (situation vs. disposition) for the emotional experience. Data from Karasawa (in press).

emotion is attributed to a personal disposition, then others tend to not have positive feelings ($r = -.17$) and express negative feelings ($r = .26$). In addition, that person is perceived as responsible for his or her feeling state ($r = .30$). Inferences about responsibility relate to (and research in the prior chapters has documented that they precede and cause) the withholding of positive feelings ($r = -.26$) and the expressions of negative emotions toward the depressed person ($r = .42$). These emotions are associated with (and I believe give rise to) an inhibition of prosocial support and rejection. The correlations between positive emotions and social support, and negative emotions and rejection, exceeded $r = .50$ (see also Sacco & Dunn, 1990)

## Conclusion Concerning Reactions to the Depressed

The pieces of the puzzle that relate depression to the social context—that is, to inferences by others of the responsibility of the depressed person for his or her feelings, now seem to be in place. When a depressed person displays unhappiness and sadness, observers tend to ascribe these feelings to something about the person who is experiencing these emotions. That is, "What is the matter with *you*?" is likely to be asked, followed by advice such as, "Go out and have a good time." As indicated, the tendency to

**TABLE 5.1.** Correlations between Causes of Another's Negative Emotions and the Subject's Judgments of Responsibility, Emotional Reactions, and Intentions Regarding Interpersonal Behaviors

|  |  | SIT | PA | NA | RESP | SUP | REJ |
|---|---|---|---|---|---|---|---|
| Dispositional attribution | (DIS) | −.55 | −.17 | .26 | .30 | −.19 | .27 |
| Situational attribution | (SIT) |  | .19 | −.27 | −.28 | .15 | −.26 |
| Positive affects | (PA) |  |  | −.32 | −.26 | .54 | −.26 |
| Negative affects | (NA) |  |  |  | .42 | −.26 | .51 |
| Assignment of responsibility | (RESP) |  |  |  |  | −.26 | .39 |
| Support | (SUP) |  |  |  |  |  | −.25 |
| Rejection | (REJ) |  |  |  |  |  |  |

*Note.* Data from Karasawa (in press).

ascribe negative emotions to the person is also true regarding opinions about "normal" people. In addition, it has been found that other symptoms of depression, including self-neglect and apathy (which have not been discussed here because of the focus on emotion), are rated among the most controllable psychiatric symptoms inasmuch as they are "passive" rather than "active" (e.g., hallucinations) (see Hooley, 1987).

Beliefs that the person caused his or her own sadness and behavioral symptoms imply that the depressed individual is responsible for his or her state. This, in turn, elicits negative feelings including anger, which instigate antisocial behavior. Inferences of responsibility also result in the absence of positive emotions, and this absence then produces a withdrawal of prosocial, supporting responses. Hence, there is the reappearance of the familiar hypothesized sequence, causal attribution → responsibility inference → emotion → action, which was expressed so frequently in the prior chapters will be repeated even more often in the chapters that follow. Regarding the present analysis, the event eliciting causal analysis is not achievement failure or a stigmatizing bodily condition but a stigma that is virtually synonymous with a negative feeling state. The attribution process is presumed to be initiated by a search for what is causing the unhappiness of another.

What is particularly destructive about this sequence for the depressed person is that social support helps to alleviate depression, while rejection produces further sadness. Indeed, Coyne et al. (1987) state that "lack of social support has a direct relationship to depression" (p. 513). Therefore, depression is characterized as embedded within a cycle in which the reaction of important others in the family may result in the maintenance and/or enhancement of the stigmatized state—that is, depression produces rejection, which in turn produces depression.

In the criminal justice system, it sometimes is said that one does not punish the insane criminal because insanity mitigates certain aversive responses. But apparently depression does not mitigate the negative reactions of others. Furthermore, the unhappiness in itself is not sufficient punishment and the individual is chastened by others for being depressed. Depression is considered a sin; as such, it results in social reprimand. Unfortunately, the social punishment of the sinner increases the degree of sin (unhappiness), so that one of the main purposes of the criminal justice system, which is to decrease the likelihood of repetition of the unwanted behavior, is not fulfilled. The "sinner" is thus not "rehabilitated."

## SCHIZOPHRENIA AND EXPRESSED EMOTIONS

Individuals might find it easier to provide causes for depression than for schizophrenia and other forms of mental illness. After all, most persons have felt "down" at times, so that the experience of sadness is shared. This personal knowledge also might foster the belief that the depressed are responsible for their state inasmuch as the vast majority of individuals do "pull themselves out of" depression, or at least do become less depressed over time. In addition, as already mentioned, "negative" or passive symptoms, such as apathy, particularly produce person ascriptions.

On the other hand, hallucinations and cognitive slippage are less frequent than, say, sadness, so that schizophrenia may seem foreign and not possible to explain. Also, the bizarre nature of schizophrenic symptoms could generate a set of perceived causative factors different from those considered for more typical or usual forms of dysfunctional behavior.

In one pertinent attributional experiment, Furnham and Rees (1988) asked adult subjects the cause of schizophrenia. Five categories of causation were revealed: (1) stress and pressure (e.g., being rejected by friends, parents having emotional extremes), (2) biology (e.g., a virus), (3) genetics, (4) low intelligence, and (5) brain damage. Evidence for both psychosocial and medical models of mental illness thus were present. Note that none of the stated causes places responsibility on the schizophrenic, who either is born that way or is made that way by society. Thus, there may be personal causality, but without controllability.

On the other hand, as indicated in Chapter 3, mental illness was once viewed moralistically, with demonic possession considered a product of sin because of intentional cavorting with the devil (see the quote by Sarbin at the start of the chapter). Thus, personal responsibility for schizophrenia also has been presumed.

In one study supporting this view conducted by Neff and Husaini (1985), more than 700 respondents from a rural area were given a description of someone with paranoid beliefs (e.g., "He has argued with men who didn't even know him because he thought they were spying on him and plotting against him"). The subjects were then asked if the person should be viewed and treated as ill (a medical view of schizophrenia, although other symptoms were not revealed), viewed and treated as morally weak, held responsible, and labeled as mentally ill. In addition, the amount of tolerance the respondents would exhibit (e.g., be willing to have a person like this join a favorite club or organization) was rated.

Nearly 40% of the sample agreed that the person was morally weak and should be held personally responsible for his behavior. In addition, there was a significant negative correlation between acceptance of the medical model and perceptions of responsibility, as well as a positive correlation between conceiving of schizophrenia as an illness and reported tolerance. Tolerance was most enhanced by the belief that the person should be labeled mentally ill.

It is evident, then, that there are a variety of beliefs about the causes of schizophrenia and that both medical and moral causation are entertained as possible explanations. Furthermore, some of the associations between perceived causality and behavioral intentions evident for other stigmas, including alcoholism, obesity, poverty, homosexuality, AIDS, and depression, have been revealed as well for schizophrenia, although the data are sparse.

Surprisingly, the most detailed evidence regarding the perceived causes of schizophrenia has been generated by a body of research that initially was unconcerned with phenomenal causality. Rather, this literature pertains to the high incidence of the return of schizophrenics to institutional settings and the determinants of coping with schizophrenia. A large number of investigations have documented that family atmosphere affects the course of schizophrenia (Vaughn & Leff, 1976). Of specific importance in this context is the finding that coping with and adjustment to this illness is facilitated by families classified as low on what is called "emotional expressiveness" (EE) toward a schizophrenic family member, whereas families scoring high on EE adversely affect the schizophrenic family member and increase the likelihood that this person will be rehospitalized (these findings also hold for depression and mania, but the research in these areas is sparse and is not considered here). Emotional expressiveness as first defined embraced a number of components including general emotional reactivity and overinvolvement, as well as the specific emotional reactions of anger, hostility, and criticism.

Given this overview, let me now turn to the expressiveness research, providing some historical perspective and more recent data relevant to a responsibility analysis of social motivation as it bears upon reactions to a schizophrenic family member.

## Research Findings

It has been reported that "in the last 10 years alone, well over 100 English-language journal articles on expressed emotion have appeared" and that this research topic "has become an international preoccupation transversing five continents" (Jenkins & Karno, 1992, p. 11). In the typical investigation, family members living with a previously hospitalized schizophrenic (the "patient") are given an extensive, semi-structured interview. Classification of family members as high or low EE is based on the comments about the patient during the interview, as well as on the general tone of these remarks. It is assumed that comments during the interview mirror the face-to-face interactions with the patient. In addition, the adjustment of the patient is assessed, as indexed by hospitalization relapse or symptom severity. As Hooley (1987) summarizes:

> Patients who return from the hospital to live with relatives who, during a semi-structured interview, talk about them in a critical, hostile, or emotionally overinvolved way, suffer elevated relapse rates in comparison with patients whose relatives do not express these negative attitudes. (p. 176)

There is rather strong agreement about the empirical association between EE and relapse and equally strong agreement about the lack of theoretical understanding of this association. To again quote Hooley (1987): "Further replications of the EE-relapse link will be less and less decisive in furthering our understanding of EE, in the absence of theoretical models to account for the empirical findings" (pp. 176–177). In a similar vein, Jenkins and Karno (1992) caution:

> Theoretical elucidation of this research construct [EE] has lagged considerably behind clinical interests. . . . The elusive theoretical and empirical bases of the construct have gone unexamined. Precisely what is inside the "black box" called emotional expression has somehow remained mysterious, as has been widely acknowledged. . . . This theoretical impoverishment provides a formidable research dilemma: *the problem of prediction without understanding.* (pp. 9–10)

What theories, then, try to account for the occurrence of hostility, criticism, emotionality and the augmentation of relapse; or, conversely stated, what theories try to account for the occurrence of low hostility, withholding criticism, modulated emotionality and their positive effects on adjustment? A number of hypotheses have been proposed. It may be that an emotionally charged atmosphere increases the general stress level in the environment and that this added stress results in the reappearance of schizophrenic symptoms. Or it may be that emotionality and criticism convey lack of respect for the patient and low expectancy of recovery and that these messages augment the likelihood of relapse. It also has been suggested that high EE is one manifestation of imposing interpersonal control, yet another antecedent of poor adjustment. But most germane in the present context is the idea that perceptions of the causes of schizophrenia constitute the key mechanism that accounts for emotional reactivity and subsequent relapse.

Hooley (1987) was among the first to propose an attributional (controllability) theory of EE, but without clear distinction between personal causality and controllability causality. She noted that "when faced with onset of the abnormal behavior of a family member, relatives have two choices [about the cause of the problem]: blaming the illness [or] blaming the patient" (p.180). As already indicated, schizophrenia has been embraced within a moral as well as a medical model (see also Medvene & Krauss, 1989). Along with Leff and Vaughn (1985), Hooley (1987) hypothesized that low EE spouses accept the legitimacy of the patient's condition (a medical model), whereas high EE spouses generally hold the patient partially responsible and "express doubts about whether the patient is genuinely ill" (p. 181)—manifestations of use of the moral model. Given disruptive behavior, Hooley (1987) quotes a member of a low EE family as stating: "It wasn't her, it was this illness. I don't think it was her fault because when she's normal, she's good." On the other hand, responses of high EE family members are illustrated by the following interview quotation: "There are times when I really feel like shaking him and saying 'pull yourself together.'" Hence, Hooley presumes unions between

Perceptions of responsibility for symptoms and behavior →
High EE (criticism and hostility) → Relapse

as well as between:

Perceptions of nonresponsibility for symptoms and behavior →
Low EE (little criticism and hostility) → Adjustment and coping

Note that here high and low EE are defined entirely by criticism and hostility rather than by general over- or underinvolvement. This is how it will be defined in the remainder of this discussion.

Two recent studies provide support for this analysis. These investigations were explicitly directed by the tenets of attribution theory and the relations between causal thinking, emotion, and action that have been proposed here (although it will be seen that the second investigation to be reported is more aware of the full theoretical principles than the first). Prior to examining this research, let us consider in somewhat greater detail than Hooley the analyses of EE from a responsibility perspective.

## A Sin–Sickness Analysis of Expressed Emotions

Given the sin–sickness, social motivation framework driving this book, anger would be expressed toward the mentally ill only under conditions of perceived personal controllability and responsibility. Hence, the phenotypic relations that have been reported as:

1. Schizophrenic family member → High EE → Poor coping (Model 1)

lend themselves to the following genotypic representation:

1A. Schizophrenic family member → Symptoms and behaviors perceived as controllable → Perception of patient is responsible → Anger, criticism (High EE) → Poor coping (Model 1A)

In addition, the phenotypic description of the family low in EE is

2. Schizophrenic family member → Low EE → Good coping (Model 2)

The representation at the theoretical level, however, is less clear. On the one hand, the conceptual representation may be

2A. Schizophrenic family member → Symptoms and behaviors perceived as uncontrollable → Perception of patient as not responsible → Low anger, low criticism (Low EE) → Good coping (Model 2A)

But, based on prior reasoning, the following alternative also can be logically proposed:

2B. Schizophrenic family member → Symptoms and behaviors perceived as uncontrollable → Patient is not responsible → Sympathy and pity (Low EE?) → Good coping (Model 2B)

In Model 2B there is a question mark following the low EE label inasmuch as there is emotional expression, which is inconsistent with the characterization of these family members as relatively nonemotional. However, the emotions conveyed are positive rather than negative. Hence, according to Model 2B, what has been captured by the high versus low EE labels are two different qualities of affective communications.

Let us, then, now turn to two studies directly influenced by attributional analyses and examine whether the data allow selection of any of the proposed models (also see Lopez & Wolkenstein, 1990). The first of these investigations was conducted by Brewin, MacCarthy, Duda, and Vaughn (1991). They examined transcripts and audiotapes of interviews with schizophrenic family members and identified causal attributions for schizophrenia. The attributions were then classified according to a number of properties, including causal controllability. An example of a controllable attribution was, "He knows I don't like him swearing, so he would continue to swear. I think he did it just to be difficult." In contrast, an attribution scored for lack of controllability was, "They [the government] stopped his money and he's got no money at all. And that's when [the onset of illness] started." In addition to the attributions for the illness, an index of disturbed behavior on the part of the patient was derived from responses to a standardized questionnaire.

Nearly 70% of the spontaneous causal attributions were scored as uncontrollable, suggesting that most family members accepted a "sickness" interpretation of schizophrenia. However, this also reveals that 30% viewed schizophrenia in "sin" terms. The most controllable attributions were expressed by those making the most critical and hostile comments (high EE), whereas low EE family members reported the least controllable ascriptions. Independent scoring of criticism and hostility revealed that both of these reactions were related to inferences of controllability. This was the case when scores on hostility were eliminated from the relation between controllability and criticism, and when scores on criticism were eliminated from the relation between controllability and hostility.

In sum, Brewin et al. (1991) identified the thought processes (causal inferences) that were related to, and theoretically gave rise to, EE (anger and criticism). Support was provided for Model 1A and Model 2A, as outlined above. Similar findings have been reported by Barrowclough, Johnston, and Tarrier (1994). However, Brewin et al. (1991) and Barrowclough et al. (1994) did not address whether perceptions of uncontrollability increase prosocial emotions such as pity and sympathy, so that high EE is linked with the negative emotion of anger, whereas low EE is related to positive emotions. This issue, however, was considered by Weisman, Lopez, Karno, and Jenkins (1993).

Weisman et al. (1993) obtained transcripts from a prior study in which the EE status of their sample already had been determined. These investigators then rated the interviews for causal ascriptions concerning patient's control over their symptoms. Weisman et al. (1993) clarify that an example of no perceived control would be the prevailing belief that the disorder and symptoms are entirely God's will, and the perception that nothing the patient can do will change fate. In contrast, an example of a great deal of perceived control would be the view that all the schizophrenic symptoms are contrived to avoid work, household chores, and other undesirable tasks. (p. 602)

In addition, all affects directly pertaining to the patient also were identified from the transcripts. The affects were coded as positive (e.g., warmth and sympathy) and negative (e.g., annoyance and hate).

The data revealed that high EE relatives expressed significantly higher beliefs in the controllability of the symptoms than did the low EE relatives, as Brewin et al. (1991) had found. In addition, high EE relatives also reported more negative affects than low EE relatives did. However, the low EE members expressed *more* positive affects toward the patient than the high EE family members did (see Figure 5.4).

This latter finding is inconsistent with prior thinking about EE and supports Model 2B previously presented. That is, low EE does not merely mean the absence of emotions, but rather is associated with the presence of positive emotions.

Unfortunately, Weisman et al. (1993) grouped together a number of positive emotions, not all of which are theoretically related to inferences of uncontrollability (e.g., love), as well as some negative emotions not theoretically associated with beliefs about controllability (e.g., frustration). In

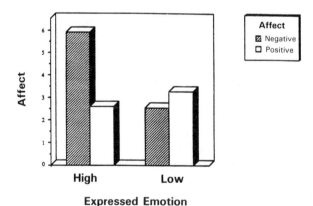

FIGURE 5.4. Components of expressed emotion (negative vs. positive) as a function of classification (high vs. low) on expressed emotion. From Weisman, Lopez, Karno, and Jenkins (1993, p. 604). Copyright 1993 by the American Psychological Association. Reprinted by permission.

addition, the researchers do not report how relapse relates to the cognitive and affective indexes. Nevertheless, this investigation provides much support for the theory being proposed here and suggests quite a different picture of the affective lives of the families of schizophrenic patients.

It also should be noted that neither Brewin et al. (1991) nor Weisman et al. (1993) consider exactly why anger and criticism result in an increased relapse rate, although there immediately come to mind some possibilities related to self-perception of inadequacy, loss of social support, fear of rejection, and the like. Specification of these mediators is needed, as well as full tests of Models 1A, 2A, and 2B with the use of path models.

## Practical Implications

In recent years, there has been a burst of studies on psychosocial interventions with families of schizophrenics. These attempts have been partially fueled by the evidence that EE predicts relapse in patients. Although not guided by attribution theory or the arguments presented in the prior pages, Lam (1991) states that the intervention attempts share the following:

> The educational component provides a model for relatives to make sense both of the patient's and their own behavior and feelings. Hence, the patient is no longer seen to be malicious and deliberately failing to control their very disturbing behavior. Relatives may also understand that delusional accusation is real to the patient and develop better ways to handle situations rather than heated arguments and counter-accusations. (p. 436)

In sum, it appears that the programs have been intuitively designed to alter attributions and/or affects—which, in turn, theoretically should result in decreased relapse. It is, therefore, now time that these interventions be consciously guided by the theoretical structure that has been suggested. This calls attention to the entire responsibility process and to positive as well as negative affects. Hence, there are immediate avenues of application suggested by the conceptual analysis (see Medvene & Krauss, 1989).

## DIVORCE AND DISTRESSED MARRIAGE

An article in *Family Circle* magazine appeared with the headline "Where's our sympathy for divorced women?" (Lear, 1991). Lear suggests that there is a general perception that "widowhood is something that happens to you. Divorce is something you cause" (p. 73). Widows, Lear argues, elicit sympathy and help; indeed, as already revealed, when the welfare system was established, its initial targets primarily were widowed women (Katz, 1986). On the other hand, in many instances divorce evokes anger and avoidance. Thus, even in our "liberated" culture, reactions to the loss of a spouse (of either gender) depend on the reason for that separation and associated beliefs about moral responsibility. Thus, reactions to divorced persons seem quite amenable to the dynamics of other stigmas examined in this book.

The determinants of divorce, in turn, depend upon many factors, including the laws and mores of the culture, the availability of spousal alternatives, poverty and wealth, and so on. In addition, particularly in the American culture, divorce is contingent upon the unhappiness or "distress" of the couples involved. And this, in turn, is subject to yet another analysis that incorporates perceptions of responsibility and emotions, namely, the couple's thoughts about the responsibility of the other for negative marriage-related events, as well as the affect that is thereby elicited. I therefore turn next to marital distress, with the apology reiterated that, although this in itself is not a stigma and certainly not a mental aberration, it deserves attention and is best placed within the interpersonal context stressed within this chapter.

Realizing that marital distress is amenable to a responsibility interpretation is an insight for which I would like to take credit. Unfortunately, that is not possible since an attributional approach to distress has been a major research thrust of Frank Fincham and his colleagues and students, particularly Thomas Bradbury (e.g., Bradbury & Fincham, 1988, 1989, 1990, 1992; Fincham, 1985; Fincham & Beach, 1988; Fincham & Bradbury, 1992). In addition, these authors make many of the distinctions that I also adopt here, including a differentiation between causality and responsibility. And they postulate a sequential or temporal series in which a hypothesized relation between responsibility for negative events and distress is mediated by other reactions, particularly what they label attributions of blame.

As was indicated in Chapter 1, there are some disagreements and divergences between the conception first offered by Fincham and my beliefs. I restrict the notion of attribution to causes and do not consider responsibility or blame to be attributions since they relate respectively to inferences about a person and to an evaluation of that person; I do not use the concept of blame because it is considered a cognitive–affective blend with components of both responsibility and anger; and positive as well as negative emotions are included within my conceptual representation of action. Finally, Fincham and his colleagues want to explain marital distress. Hence, they are likely to include many other variables, as needed, to shed light on this phenomenon. On the other hand, my colleagues and I are attempting to develop a general theory of social motivation that captures the distinction between sin and sickness (see Weiner, 1993b). When formulating general laws, there must be a search for what is common across domains and an ignoring of the unique factors that enhance predictions of any particular phenomenon. Thus, my attention is confined to perceptions of responsibility and the antecedents and consequences of this inference.

Let me, then, examine in detail the responsibility-related work of Bradbury, Fincham, and their associates. Much that is written in the next few pages is directly extracted from their work and writings; there is little I can add to their thorough analysis other than to bring their thoughts and research to the attention of the readers of this book who may be unaware of this body of work and to show how it fits within a larger theoretical context.

Research on marital distress, although having a short history, already has progressed through various phases (see review in Bradbury & Fincham, 1990). Initially, many survey studies were conducted by sociologists examining the correlates of marital satisfaction, particularly demographic, personality, and family structure variables. The focus then shifted to research concerning the overt behavior of couples engaged in some sort of conflict-related conduct in a laboratory setting. These investigations revealed the comparatively poor problem-solving strategies, the high rates of negative behavior and reciprocated negative behavior, and the rigidity that couples in marital disharmony exhibit. More recently, these behavioral studies became supplemented (or perhaps even supplanted) with an attempt to address the affective and cognitive components of marital interaction. This broad concern gave rise to the study of causal attributions that spouses make for the events in their marriage.

## Hypotheses and Empirical Research

The basic quest in the empirical studies is relatively straightforward—determining if there is an association between reported marital satisfaction and attributions for the causes of positive and negative marital events. Bradbury and Fincham (1990) report the following about the interconnection between behavioral and cognitive approaches to the study of marital satisfaction:

> The common tendency in distressed marriages for a negative behavior of one spouse ("You really should be more pleasant around my parents") to be followed by a negative behavior by the partner ("Don't tell me how to behave") may be due to the attribution that the partner makes for the couple's behavior ("He bosses me around because he doesn't care about me or my feelings"). (p. 4)

Specifically, it has been hypothesized that dissatisfied spouses, compared to spouses satisfied in their marriage, offer explanations for negative partner behavior that hold the partner responsible and offer attributions for positive behavior that do not implicate the positive, intentional role of the partner. As Bradbury and Fincham (1992) illustrate for negative and positive events:

> A happily married wife might ascribe her husband's lack of interest in sex to pressures on him at work, whereas a distressed wife might attribute this same behavior to her husband's lack of love for her. Moreover, a satisfied husband might attribute an unexpected gift from his wife to her wanting to do something special for him, while a dissatisfied husband might view the same act as an attempt on her part to justify spending money on herself. (p. 613)

The attributions made in a marriage typically are studied by presenting a spouse with a real or a hypothetical marital event and then ascertaining opinions about the causes of that event. Often various properties or dimensions of that cause are assessed, including locus (whether the cause is internal or external to the spouse), the endurance of the cause over time, and causal generality across situations. In addition, ratings of responsibility of the partner and blame also are ascertained. Two other issues are addressed that will be briefly considered a few pages later, namely, (1) ascertaining whether the attributions for marital problems cause marital distress (as opposed to marital distress giving rise to beliefs about spousal causality) and (2) examining the sequential ordering of the concepts of causation, responsibility, blame, and marital distress.

The following research investigation is illustrative of the type of studies that have been conducted. Bradbury and Fincham (1992) first recruited couples from all walks of life to participate in their research. The couples initially were given a measure of marital satisfaction and classified as satisfied or dissatisfied. The spouses then were separated and asked to reveal the extent to which they experienced a number of common marital problems. They also revealed their causal attributions and inferences about responsibility for these problems. The participating couples were then reunited and instructed to "try and work toward a mutually agreeable solution" to an issue that they both had identified as a problem. The conversation was tape recorded and scores on a variety of behavioral indexes related to problem solving (e.g., mutual concern displayed, number of problem solutions offered, etc.) were determined.

The data documented an oft-confirmed finding—namely, that poorer problem-solving skills were demonstrated by the maritally distressed than by the satisfied couples. In addition, higher levels of distress related to perceptions of spousal responsibility, or the tendency to perceive the partner as blameworthy and as behaving intentionally in regard to this problem. Finally, problem-solving deficiencies were associated with causal perceptions (which include ascriptions of the problem to the spouse) as well as with inferences concerning partner responsibility.

Reviewing a vast literature that includes causal assessment regarding both positive and negative marital events, Bradbury and Fincham (1990) concluded:

> It would appear that an association exists between marital dissatisfaction and the tendency to view positive partner behaviors as . . . less positive in intent, motivated by selfish concerns, and less worthy of praise. . . . Evidence also emerges for an association between marital dissatisfaction and ascribing negative events to the partner and . . . a tendency to infer more . . . negative intent for negative relationship events. (pp. 13–14)

## Is the Relation between Responsibility and Marital Dissatisfaction Causal?

As reviewed above, there is an association between attributional thinking and marital happiness. But do cognitions determine the goodness of the relationship, or does the goodness of the relationship determine how the spouse is perceived? Research also has examined this question.

To supply an answer, longitudinal studies have been conducted with the measurement of variables at two or more points in time. For example, Fincham and Bradbury (1987) examined the association between causal beliefs and marital satisfaction in 34 couples, with measurements taken twice, one year apart. The researchers reported that wives' relative distress was greater at Time 2 to the extent that they made unfavorable responsibility attributions for their husbands' behavior at Time 1 (see also Fincham & Bradbury, 1993). After reviewing numerous research investigations, Bradbury and Fincham (1990) concluded: "The findings of the experimental and longitudinal investigations reviewed here are consistent with the pervasive assumption that attributions exert a causal influence on judgments of relationship quality" (p. 22).

If it is indeed the case that cognitive inferences in regard to causality and responsibility determine relationship satisfaction, then it follows that interventions may be possible that improve marriages by altering inferences about responsibility. This is conceptually identical to EE research in which families are taught that schizophrenic behavioral patterns do not signal sin, or intentional misbehavior.

Some findings supporting the efficacy of intervention have been reported. For example, Margolin and Weiss (1978) gave marital counseling in part to help spouses "abandon blaming attributions, accept greater personal responsibility for relationship failure, and to be more accepting of their partners' positive efforts" (p. 1485). Following the training period, the marital satisfaction for the group receiving this treatment increased. However, according to Bradbury and Fincham (1990), the intervention studies thus far have yielded mixed results, and very few have been undertaken. Hence, this remains a direction for future research.

## The Temporal Sequence Issue

It already has been reported that Fincham and his colleagues have proposed that there are three general classes of attributions of significance in marriage: causality, responsibility, and blame. Furthermore, these are represented in a sequential order so that the presence of blame presupposes that there will be an attribution of responsibility, just as an attribution of responsibility presupposes that there will be an attribution of personal causality. And also as already indicated, much within this set of presumptions has been incorporated into my thinking.

One test of this sequential process, and its relation to marital distress, was reported by Lussier, Sabourin, and Wright (1993). These investigators were able to enlist the aid of 206 couples. The couples reported their marital satisfaction or adjustment, causal attributions for general marital conflict (e.g., "Conflicts in our relationship are due to the things my partner says or does), responsibility (e.g., "I hold my partner responsible for the conflicts that occur between us"), and blame (e.g., "My partner is to blame for the conflicts that occur between us"). Path analyses were then employed to ascertain the relation between these variables and marital satisfaction.

The pertinent data for husbands and wives (the female data are in parentheses) are shown in Figure 5.5. Figure 5.5 reveals strong relations between causality and responsibility (average $r = .55$), responsibility and blame (average $r = .74$), and blame and marital happiness (average $r = -.39$). Furthermore, marital happiness is directly related only to blame, not to causal beliefs or inferences about responsibility. From my perspective, inasmuch as blame includes the affective response of anger, these data also provide supporting evidence for the causality → responsibility → anger → action sequence that has been proposed throughout this book. Indeed, the relation between responsibility and blame is so high as to strongly suggest that these are not independent constructs. Recall that it has been contended that blame is a blend of both inferences of responsibility and negative effect.

In sum, the investigation reported by Lussier et al. (1993) provides

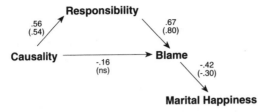

FIGURE 5.5. Path model relating perceptions of causality for a negative event, responsibility inferences, and blame to marital happiness. From Lussier, Sabourin, and Wright (1993). Copyright 1993 by the American Psychological Association. Reprinted by permission.

substantial support for the responsibility approach to social motivation, although there are few studies that have examined the applicability of the entire sin–sickness theory to marital distress. Again, this obviously is a direction that I would hope emerges in future research.

## GENERAL SUMMARY OF STIGMATIZATION

The prior three chapters have considered an array of stigmas: in Chapter 3, alcoholism, obesity, and poverty; in Chapter 4, AIDS and homosexuality; and in Chapter 5, depression and schizophrenia. In addition, many stigmas have been commented upon in less detail, including heart problems, cancer, and others. And in later chapters additional stigmas will be the topic of discussion, particularly poverty (again) and those who abuse children and spouses. Hence, reactions to the stigmatized certainly play a central role in the present understanding of social motivation. This is in part because perception of others, or social perception, and action related to those others, or social motivation, are joined or interconnected.

The research related to these diverse stigmas is distinct and unique, with each stigma yielding a different set of observations. For example, in this book I have reported research concerning employment discrimination against the obese, criminal sentencing when the offender was drunk while committing the offense, the attitudes of conservatives toward the poor, medical care toward those with AIDS, "gay bashing," reactions to sadness, the family atmosphere of the schizophrenic, etc. Yet this array of facts is subject to relatively simple understanding and interpretation: Others are judged as responsible or as not responsible for their plights, that is, they are sinners or sick (see Weiner, 1993b). This inference gives rise respectively to anger or sympathy, which then generates negative or positive interpersonal reactions. Hence, if obesity is due to overeating, if AIDS was contracted by promiscuous sex, if the schizophrenic person is perceived as being obstinate, and if the spouse intended the negative act, then there will be retribution to gain social justice and to dispense "just deserts." On the other hand, if obesity is due to a thyroid problem, if the virus associated with AIDS was spread with contaminated blood, if the schizophrenic person was "born that way," and if the spouse did not do the negative act "on purpose," then the reactions of others will be positive or at least not antagonistic. In the last four examples, either there was impersonal causality, the cause was not controllable, or circumstances were mitigating, so that the stigmatized individual was not held responsible. Affective reactions are then either sympathy, or there is a reduction of anger.

Of course, each particular stigma is associated with a unique set of issues, determinants, and reactions. But over and above this specificity is the general lawful sequence of causal thinking → inference of responsibility → emotional response → action.

When the reactions of the family influence the course of the illness or problem, as is the case for depression, schizophrenia, and marital distress, then causal inferences and their consequences are of special importance. In the family, episodes of anger, rejection and avoidance are repeated over and over, so that they extract a toll on the recipient of these communications. Because of this practical importance, it is essential to provide conceptual analyses of the involved processes, for these theories can then direct intervention. Family interventions for depression, schizophrenia, and fragile marriages have been undertaken but are not well guided by general theory. I hope these chapters have provided some guidelines to redress this shortcoming.

# 6

---

# Helping Behavior

I'm one of the undeserving poor; that's what I am. Think of what that
means to a man. It means that he's up agen middle class morality all
the time. If there's anything going, and I put in for a bit of it, it's
always the same story: "You're undeserving; so you can't have it." But
my needs is as great as the most deserving widow's that ever got
money out of six different charities in one week for the death of the
same husband.

—George Bernard Shaw, *Pygmalion* (Act Two)

The study of social motivation embraces many topics. Surely included are
affiliative needs; group behavior; a variety of relationships that involve
interpersonal power, including dominance, submission, and dependence;
and so on. But at the very heart of the domain of social motivation are
helping behavior—going toward others to administer aid and support—
and aggression—going against others to "eliminate" them by imposing
something negative or withholding something positive. Help and aggression, which are likely to alter one's own "survival fitness," form the back-
bone of evolutionary approaches to social conduct.

In the following two chapters, I turn to these opposing aspects of
social behavior. If a theory of social motivation is to have validity and
generality, then it must address helping and aggression, using the same
principles and concepts to explain these contrasting actions. I will first
consider help giving, inasmuch as there is growing evidence documenting
the role of perceived responsibility as a determinant of helping behavior.
Furthermore, the research that has been undertaken from this perspective

has systematically progressed, so that it now fully incorporates the conceptual analysis that has been presented in this book. Because much of this research has been theory driven, it has provided not only a testing ground for the theory but also the opportunity for theoretical alteration. In addition, some researchers have been able to apply the conceptual understanding of help giving to public policy issues, as will be examined later in the chapter, thus documenting the important role of theory construction in applied contexts.

The determinants of help giving, as is the case for the continuation of depression, the reoccurrence of the symptoms of schizophrenia, and the decision to divorce, are too numerous to list. The kinship relationship between the helper and the help receiver, their mutual liking, the number of others available to help, the severity of the need for aid, the mores of the culture, and personal costs and benefits are just some of the many determinants of help and neglect, with the particular circumstances or situation likely to make one or another of these antecedents primary in influencing behavior. For example, one may aid one's mother regardless of many other possible inhibitors of this behavior, while agreeing to help another fix a flat tire may greatly depend on how busy the person is at the time when asked and may depend on what he or she is wearing. In the present context, the multitude of determinants of help are neglected and one variable and its emotional consequences are focused upon: perceptions of responsibility for the need and the affects of anger and sympathy. This approach reflects my belief that a theoretical psychologist should not focus on a theory for a specific motivational domain, such as a theory of achievement or aggression or helping, for it is not possible to construct such a theory with any hope of capturing the many determinants of action. Rather, it may be more fruitful for conceptual advancement to take one mechanism or process and examine how it contributes to a variety of psychological domains, where each domain also is associated with other variables (some unique) that contribute to the behavior in question.

Perhaps more than any other area within the field of social motivation, investigators also have documented that emotions play an important motivational role in helping behavior (see review in Carlson & Miller, 1987). For example, it has been suggested that helping behavior is mediated by the emotions of discomfort, distress, empathy, gratitude, guilt, and yet others. Again, in any given situation one or the other of these may account for help giving. In the present context, the multitude of affective determinants of help giving also are neglected, while, as indicated, two emotions that are important in other domains of social motivation assume central importance—namely, anger and sympathy (the latter is used interchangeably with pity, although, as I have suggested, there are very valid reasons to differentiate between sympathy and pity). As already indicated, it is not presumed here that perceptions of responsibility and the affects that this elicits are involved in all situations in which help is given or withheld. However, the role of causal beliefs and the associated emotions of anger and sympathy may be more relevant than has been recognized.

Consider, for example, a well-known experiment conducted by Langer, Blank, and Chanowitz (1978) that typically is discussed under the rubric of compliance, but also can be considered as illustrating "passive" helping. Langer et al. (1978) had an experimental confederate approach a person who was about to use a copying machine and ask for permission to use the machine first. In one condition, the requester said: "Excuse me, I have 5 pages. May I use the Xerox machine?" In a second, so-called placebic information condition, the requester asked: "Excuse me, I have 5 pages. May I use the Xerox machine because I have to make copies?" Langer et al. (1978) contend that these two conditions are identical because "what else would one do with a copying machine except to make copies of something?" (p. 48). However, there was greater compliance (or passive helping) in the placebic information than in the request-only condition. This suggested to Langer et al. (1978) that when an event is not important, individuals may be unaware of the information provided by others and behave "mindlessly." This implies that causal attributions, inferences of responsibility, and affects will play little role in help giving in many life situations.

Folkes (1985) then examined the Langer et al. proposition by varying the information communicated to the potential "helper." In this investigation, the communicated messages differed in the controllability of the cause for wanting to get to the front of the Xerox line. In the controllable condition, subjects stated: "I don't want to wait" or "I want to go see my boyfriend." Conversely, in the uncontrollable condition the confederate explained by adding the clause, "because I feel really sick." In four studies, Folkes (1985) found less help (compliance) in the controllable than in the uncontrollable causal condition. Behavior in this context, then, is not as mindless as Langer et al. (1978) would have us believe. Ratings of responsibility and affective reactions were not assessed, but I do think they would be the mediating variables in this context.

## HELP FOR THE STIGMATIZED

Helping behavior and the influence of perceptions of controllability and responsibility were already examined in this book when I considered reactions to the stigmatized. Let me review some of these findings briefly, for they obviously are pertinent to this chapter. In Chapter 3, I presented an investigation by Weiner et al. (1988), and asked the reader to complete a similar experiment, in which ten stigmas (e.g., AIDS, Alzheimer's disease, blindness, cancer) were rated according to perceptions of responsibility for the stigma, anger and sympathy toward persons with this problem, and the tendency to give personal aid as well as to advocate welfare for these individuals. As shown in Tables 3.2–3.4, higher responsibility for a stigma was associated with greater anger and reduced helping, whereas low responsibility was related to heightened sympathy and increased judgments to help. In Chapter 4, it was revealed in greater detail that when HIV infection is ascribed to a blood transfusion (an uncontrollable cause) as opposed to the more prevalent, controllable causes of sexual activity and drug use, then prosocial responses are increased. And as reviewed in Chapter 5, there is a tendency for individuals to withhold social support from the depressed, in part because they are perceived as personally responsible for their problems.

But in the context of judgments of responsibility and affective reactions the most detailed analysis of help giving was presented when I considered reactions to poverty. The data from the reviewed research are depicted in Figure 3.4 and will be returned to in detail later in the chapter. It is evident from Figure 3.4 that beliefs about responsibility and affective reactions mediate between the need for aid and help-giving judgments.

My intent in this very cursory review is to have the reader recall that helping behavior has been examined in many prior places in the book and that a theoretical sequence has proved fruitful that includes need for help → causal attribution → judgment of causal controllability → responsibility inference → anger and sympathy → social conduct. In this chapter, other contexts in which this is the case, and a closer theoretical examination of the data, are of main concern.

## MODELS OF HELPING BEHAVIOR

In Chapter 1, it was contended that the responsibility process is set in motion by an event in need of explanation. If there is a perception of personal causality, then it is determined if the cause was or was not controllable. In the absence of mitigating circumstances, controllable causality gives rise to an inference of responsibility. However, it also was acknowledged that at times inferences of responsibility precede judgments of personal controllability (which is merely skipped over) and that the salience of mitigating circumstances (e.g., the wrongdoer is an infant) may make the gathering of information pertinent to controllable causality of little importance. Thus, the process (sequence) leading to inferences of responsibility is not invariant across situations.

In a similar manner, throughout this book a particular motivational sequence has been advocated: The assignment or nonassignment of responsibility generates the affects of anger or pity, respectively, and these feelings determine social conduct. Hence, a thinking–feeling–acting sequence is postulated, with thinking the distal determinant of action and feelings proximal.

But here again, it would be foolhardy and unnecessarily rigid (as well as incorrect!) to presume that this is an invariant order. There are, of course, bidirectional relations; it is known, for example, that feeling states influence what one thinks and that what one does alters feelings. And of greater importance in the present context, there intuitively seem to be instances in which thoughts, rather than emotions, directly affect action, or together with emotions determine what one does. This possibility was not acknowledged in earlier chapters in order not to introduce too much complexity at an early stage.

Indeed, many different motivational processes that include thinking, feeling, and action are possible. A few of these are depicted in Figure 6.1. Model 1 in Figure 6.1 repeats what has been advocated thus far. In Model 2 thoughts directly as well as indirectly influence action. Then Model 3 adds a relation between anger and sympathy (pity)—perhaps these affects are mutually inhibitory or hedonically incompatible. Model 4 includes both a direct influence of thoughts to action as well as a relation between the two affects. And finally, in Model 5 the eliciting stimulus itself affects the behavioral response. For example, it may be that a failing student elicits more help than a drowning person because less personal cost is involved. Or a teacher may help an "unworthy" student because it is part of his or her role. Of course, these are only some models that may be postulated (for a more complete discussion of these models, see Reisenzein, 1986).

Thus far in this book, I have not undertaken a comparison of the validity of these models of social conduct in part because there has not been a sufficient collection of data to allow a pertinent analysis of the relative merits of the different conceptual models. Indeed, the vast majority of investigations have merely examined affective or behavioral reactions to various events, states, or plights that could be considered under or not under the personal control of the individual involved (i.e., the person was or was not responsible for the condition). However, there are a sufficient number of studies of help giving from a responsibility–affect mediational perspective that enable comparisons between the various models, and this issue is addressed (but surely not fully resolved) in this chapter.

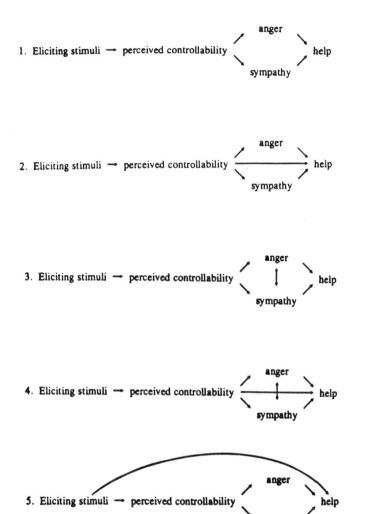

**FIGURE 6.1.** Various models of helping behavior relating the eliciting stimulus, responsibility inference, and affective reactions to help giving.

## AN EXPERIMENTAL DEMONSTRATION

Prior to continuing with the reading, it is again time for you to take part in an experiment and engage in "experiential learning." In this case, the investigation involves help giving in an achievement context. In Experiment 6.1, two vignettes, or two experimental conditions, are created. In both, a student asks to borrow your class notes (for some of the readers, there will have to be a return—I hesitate to say a regression—to an earlier stage of career development). Beliefs about the controllability of the cause of the need, affective reactions of anger and sympathy, and behavioral reactions are asked for (responsibility is not assessed since this was not done in prior research using this paradigm). Obviously, the data will enable us to examine the relations between thinking (causal controllability and, by implication, personal responsibility), feeling, and doing. As will be evident, the two vignettes provide different causes for the need of the notes. It will not be difficult to discern what is being varied between the vignettes. You should try to put yourself in this situation and reveal as truthfully as possible how you might feel and what you might do were this a real situation rather than a role-playing enactment. Please do this now.

The results of Experiment 6.1 will be returned to later in the chapter. First, I turn to some early studies of help giving, examining them from a perspective of responsibility. The reader is warned that in contrast to the prior discussions in the book, in this chapter specific research investigations are examined in detail to determine, on the one hand, if there is support or disconfirmation of the general conceptual framework advocated and, on the other hand, to select which of the various models outlined in Figure 6.1 best captures the data. The chapter thus has a "tone" or "flavor" different from the prior chapters in the book and is necessarily redundant (but not unpleasantly so) with studies reporting similar findings.

## PERTINENT EARLY STUDIES OF HELP GIVING

A few early studies that were concerned with the determinants of help giving included the responsibility of the needy individual as a manipulated factor, although the experimenters were not necessarily aware that this factor was being varied (as first pointed out by Ickes & Kidd, 1976; see also Barnes, Ickes, & Kidd, 1979). Therefore, the interpretations of this research were not couched within a framework of responsibility. Two of the experiments (Berkowitz, 1969; Schopler & Matthews, 1965) in part varied the presence or absence of personal agency as the cause of the need for help. These investigators were interested in the effects of locus of causality on helping—that is, whether the cause of the need was internal or external to the needy individual. However, since personal agency has been suggested to be the first differentiation in the responsibility process, the manipulation of causal locus is confounded with (produces) a variation in perceptions of personal responsibility.

Schopler and Matthews (1965) conducted the first of the two locus

## EXPERIMENT 6.1
## Helping in an Achievement Context

The following stories concern a student's attempt to borrow your class notes. In each instance the story will describe this event and indicate why he is seeking help. Afterwards you will be asked to relate your thoughts and feelings about the person involved and what you might do.

> At about 1:00 in the afternoon you are walking through campus and a student comes up to you. He says that you do not know him but that you are both enrolled in the same class, where he happened to notice you. He asks if you would lend him the notes from the classes last week. He indicates that he needs the notes because he was having difficulty with his eyes; a change in glasses was required, and during the week he had difficulty seeing because of eyedrops and other treatments. You note that he is wearing a patch over one eye.

Please answer the following questions about the incident:

1. How much anger and annoyance do you feel toward this person?

| 1 | 2 | 3 | 4 | 5 | 6 | 7 |
|---|---|---|---|---|---|---|

A great deal of anger and annoyance           No anger and annoyance

2. How much sympathy do you have for this person?

| 1 | 2 | 3 | 4 | 5 | 6 | 7 |
|---|---|---|---|---|---|---|

A great deal of sympathy           No sympathy

3. How likely is it that you would lend your class notes to this person?

| 1 | 2 | 3 | 4 | 5 | 6 | 7 |
|---|---|---|---|---|---|---|

Definitely *would* lend the notes           Definitely would *not* lend the notes

4. How controllable is this person's reason for not taking notes? That is, is the reason that he does not have the notes subject to personal influence? One might think that he should have been able to control the amount that he was affected by the problem.

| 1 | 2 | 3 | 4 | 5 | 6 | 7 |
|---|---|---|---|---|---|---|

Under personal control           Not under personal control

At about 1:00 in the afternoon you are walking through campus and a student comes up to you. He says that you do not know him but that you are both enrolled in the same class, where he happened to notice you. He asks if you would lend him the notes from the classes last week. He indicates that he needs the notes because he skipped class to go to the beach and "take it easy."

Please answer the following questions about the incident.

1. How much anger and annoyance do you feel toward the person?

| 1 | 2 | 3 | 4 | 5 | 6 | 7 |
|---|---|---|---|---|---|---|

A great deal of anger and annoyance      No anger or annoyance

2. How much sympathy do you have for the person?

| 1 | 2 | 3 | 4 | 5 | 6 | 7 |
|---|---|---|---|---|---|---|

A great deal of sympathy      No sympathy

3. How likely is it that you would lend your class notes to this person?

| 1 | 2 | 3 | 4 | 5 | 6 | 7 |
|---|---|---|---|---|---|---|

Definitely *would* lend the notes      Definitely would *not* lend the notes

4. How controllable is this person's reason for not taking notes? That is, is the reason that he does not have the notes subject to personal influence? Are such distractions as going to the beach under personal control?

| 1 | 2 | 3 | 4 | 5 | 6 | 7 |
|---|---|---|---|---|---|---|

Under personal control      Not under personal control

studies related to helping. In these studies, subjects were led to believe that they were paired with another participant, with the "true" subject designated as the "director" of the other (who was, in fact, nonexistent). The task was to complete crossword puzzles, and the second (fraudulent) subject was dependent on the director for the receipt of needed letter clues. In the external locus condition, it was communicated that this second participant had no choice but to ask the director for these letters. This impeded the director's own performance. In the internal condition, it was made known that the second subject had a choice to receive letters or to make this request of the director and the subject selected the latter alternative. The data revealed that the director-designated subjects gave more letters in the external (no choice) rather than in the internal (choice) condition. Schopler and Matthews (1965) explain:

> Perception of the locus of the partner's dependence seems clearly to relate to the extent of help that he can obtain. If the partner is seen as a victim of circumstance, he will be helped more than if he is seen as being dependent on his own . . . The criminal who is seen as a victim of circumstances is more likely to elicit sympathetic, helping responses than one who is judged to have voluntarily committed the deviant act. (pp. 611–612)

It is evident that the alleged subject who freely chooses to be dependent on the director will be perceived as more responsible for this imposition (rather than for the need itself) than the subject who is forced to be dependent. However, in this investigation not only were locus and responsibility not disentangled, but there was another confounding in that helping hurt the lender.

In the second pertinent study that apparently manipulated the locus of causality of a need (or a behavior), Berkowitz (1969) also led subjects to believe that they were supervising others. To avoid the shortcoming in the study by Schopler and Matthews (1965), the alleged supervisor was not eligible for rewards given for task completion. One of the supposed workers at the task then asked the supervisor for help, either because "the experimenter gave me the wrong paper" or because "I took it sort of easy." Helping was observed to be greater in the external than in the internal causation condition. Obviously, from the perspective of this book, this manipulation also blends internal causality with personal responsibility— as indicated many times, particularly in Chapter 2, lack of effort is the prototypical antecedent for inferences of responsibility.

A third early experiment related to a responsibility analysis of helping was conducted by Piliavin, Rodin, and Piliavin (1969). These investigators left the laboratory and examined help giving in a real life context. A confederate fell to the floor on the subway while other experimenters observed the spontaneous tendencies of the riders to help the victim. In one condition, "the victim smelled of liquor and carried a liquor bottle wrapped tightly in a brown bag," while in a second condition the victim "carried a black cane" (p. 219). Piliavin et al. (1969) state that "it was assumed that people who are regarded as partly responsible for their plight would receive less sympathy and consequently less help than people seen as not responsible for their circumstance" (p. 290). While Piliavin et al. (1969) merely "assumed" this, we know from the reviews in the prior chapters that an ill person is perceived as less responsible for his or her plight and receives more sympathy than an individual who is drunk (see also Weiner, 1980a).

In part guided by this responsibility–affect analysis, Piliavin et al. (1969) predicted that persons carrying the cane would be helped more than the drunk individuals. However, they did not emphasize this intervening process and instead offered other reasons for their predictions, focusing on the greater costs (e.g., potential violence) involved in helping a drunk person. The data strongly supported the hypothesis: The victim with the cane received help on about 95% of the occasions in which he fell. On the other hand, the drunk was only helped approximately half the times that he fell. Furthermore, the aid was given sooner to the cane-carrying victims.

## Planned Manipulations of Responsibility

The initial investigation that purposively manipulated individual responsibility for a need state was conducted by Barnes et al. (1979), although they labeled their manipulated variable "intentionality," which I recognize as one determinant of responsibility. Barnes et al. (1979) had experimenters pretend to be classmates of other students whom they called to borrow class notes. Hence, like Piliavin et al. (1969), these investigators left the laboratory setting. In what was considered the unintentional condition, the experimenter said, "I just don't seem to have the ability to take good notes. I really try, but I just can't do it." In an intentional condition, the confederate said: "I just don't seem to have the motivation to take good notes. I really can take good notes, but just don't try" (p. 369). Recall from Chapter 2 that lack of ability as a cause of achievement failure (or need) absolves the person from responsibility because low ability is construed as uncontrollable, whereas lack of effort as a cause of a need results in a person's being held responsible because trying is subject to volitional alteration.

Barnes et al. (1979) report that there was a much higher rate of agreement to help the needy student in the low-ability rather than the lack-of-effort condition. The experimenters also note that both ability and effort are internal to the needy person, so that the locus explanation of help provided by Schopler and Matthews (1965) and Berkowitz (1969) can be more correctly incorporated within an interpretation that is based on the concept of intentionality (or, more appropriately, responsibility).

## Summary of Initial Research

On the basis of the results of the four experiments just reviewed (in chronological order: Schopler & Matthews, 1965; Berkowitz, 1969; Piliavin et al., 1969; Barnes et al., 1979), it can prudently be suggested that perceptions of responsibility for a need influence the decision of the potential help provider. These experimenters manipulated and/or measured locus, controllability, and intentionality—all considered determinants of responsibility. Two of these studies took place within a laboratory setting, and two examined reactions in real-life contexts, but all did involve actual behavioral observations. Although the results of each individual experiment perhaps can be accounted for without making use of the concept of responsibility, a responsibility perspective appears to be the only one that can incorporate the data from all of these diverse manipulations.

In none of the studies, however, was there an assessment of perceptions of responsibility. In addition, affects were unmeasured and, for the most part, ignored. The next phase of this research history, to which I now turn, was consciously guided by the belief that perceptions of responsibility and the affects elicited by this appraisal play key roles in help giving (although again responsibility often was not assessed).

## INVESTIGATIONS ASSESSING RESPONSIBILITY AND EMOTIONS

Many of the research investigations that include the assessment of controllability and/or responsibility as well as the emotional consequences of these appraisals are similar to Experiment 6.1, already performed by the reader. Let us therefore return to this experiment before examining the pertinent empirical literature.

In Experiment 6.1, two vignettes were created that depicted a student in need of class notes. In one of these vignettes, the student had "difficulty with his eyes." In the second vignette, the notes were not taken because the student "went to the beach." From the many prior discussions it should be evident that "going to the beach" is subject to volitional control and is causally equivalent to lack of effort. On the other hand, eye problems, just as other stigmatizing physical conditions, are expected to be perceived as not subject to volitional alteration. The person needing the notes because of going to the beach therefore would be responsible for his plight, whereas this is not the case with eye problems. (Recall that, to be consistent with prior research, control rather than responsibility was measured. However, in this context, where mitigating information is not given, control and responsibility can be taken as nearly comparable concepts.)

Inasmuch as responsibility has been hypothesized as giving rise to anger, and lack of responsibility for a need as giving rise to pity, it follows that anger should be directed at the student who went to the beach, whereas sympathy will be expressed for the student who had eye problems. Furthermore, since anger is believed to initiate antisocial responses, the person needing notes because he went to the beach is expected to elicit neglect. Conversely, sympathy evokes altruistic behavior, so that a positive response to the student with eye problems is anticipated. It is therefore hypothesized that the data will fall into two patterns or groupings of responses:

1. No notes because of going to the beach; controllability/responsibility; anger, no sympathy; no help
2. No notes because of eye problems; uncontrollability/nonresponsibility; no anger, sympathy; help

You might now compare your ratings for these two conditions and determine if the patterns outlined above are displayed. I am confident that this will indeed be the case. But these are only groupings of associations; without a more sophisticated statistical treatment of data from many respondents, temporal sequences cannot be proven.

I next consider a succession of investigations that directly tested whether inferences of controllability (responsibility) and affective consequences mediate between the perceptions of a need and the willingness to provide help. These studies share a similar methodology: The situations are hypothetical rather than real, and in almost all of the investigations the dependent variables include the judgment or intent to help rather than their actual help giving, as was observed in some of the studies just reviewed (e.g., Berkowitz, 1969; Piliavin et al., 1969; etc.). The implicit position of the researchers is that "role-enactment strategies . . . can help us to spread a broad net, to generate hypotheses, and to build heuristic models of human social behavior" (Cooper, 1976, p. 609). One specific manner in which role methodologies allow for the building of heuristic models is that ratings of the relevant mediating variables, including inferences of controllability, responsibility, and affective reactions, can be readily obtained. This was not possible in the research, for example, conducted by Piliavin et al. (1969), where it would not be reasonable to obtain ratings of sympathy and anger among the passengers who watched the drunk or ill person fall. In addition, the researchers who have employed this methodology have used the situations crafted by Piliavin et al. (1969) and Barnes et al. (1979), where it is known what the actual behavioral responses were as a function of the experimental manipulations.

## The Partial Correlation Approach

The first series of studies to be examined are ones that I published (Weiner, 1980a, 1980b). These are the initial experiments testing the controllability (responsibility)–emotion mediational approach (along with the investigation by Meyer & Mulherin, 1980) and were the least sophisticated in terms of statistical treatment.

Weiner (1980a) reports on six experiments. To ascertain that there are affective reactions to the needy, in one study the situation created by Piliavin et al. (1969) was described. The subjects read each vignette and were told: "Try to assume that you actually are on the subway and try to imagine this scene. Describe your feelings in this situation" (Weiner, 1980a, p. 190). It was found that 27% of the affects directed toward the drunk person were negative, whereas this was the case for only 3% of the feelings regarding the ill person. On the other hand, 46% of the affects elicited by the ill individual were sympathy and concern, whereas these were expressed in only 30% of the reports concerning the drunk. Thus, in this free-response context the anticipated affects in the two scenarios were expressed.

In a subsequent investigation, these scenarios again were presented, but now the subjects rated the controllability of the cause of the need, their feelings of sympathy and concern, their emotions of disgust and distaste (the last two being the closest descriptive category for the negative affects expressed in the prior study), and their likelihood of providing help. Table 6.1 shows the correlations between these ratings. It is clear that the anticipated patterns are exhibited: Controllability correlates negatively with sympathy, positively with the unpleasant emotions, and negatively with intentions to help. In addition, sympathy correlates positively with help, whereas the negative affects were inversely associated with reports of help giving.

The next step in the statistical analysis is crucial to an examination of the ordering of the hypothesized mediating variables. If the sequence of the motivational variables is need → controllability (responsibility) → emotion → action and if emotion is partialled from (taken out of) the thinking–help relation, then that association should be greatly reduced. This is because

**TABLE 6.1.** Correlations between the Judgments of Control, Affect, and Help, Including Both the Drunk and Ill Conditions

| Variable | Control | Sympathy | Disgust | S-D | Help |
|---|---|---|---|---|---|
| Control | | −.77 | .55 | −.73 | −.37 |
| Sympathy (S) | | | −.64 | .90 | .46 |
| Disgust (D) | | | | −.91 | −.71 |
| S-D | | | | | .65 |
| Help | | | | | |

*Note.* From Weiner (1980a, p. 192). Copyright 1980a by the American Psychological Association. Reprinted by permission. All correlations are significant at $p < .01$.

emotion is presumed to bridge thinking and action. On the other hand, if controllability/responsibility is partialled from the emotion–action relation, then that association should not be altered. This is because it is presumed that thinking precedes feelings.

The partial correlations of these data are presented in Table 6.2. The top row of Table 6.2 merely repeats the correlations already given in Table 6.1 between both the controllability and the emotion ratings and the judgments of help giving. Column 2 in that table shows the correlations between controllability and help when each of the affects is partialled from that association. As can be seen, for example, the correlation of control with helping is only $r = -.02$ when sympathy is the partialled variable. On the other hand, when ratings of controllability are eliminated from the correlations between emotions and helping (see row 2), those associations are barely reduced (e.g., from $r = -.71$ to $r = -.66$ for the negative affect). This pattern of data strongly suggests that controllability is the distal, and affect the proximal, determinant of helping judgments (and, presumably, of actual helping behavior).

I then repeated these investigations (Weiner, 1980b), this time describing the settings created by Barnes et al. (1979) of a student wanting to borrow class notes. When asked to express their feelings toward individuals needing notes because "they went to the beach," 40% of the reports were negative, characterized as anger (which has been the anticipated negative emotion to responsibility, as opposed to disgust, which may be unique to the scenario with the drunk). This was the case in only 4% of the free-response affects directed toward the student who needed class notes because of eye problems. Conversely, only 6% of the affects toward the

**TABLE 6.2.** Correlation of Variables with Judgments of Helping, Including Both the Drunk and Ill Conditions, with Individual Variables Statistically Partialled from the Analysis

| Partialled variable | Dependent variable correlated with helping judgment | | |
| | Control | Sympathy | Disgust |
|---|---|---|---|
| None | −.37* | .46** | −.71*** |
| Control | — | .30 | −.66*** |
| Sympathy | −.02[a] | — | −.61*** |
| Disgust | .04 | .01 | — |

*Note.* From Weiner (1980a, p. 192). Copyright 1980a by the American Psychological Association. Reprinted by permission.
[a]Indicates the correlation between perceptions of control and helping ratings, with sympathy ratings partialled out.
*$p < .05$. **$p < .01$. ***$p < .001$.

student who went to the beach were sympathy and concern, whereas these emotions were expressed in 33% of the affective reactions elicited by the student with eye problems.

In a second investigation, these scenarios were described and perceptions of the controllability of the cause of the need, feelings of sympathy and anger, and intentions to help were ascertained. The correlations between these variables are shown in Table 6.3, which documents the usual patterns of high controllability, low sympathy, high anger, and lack of helping (and, therefore, low controllability, high sympathy, low anger, and intentions to help). Partial correlation analyses were then performed. Table 6.4 reveals that when sympathy and anger are taken from the correlation between control and helping ($r = -.40$), that correlation then drops to $r = -.10$. On the other hand, when perceptions of controllability are partialled from the correlations **between** sympathy and helping ($r = .59$) and anger and helping ($r = -.49$), then those associations are only weakly reduced to, respectively, $r = .48$ and $r = -.41$. Again, therefore, emotions are more proximal to helping than thoughts are.

## The Structural Equation Approach

The next set of investigations, represented by the research of Meyer and Mulherin (1980), Reisenzein (1986), Schmidt and Weiner (1988), Betancourt (1990a), Matsui and Matsuda (1989), Kojima (1992), and Dooley (1995), used very similar methods to the ones already introduced, with the introduction of some new helping settings, added variables, and alternative operational measures of the dependent variables. These researchers advanced the prior studies by employing path analytic or structural equation techniques. In these statistical treatments of the data, relations between variables are ascertained with all other pertinent variables held constant, which might be considered a series of simultaneous multiple regression or partial correlational analyses. Causal sequences, therefore, can be more

TABLE 6.3. Correlations between the Dependent Variables

| Variable | Sympathy | Anger | Lending |
|---|---|---|---|
| Control | −.54* | .36* | −.40* |
| Sympathy | | −.50* | .59* |
| Anger | | | −.49* |
| Lending | | | |

*Note.* From Weiner (1980b, p. 679). Copyright 1980b by the American Psychological Association. Reprinted by permission.
*$p < .001$.

**TABLE 6.4.** Correlations between Lending and Other Dependent Variables, Holding Control or Affect Constant

| Partialled variable | Dependent variable correlated with lending | | |
| | Control | Sympathy | Anger |
| --- | --- | --- | --- |
| None | −.40* | .59* | −.49* |
| Control | — | .48* | −.41* |
| Sympathy | −.12 | — | — |
| Anger | −.28* | | |
| Sympathy and Anger | −.10 | | |

*Note.* From Weiner (1980b, p. 680). Copyright 1980b by the American Psychological Association. Reprinted by permission.
*$p$ < .001.

meaningfully inferred. However, again either causal controllability or responsibility, but not both, was assessed.

As already indicated, the investigation by Meyer and Mulherin (1980) was undertaken about the same time as the ones by Weiner (1980a) and appeared in the same journal volume. Meyer and Mulherin also created hypothetical scenarios, in this case involving a request by an acquaintance to borrow money because the acquaintance was out of work. The causes of unemployment were varied: Some causes were internal and controllable (e.g., the needy person did not like to work or was laid off because of lack of effort on the job), while other causes were uncontrollable (e.g., the needy person could not work for health reasons or could not work because of high unemployment). For each of these causes (situations), subjects rated their presumed intensity of affective experience for 25 emotions as well as the likelihood of their helping this friend, assuming that they themselves had sufficient funds.

A factor analysis of the affective ratings yielded a bipolar factor labeled anger versus concern (which were treated as separate variables in the Weiner 1980a, 1980b studies). This factor loaded positively on affects including anger and irritation and loaded negatively on concern and sympathy. In addition, a second unipolar factor emerged that was labeled "empathy." This factor loaded on feelings, including troubled and miserable, that might have been experienced by the stimulus person, as well as on the emotions of pity and sympathy.

A path analysis that includes the scores on the two affective factors is depicted in Figure 6.2. In that figure, the values in parentheses are the correlations between the variables, while the values before the parentheses are the path coefficients, or the associations between the variables with all other variables held constant or partialled. Figure 6.2 reveals that percep-

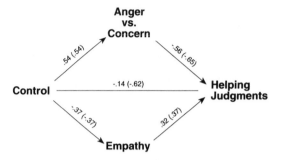

**FIGURE 6.2.** Simplified attributional model of helping behavior with results of path analysis. The correlations are in parentheses. From Meyer and Mulherin (1980, p. 207). Copyright 1980 by the American Psychological Association. Reprinted by permission.

tions of controllability relate positively with anger and negatively with empathy. Anger, in turn, is associated with lack of help, whereas empathy increases reports of help giving. Meyer and Mulherin (1980) note:

> Control is highly correlated with the two affective factors and . . . all three of these variables are correlated significantly with helping judgments. Thus, the control variable has both direct and indirect (through the affect scores) effects on helping judgments. . . . However, it is evident that the direct effects of emotion were greater than the direct effect of control . . . and that the indirect effect of control . . . was much larger than the direct effect. (p. 207)

These findings strongly support the general mediational hypothesis and are most consistent with Model 2 in Figure 6.1, which also includes a direct path from thinking to action. In addition, the data are quite systematic and consistent with the prior research, particularly that reported by Weiner (1980b), which provided additional evidence of a weak yet present association between perceptions of control and action when affects were partialled from this relation (see Table 6.4).

Reisenzein (1986) then continued this pursuit, again using hypothetical vignettes and assessing beliefs about causal controllability, the affects of anger and sympathy, and intentions to help. In distinction to Meyer and Mulherin (1980), the various models depicted in Figure 6.1 were tested and compared. In addition, structural modeling rather than path analysis was the measurement technique employed. Although this procedure is conceptually similar to path analysis, it has other positive aspects that need not be examined here, including the use of multiple indicators of each construct so that factor analysis also is incorporated within the procedure.

Reisenzein (1986) had subjects respond to both the subway scenario based on Piliavin et al. (1969) and the class notes scenario based on Barnes et al. (1979), which had respectively been used in Weiner (1980a, 1980b). The correlational data (for the subway scenario only) are displayed in Table 6.5, combined over the three indicators of each variable (e.g., controllability was measured with scales labeled "controllability," "responsibility," and "fault"; sympathy was measured with items labeled "sympathy," "pity," and "concern"; and so on). Table 6.5 displays the usual associations: controllability relates negatively with sympathy, positively with anger, negatively with help, and so on.

Structural equation analyses were then conducted (see Figure 6:3). Figure 6.3 reveals that Model 5 in Figure 6.1, which has no direct path from controllability to helping but does include a direct path from the situation to help giving, best accounts for the results. As shown in Figure 6.3, sympathy relates positively ($r = .36$) and anger negatively ($r = -.30$) to judgments of helping. In contrast to the findings reported by Meyer and Mulherin (1980), adding a path from controllability help did not increase the prediction of help giving.

The next study presented in this series was undertaken by Schmidt and Weiner (1988). I will not dwell on it, for it was a replication of the research already reviewed. One new variable was introduced: Prior to reading the class notes scenario, different experimental sets were introduced. Subjects were asked, for example, to be as objective as possible, or to imagine themselves as the recipient of this request. None of these instructional sets had any effects, so that the data were combined into one analysis that included almost 500 participants.

The structural equation data for the "lending class notes" vignette are shown in Figure 6.4. The best-fitting model exactly replicates the conclusions of Reisenzein (1986), supporting Model 5 in Figure 6.2, in which there is a direct path from the stimulus to helping, representing the determinants of help unrelated to perceptions of responsibility; a direct path

TABLE 6.5. Input Correlation Matrix for Subway Scenario

| | Control | Sympathy | Anger | Help |
|---|---|---|---|---|
| Control | | −.48 | .51 | −.44 |
| Sympathy | | | −.30 | .45 |
| Anger | | | | −.43 |
| Help | | | | |

*Note.* From Reisenzein (1986, p. 1128). Copyright 1986 by the American Psychological Association. Reprinted by permission. All correlations are significant at $p < .01$.

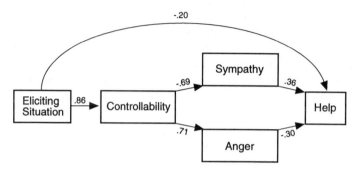

**FIGURE 6.3.** Simplified structural analysis of the determinants of help giving in the subway scenario. Data from Reisenzein (1986).

from affect to helping; and no direct connection between thinking and action.

Weiner and Graham (1989) then continued in this tradition but asked if the proposed linkages between cognitions, affects, and behavior are influenced by cognitive development. It could be, for example, that the hypothesized cognition–emotion linkages appear earlier (or later!) developmentally than do the relations between emotion and action.

To examine this issue, subjects were recruited who ranged in age from

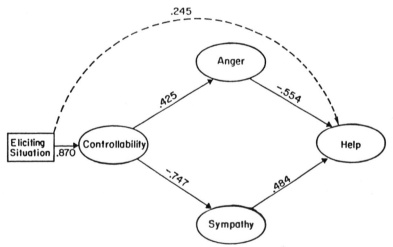

**FIGURE 6.4.** Structural model of helping, combining subjects in all conditions. From Schmidt and Weiner (1988, p. 618). Copyright 1988 by Sage Publications, Inc. Reprinted by permission.

5 to 95. Stories were designed that could elicit either pity or anger among all the respondents. For example, in one vignette the participants imagined that a neighbor had agreed to take care of their plants (or goldfish, for the children) but failed to keep this promise. The causal information revealed that the neighbor did not fulfill the agreement because she became ill (uncontrollable condition) or because she was busy and forgot all about it (controllable condition). Table 6.6 impressively shows the familiar pattern of correlations for all of the age groups—that is, control relates negatively with pity and help and positively with anger; whereas pity relates positively, and anger negatively, with help. Table 6.7 then gives the partial correlations between perceptions of control and judgments of help, with affective variables partialled from the association, and between affect and help, with controllability partialled. It is evident from Table 6.7 that when either the emotion of pity or anger is taken from the relation between controllability and help, that association dramatically decreases. On the other hand, when control is taken from the association between either of the affects and help giving, that relation remains quite substantial.

Finally, path analyses were performed for each age group. All the paths were virtually identical, going from cognition to affect to help giving; the average path between control and the emotions was $r = .62$, and the average path between emotions and help giving was $r = .45$. There was no direct association between thinking and acting. These findings were consistent across all ages, which is a rather dramatic result.

## Theoretical and Empirical Extensions

It was stated some pages ago that there are many, many determinants of helping and that I identify just one mediational process—namely, that of

**TABLE 6.6.** Correlations between Controllability, Affects of Pity and Anger, and Judgments of Help, within Each Age Group

|  | Age group | | | | | |
|---|---|---|---|---|---|---|
|  | 5–6 ($n = 42$) | 10–12 ($n = 39$) | 18–20 ($n = 119$) | 30–45 ($n = 70$) | 60–74 ($n = 55$) | 75–95 ($n = 45$) |
| Control × Pity | −.49 | −.58 | −.68 | −.67 | −.50 | −.43 |
| Control × Anger | .34 | .53 | .58 | .66 | .58 | .40 |
| Control × Help | −.30 | −.12 | −.19 | −.32 | −.40 | −.24 |
| Pity × Help | .51 | .25 | .27 | .41 | .43 | .43 |
| Anger × Help | −.58 | −.28 | −.33 | −.41 | −.51 | −.29 |

*Note.* From Weiner and Graham (1989, p. 416). Copyright 1989 by Lawrence Erlbaum Associates, Inc. Reprinted by permission.

TABLE 6.7. Zero-Order and Partial Correlations between Controllability, Affects of Pity and Anger, and Judgments of Help within Each Age Group

|  | Age group | | | | | |
|---|---|---|---|---|---|---|
|  | 5–6 ($n = 42$) | 10–12 ($n = 39$) | 18–20 ($n = 119$) | 30–45 ($n = 70$) | 60–74 ($n = 55$) | 75–95 ($n = 45$) |
| Control × Help[a] | −.30 | −.12 | −.19 | −.32 | −.40 | −.24 |
| Control × Help.P[b] | .07 | .04 | .00 | −.07 | −.24 | −.07 |
| Control × Help.A[c] | −.13 | .04 | .01 | −.08 | −.15 | −.14 |
| Pity × Help[a] | .51 | .25 | .27 | .41 | .43 | .43 |
| Pity × Help.C[d] | .44 | .22 | .20 | .28 | .29 | .37 |
| Anger × Help[a] | −.58 | −.28 | −.33 | −.41 | −.51 | −.29 |
| Anger × Help.C[e] | −.54 | −.26 | −.27 | −.27 | −.37 | −.22 |

*Note.* From Weiner and Graham (1989, p. 416). Copyright 1989 by Lawrence Erlbaum Associates, Inc. Reprinted by permission.
[a]Zero-order correlation.
[b]Partial *r* between control and help, holding pity constant.
[c]Partial *r* between control and help, holding anger constant.
[d]Partial *r* between pity and help, holding control constant.
[e]Partial *r* between anger and help, holding control constant.

controllability (and, by implication, responsibility) followed by emotion. Betancourt (1990a) points out, however, that this narrow focus leads to an overfragmentation of the approaches to helping. He argues instead that various determinants of action should be integrated within one conceptual structure.

In his attempt to combine theoretical perspectives, Betancourt proposed that the empathy approach advocated by Batson and his colleagues (e.g., Batson, Duncan, Ackerman, Buckley, & Birch, 1981) could be integrated within the attributional conception. This approach focuses on the capacity of the lender to vicariously experience what the needy person is feeling. Thus, an empathic perspective is conceived by Betancourt (1990a) as an "observational set characterized by a concern for another person's situation" (p. 575). Betancourt (1990a) reasoned that

> subjects who are given an uncontrollable cause are likely to experience more pity than those given a controllable cause, just as those adopting an empathic set are likely to experience more interpersonal feelings, such as sympathy and compassion, than those not taking the empathic perspective. (p. 576)

Hence, the attributional and the empathy viewpoints have conceptual overlap in that each is anticipated to influence help-related emotions.

Betancourt then offered the following model of help giving (see Figure 6.5). Figure 6.5 reveals that both ascriptions (A) for a person's need and perspective (P) influence perceptions of causal controllability (C). Specifically, it was hypothesized that taking an empathic perspective will tend to result in the perception of causes as uncontrollable. In addition, an empathic perspective as well as perceptions of uncontrollability are anticipated to increase feelings of sympathy and pity (EE, or empathic emotions). Finally, ascriptions of uncontrollability as well as sympathy and pity are predicted to augment help giving (H). Thus, Betancourt (1990a) is an advocate of Model 2 in Figure 6.2 inasmuch as causal thoughts are both indirectly and directly linked to behavior.

Two experiments were conducted to test the model shown in Figure 6.5. In each investigation, an empathic set was induced by asking subjects to take the perspective of the person in need of help and to "imagine how the person feels about what has happened" Betancourt (1990a) expanded this instruction so that it had a greater effect than a similar approach used in Schmidt and Weiner (1988). Subjects then read one of the five stories that varied the controllability of the need for academic help (ranging from going out of town with friends for fun, the most controllable cause, to having an accident that resulted in hospitalization and an inability to read, the most uncontrollable causal scenario). Subjects evaluated the controllability of the need, reported their affects of sympathy and anger, and their intentions to help. In one of the two studies conducted by Betancourt (1990a), the intention to help was an answer to a personal request and required one to leave his or her phone number and the amount of time volunteered to be spent in helping the person in need. Hence, this operationalization of intention to help was much more than a hypothetical report.

The data from the two experiments were quite similar. Table 6.8 gives

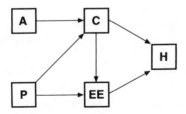

**FIGURE 6.5.** A model representing helping behavior (H) as a function of causal attributions for a person's need (A), a potential helper's psychological perspective (P), perceived controllability of the attributions (C), and empathic emotions (EE). From Betancourt (1990a, p. 577). Copyright 1990a by Sage Publications, Inc. Reprinted by permission.

TABLE 6.8. Correlations between Relevant Variables of Experiment 6.1.

|  | Perspective | Control | Empathic emotion |
|---|---|---|---|
| Perspective |  |  |  |
| Controllability | −.19* |  |  |
| Empathic emotion | .41** | −.40** |  |
| Helping | .31** | −.43** | .45** |

*Note.* Adapted from Betancourt (1990a, p. 582). Copyright 1990 by Sage Publications, Inc. Reprinted by permission. Higher levels correspond to higher empathy, perceived controllability, empathic emotions, and help offered ($N = 150$).
*$p < .01$. **$p < .001$.

the correlation matrix for the data in the first investigation. It is evident from Table 6.8 that an empathic perspective decreases perceptions of controllability and increases empathic emotions (defined as sympathy minus anger), as well as fostering help. These relations were as predicted. In addition, the remaining correlations are consistent with the results of prior studies. Finally, the model shown in Figure 6.5 (and therefore Model 2 in Figure 6.1) provided the best fit with the data. Thus, Betancourt (1990a) achieved his goal of incorporating an additional variable that lent itself to an attribution-emotion mediational interpretation of help giving.

## Cross-Cultural Replications

In the examination of reactions to stigmas presented in Chapter 3, a study conducted in the People's Republic of China was presented that displayed the same pattern of data found in responses from American college students. Such cross-cultural replication increases the confidence one has that general psychological processes are being identified and that general laws are being formulated. In a similar manner, the findings reported by Weiner and Kukla (1970), discussed in Chapter 2, regarding the evaluative consequences of ability and effort ascriptions, have been replicated in numerous cultures. Indeed, my implicit (and at times explicit) position throughout this book is that the hypothesized processes and mechanisms under examination are pancultural, surely not restricted to American respondents.

In an investigation undertaken by Matsui and Matsuda (1992), there was an attempt to find evidence for the responsibility–emotion mediational model among Japanese respondents. Again the class notes scenario from Weiner (1980b) was used. Matsui and Matsuda (1992) elaborated their investigation by introducing an additional variable—namely, whether the person seeking to borrow class notes was liked or disliked. The typical variables of causal controllability, anger, sympathy, and judgments about helping were assessed (using the same indicators as Reisenzein, 1986), and there also was assessment of the degree to which the lender liked the person in need.

A path analysis of these data was performed, with the best-fitting model depicted in Figure 6.6. As Figure 6.6 illustrates, liking influences perceptions of controllability: If one is liked, then there is a tendency to perceive the cause of a need as uncontrollable (reminding one of the findings reported by Betancourt (1990a) that empathy increases perceptions of causal uncontrollability). Controllability, in turn, relates negatively to the resultant affect (sympathy minus anger), while this emotional composite score is directly associated with judgments to help. Perceptions of control had no direct influence on helping, but the degree of liking did relate to judgments about helping. Hence, this pattern of data is most closely captured by Model 5 in Figure 6.1.

In a related study also undertaken in Japan (Kojima, 1992), the person who was asking to borrow the class notes was either a stranger (as in Weiner, 1980b, and most other studies of helping) or someone with whom the lender was familiar. In addition to the usual correlational and path analytic techniques for determining the relations between causal controllability, emotion, and help giving, Kojima partitioned how well the variables predicted help giving by examining whether the relations were direct or indirect (mediated through other variables). That is, he determined how much of the variability in the helping judgments was due to familiarity, controllability, and feelings, and whether those relations were direct or were mediated by other variables. These findings are shown in Table 6.9.

Table 6.9 reveals that familiarity is directly linked to helping judgments and is strongly associated with help giving (we are more likely to help those we know). Attributions of causality (controllability) have both

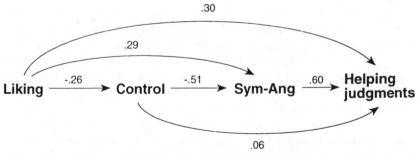

**FIGURE 6.6.** Path analysis of the effects of liking, perceptions of control, and affective reaction (sympathy minus anger) on judgments of helping. From Matsui and Matsuda (1992). Reprinted by permission of the authors.

TABLE 6.9. The Effects of Familiarity, Attribution, and
Affects on Helping

| Variable | Effects of independent variable | | |
| --- | --- | --- | --- |
| | Direct | Indirect | Total |
| Familiarity | .37 | .08 | .45 |
| Attribution | .16 | .28 | .44 |
| Affects | .40 | — | .40 |

Note. Data from Kojima (1992, p. 75).

direct and indirect linkages with helping judgments, but they primarily
influence helping indirectly (through an association with emotion). And
affect has only a direct influence on help giving. This partitioning of the
variance or the predictability of the helping judgments clearly is consistent
with the position that not all of the determinants of helping are mediated
through thoughts about responsibility and emotions and that responsibility
has some effects on helping that are independent of anger and sympathy.

## AIDS and Helping

Help giving to persons with AIDS was examined in Chapters 3 and 4, but
without considering the complexity that can be uncovered with path analytical and structural equation techniques. Dooley (1995), guided by the
responsibility–affect analysis of helping, did use path methodologies to
ascertain the determinants of help giving to those with AIDS.

In her study, Dooley presented subjects with four scenarios that described individuals who differed in the cause of their HIV infection. The
causes represented were blood transfusion, heterosexual behavior, homosexual behavior, and drug use (see also Graham et al., 1993, as discussed
in Chapter 4 and Experiment 4.1). In addition, there was a control condition in which no causal information was provided.

The subjects then rated, on multiple-item scales, the controllability of
the infection, their feelings of anger and pity, and their desire to help the
ill individual. In addition, Dooley (1995) assessed knowledge about HIV
transmission and the gender of the respondents.

Dooley reported the usual relations between the causes of the illness,
perceptions of controllability, and feelings of pity and anger. Greatest
controllability was inferred with drug use and homosexual behavior, and
these causes augmented anger and reduced pity. Conversely, the least
controllability and anger and the most pity were reported toward those

infected with the HIV virus because of a blood transfusion.

The model best fitting these data was then determined (see Figure 6.7). As the figure reveals, knowledge about HIV transmission directly increases the reports of helping ($r = .21$). In addition, women are more likely than males to state that they would help ($r = .23$). Again, these are non-responsibility mediated determinants of help. Most germane to the present discussion, the onset controllability of the disease relates negatively with pity ($r = -.44$) and positively with anger ($r = .32$). In a structural equation analysis, pity emerged as the primary determinant of judgments to help ($r = .42$). As others have reported, perceptions of controllability only indirectly influenced behavior through its effects on pity. However, inconsistent with the vast majority of pertinent literature, in this investigation anger had no direct effect on reports of helping.

## Summary

Tables 6.10 and 6.11 include a summary of the studies already examined, as well as other research not discussed because it was examined in prior chapters. The summary in these tables includes the investigator and the

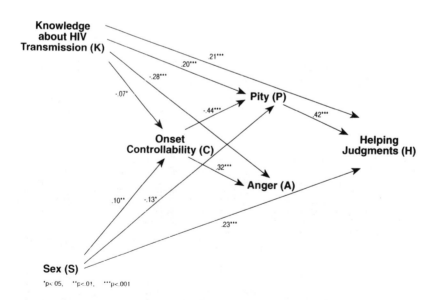

FIGURE 6.7. Structural equation analysis of the determinants of giving help to those with AIDS. Adapted from Dooley (1995). Copyright 1995 by Bellwether. Adapted by permission.

**TABLE 6.10.** Summary of Relevant Investigations of Help Giving: Correlation Coefficients

| Investigator | N | Subjects | Situation | Additional information | Correlation coefficients | | | | | | |
|---|---|---|---|---|---|---|---|---|---|---|---|
| | | | | | C×S | C×A | C×H | S×H | A×H | C×(S−A) | (S−A)×H |
| Weiner (1980a) | 28 | American college students | Help drunk vs. ill person on subway | Measured disgust, not anger | −.77 | .55 | −.37 | .46 | −.71 | | |
| Weiner (1980b) | 116 | American college students | Request to lend class notes | | −.54 | .36 | −.41 | .59 | −.49 | | |
| Meyer & Mulherin (1980) | 80 | Canadian college students | Request to lend money | Eight causes of the need for money | −.37 | .64 | −.14 | .37 | −.65 | | |
| Reisenzein (1986) | 138 | American college students  Request to lend class notes | Help drunk vs. ill person on subway | Same subjects in both situations | −.49 | .51 | −.44 | .45 | −.43 | | |
| Schmidt & Weiner (1988) | 496 | American college students | Request to lend class notes | Combined across four conditions; varied experimental set | −.64 | .35 | −.29 | .47 | −.58 | | |
| Weiner, Perry, & Magnusson (1988) | 59 | American college students | Help the stigmatized (Charity, personal assistance) | Combined across ten stigmas | | | −.38 | | | −.44 | .65 |
| Weiner & Graham (1989) | 370 | American, age 5–95 | Varied | Results combined across age groups | −.56 | .52 | −.26 | .38 | −.35 | | |

| Study | N | Population | Help measure | Notes | C–S | C–A | C–H | S–H | A–H |
|---|---|---|---|---|---|---|---|---|---|
| Betancourt (1990) | 150 | American college students | Help a failing student | Five causes of the need for help, manipulation of empathic set; help was not simulational | −.41 | | −.43 | .45 | −.52 |
| Matsui & Matsuda (1992) | 100 | Japanese college students | Request to lend class notes | Varied degree of liking of student | −.51 | .61 | −.52 | .53 | −.52 |
| | 80 | Japanese college students | Request to lend class notes | Composite index: Affect = sympathy–anger | −.42 | .57 | −.38 | .54 | .65 |
| Kojima (1992) | 112 | Japanese college students | Request to lend class notes | Composite affect index for some analyses | −.71 | .61 | −.47 | .51 | −.61 |
| Zucker & Weiner (1993) | 122 | American college students | Personally help the poor | Fifteen causes of poverty; differentiate two types of helping | −.31 | .44 | −.28 | .61 | −.45 |
| | | | Welfare for the poor | | | | −.39 | .43 | −.34 |
| | 47 | American adults | Personally help the poor | | −.53 | .17 | −.61 | .77 | −.19 |
| | | | Welfare for the poor | | | | −.56 | .79 | −.32 |
| Dooley (1995) | 225 | American college students | Help person with AIDS | Four causes of AIDS | | | | | |
| Mean | | | | | −.52 | .48 | −.38 | .51 | −.51 |

*Note:* C = Controllability/Responsibility; S = Sympathy; A = Anger; H = Help.

TABLE 6.11. Summary of Relevant Investigations of Help Giving: Partial Correlation Coefficients and Path or Regression Coefficients

| Investigator | N | Situation | Partial correlation coefficients | | | | | | Path or regression coefficients | | | |
|---|---|---|---|---|---|---|---|---|---|---|---|---|
| | | | C × H/S | C × H/A | C × H/ (S−A) | S × H/C | A × H/C | (S−A) × H/C | C × H | S × H | A × H | (S−A) × H |
| Weiner (1980a) | 28 | Help drunk vs. ill person on subway | −.02 | .04 | .21 | .31 | −.66 | | | | | |
| Weiner (1980b) | 116 | Request to lend class notes | −.12 | −.28 | −.10 | .48 | −.41 | | | | | |
| Meyer & Mulherin (1980) | 80 | Request to lend money | | | | | | | −.14 | .32 | | −.56 |
| Reisenzen (1986) | 138 | Help drunk vs. ill person on subway | | | | | | | NS | .36 | | −.31 |
| | | Request to lend class notes | | | | | | | NS | .71 | | −.44 |
| Schmidt & Weiner (1988) | 496 | Request to lend class notes | | | | | | | NS | .48 | | −.55 |
| Weiner, Perry, & Magnusson (1988) | 59 | Help the stigmatized (charity, personal assistance) | | | | | | | .14 | | | .68 |

| Study | N | Situation | | | | | | | | | | |
|---|---|---|---|---|---|---|---|---|---|---|---|---|
| Weiner & Graham (1989) | 370 | Varied | −.07 | −.07 | | .31 | −.32 | | NS | | | .45 |
| Betancourt (1990) | 150 | Help a failing student | | | | | | | −.31 | .36 | | |
| Matsui & Matsuda (1992) | 100 | Request to lend class notes | | | | | | | −.11 | | | .49 |
| | 80 | Request to lend class notes | | | | | | | .06 | | | .41 |
| Kojima (1992) | 112 | Request to lend class notes | | | −.07 | | | .42 | −.16 | | | .41 |
| Zucker & Weiner (1993) | 122 | Personally help the poor | | | | | | | NS | .48 | −.28 | |
| | | Welfare for the poor | | | | | | | −.34 | .21 | −.02 | |
| | 47 | Personally help the poor | | | | | | | −.36 | .55 | .12 | |
| | | Welfare for the poor | | | | | | | −.23 | .48 | −.02 | |
| Dooley (1995) | 225 | Help person with AIDS | | | | | | | NS | .42 | NS | |

Note. C = Controllability/Responsibility; S = Sympathy; A = Anger; H = Help; / = the variable after this symbol was partialled out.

year of the investigation(s), the number and type of research subjects, the experimental situation, other information about the research, and pertinent statistical figures (the strengths of the germane correlation, partial correlation, path, and/or regression coefficients).

Examination of Table 6.10 reveals some of the shortcomings of this research: with two exceptions, the subjects were college students; the research paradigm was role-playing or simulation, with only one investigation without judgments of helping or attitudes toward welfare as the main dependent variable; controllability or responsibility was not assessed or were reported as a combined index; the two situations previously introduced by Piliavin et al. (1969) and Barnes et al. (1979) that involved falling on a subway train and asking to borrow class notes predominated (although in role-playing contexts); and I was personally involved in about half of the investigations. These liabilities weaken the generality of the findings and the conclusions that one would like to draw. On the positive side, the situations did include the lending of money and the nonspecific helping of persons who had AIDS, were poor, or had a variety of stigmas, and there were other situations pertinent to helping among children; subjects from another culture in addition to the United States (Japanese students) were represented, as were children; and nearly 2,500 subjects were tested.

Table 6.10 reveals consistent, systematic, and supportive data in the published investigations. Examining the correlational data shows that all of the studies reporting these figures find negative associations between controllability/responsibility and sympathy (average $r = -.52$) and positive associations between controllability/responsibility and anger (average $r = .48$). These data strongly support the postulations first introduced in Chapter 1 regarding appraisal–emotion linkages.

Turning next to the associations between thought and feelings, on the one hand, and judgments of helping, on the other, it is evident that in all of the studies the correlations between controllability and helping are negative (average $r = -38$), while the correlations between emotions and helping are negative for anger (average $r = -.51$) and positive for sympathy (average $r = .51$). These associations also are in the anticipated directions and encourage the belief that affects may be more significant determinants of helping (or, in this case, helping judgments or intentions) than thoughts are.

More sophisticated analyses involving partial correlations, regression, and/or path analyses shown in Table 6.11 provide more exacting tests of the models shown in Figure 6.1. In virtually all of the investigations that provide appropriate data, affects are the more proximal and more important determinants of behavior than thoughts are.

What, then, can be concluded at this point regarding a responsibility–affect approach to helping, based on the reviewed studies?

1. There is an interrelation between thoughts about controllability of a need (and, by implication, responsibility), affective reactions of anger and sympathy to this causal inference, and intentions to help (and, by implication, actual helping behavior).
2. Affects are proximally linked to help giving.
3. The affects of sympathy and anger have a stronger and more direct influence on judgments of helping than do causal ascriptions and responsibility inferences.
4. It is uncertain whether causal thoughts have a direct as well as an indirect influence on helping. Some investigations find this proximal union, others do not.
5. The stimulus situation itself and other factors influence help giving, independent of the responsibility–emotion mediational input. Variables such as the degree of elicited empathy, the gender of the respondent, liking of the needy person, familiarity, and so on will in part determine if help is provided, regardless of perceptions of responsibility for the need and the affective reactions that this evokes.
6. Based on the evidence gathered thus far, Model 5 in Figure 6.1 and Model 2 are best supported by the data. Model 5 includes a direct path from the stimulus to help and from emotions to help, but only an indirect path from controllability to help via the emotions. Model 2, on the other hand, also includes a direct path from controllability to help. I therefore propose the following model (referred to as Model 6) as thus far providing the closest fit to the data:

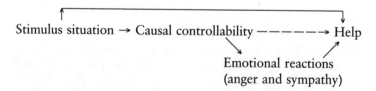

In this diagram, the dashed line from controllability to help indicates that the relationship is weak and/or tentative.

7. As with virtually all psychological conclusions, more investigations are needed, using a variety of methodologies, to test these propositions further. The body of evidence is weakened because of the similarity of many of the studies.

## ADDITIONAL CONCEPTUAL ADVANCES

The 7-point summary of the preceding literature review may have left the impression that there is little more of importance to accomplish *from this perspective* in regard to helping behavior, other than to determine if there is or is not a direct path from causal thinking to action and to replicate the reported findings with other methodologies. However, this is far from the truth.

A theoretical variation of the model that was just depicted (and referred to as Model 6) is now introduced that points out some limitations or limiting conditions of that model, as well as a new conceptual direction. Indeed, rather than conclude that the issues are "resolved," one of the main virtues of the responsibility–affect mediational approach is that it lends itself to further development and theoretical elaboration.

### "Hot" versus "Cold" Theory

Psychologists often label cognitions as "cold" and emotions as "hot," thereby mirroring everyday metaphors that consider "hot-headed" action as driven by emotion, whereas one who is cold acts "without a heart," or without emotions. The theory proposed throughout this book merges the head with the heart in that emotions arise from thoughts (e.g., sympathy is evoked by perceptions of an uncontrollable plight, anger by a controllable need). But it has been emphasized that conduct is "hot" in the sense that emotions are more proximal to action than cognitions are.

It might be contended, as previously suggested, that often actions are "heartless" and that behavior is primarily guided by higher-order cognitions and rationality. If this is so, then Model 6 that has been offered is unduly restrictive by presuming that emotions are invariantly the immediate and more important determinants of action. Perhaps this "error" was made because of the particular selection of experimental conditions or scenarios that gave rise to the empirical findings.

If indeed at times emotion, and at times thought, is the proximal and more important determinant of action, then the question that immediately arises is under what conditions is each of these alternatives dominant? That is, when will thinking and rationality be primary, and when will feelings most influence what one does? And an answer to this question also immediately comes to mind, namely, the more one is "involved" in the situation and the more significant or consequential the context, then the greater the contribution of emotions relative to thought in determining behavior. Thus, for example, when your child commits a misdeed it will elicit more feeling-directed behavior than when a neighbor's child misbehaves; if your mother falls on the subway, your actions are more emotion-instigated than they would be if a stranger had fallen; the decision to help a friend in need of money is more likely to be influenced by emotion than is the decision to help a stranger with financial need; and a resolution to personally help a stranger will be more affect guided than a judgment of how the government should distribute funds to the needy.

The situations crafted in the investigations of help giving were not particularly "hot" in that they most often involved aid to strangers. However, affects would be presumed to be evoked in that subjects are asked personally to lend class notes or money or to pick up someone in a subway. This may account for the priority of emotions as behavioral determinants in those investigations.

A study I conducted with Zucker (Zucker & Weiner, 1993) examined conditions that were anticipated to influence whether help giving is more mediated by cold thoughts or by hot emotions. That investigation was described in detail in Chapter 3, but in order not to introduce too much new information at that time, not all of the experiment was presented. In that research, subjects rated 13 causes for importance in bringing about poverty (laziness, lack of jobs, etc.) In addition, the subjects rated how responsible the poor were for being impoverished, their feelings of sympathy and anger toward the poor, and judgments were made regarding aid for the poor. Measures of political ideology also were obtained.

Of key importance in this context is that two types of helping were distinguished. One question asked how much the subject would be personally willing to help the poor, in accordance with the helping question in most prior research. A second index of helping concerned the degree to which the government should provide welfare to the poor. Although neither of these indexes involve actual helping, and although the respondents did not personally know to whom help was being given, they were, nonetheless, providing help in one condition, whereas in a second condition they were merely bystanders. It therefore was anticipated that judgments to personally help would be more characterized as "hot," or driven by emotions, than would the opinions about governmental aid, which would be more characterized as "cold," or guided by inferences of responsibility.

The structural equation analysis of these data is depicted in Figure 6.8 (which is an elaboration of Figure 3.4). Examination of Figure 6.8 reveals that personal intentions of helping are determined by the affects of pity and anger and that political ideology and beliefs about responsibility only influence helping judgments indirectly, via their effect on emotions (see also the discussion in Chapter 3). On the other hand, welfare judgments are directly linked not only to beliefs about how responsible the poor are for

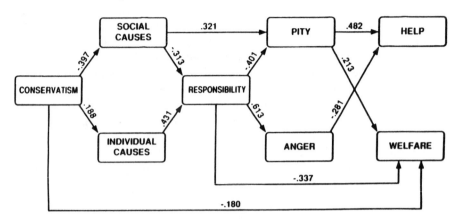

**FIGURE 6.8.** Structural equation analysis of the determinants of help for the poor. From Zucker and Weiner (1993, p. 937). Copyright 1993 by V. H. Winston & Sons. Reprinted by permission.

being poor but also to conservatism—that is, the more the poor are thought to be responsible for their fate and the more extreme the conservatism of the respondent, the less the belief in aid through welfare. Note that welfare judgments are weakly influenced by affects, and then only by pity.

It may not be entirely accurate to label the influence of political ideology on welfare as "cold," inasmuch as this attitude is linked with great emotionality in relation to many issues (consider, for example, a pro- or antiabortion attitude linked with political ideology). But it is the case that the affective component of political ideology is more diffuse or less specific than the report of the amount of pity and anger that are directly elicited by the poor. Furthermore, ideology also had a small influence on welfare judgments relative to beliefs about responsibility. In sum, as I previously had written (Weiner, 1986):

> The amount of variance in helping behavior (and helping judgments) that is directly accounted for by thought (attributions) as opposed to emotion will in part depend on the emotion-arousing properties of the situation. . . . As one becomes increasingly involved in a situation, perceptions of controllability will have a lessening direct influence on the decision to help or neglect. On the other hand, as situations become increasingly remote or trivial to an actor, "cold" thoughts will play a large, direct part in helping, with emotions relegated to a less important role. (p. 204)

Again, therefore, many issues remain to be resolved. The mediational models presented in Figure 6.1—and what I offered as the "best" representation of the data, Model 6—provide structural guidelines rather than a definitive conclusion.

## CONCEPTUAL DEVELOPMENT AND PRACTICAL APPLICATION

In many of the studies that have been presented, subjects were asked if they would provide help to a particular person who, for example, falls in the subway, misses class, is unemployed, and the like. In other research investigations, the respondents were asked if they, or the government, would (should) help a class of needy individuals, such as the poor, the sick, persons with AIDS, and so on. However, in many instances the decision to be made is not if help should or should not be provided (as might be the case in the subway and class notes scenarios) but rather to whom and how much help should be given. For example, government policy makers must decide to allocate resources to persons with AIDS or to the mentally handicapped, to Vietnam War veterans or to the unemployed, and so on. And these decisions must be made in the face of limitations in the amount of available resources, space, time, and so on. In these situations, what determines the allocation of help giving? That is the issue that Skitka, Tetlock, and their colleagues have tackled (see Skitka, McMurray, & Burrows, 1991; Skitka & Tetlock, 1992, 1993a, 1993b). They have used this practical setting to both document the use of the responsibility–affect mediational model and to further their conceptual analysis.

To answer the question of allocation distribution, Skitka and Tetlock (1992, 1993a) have proposed a four-stage model in which perceptions of responsibility play a key role. This model is reproduced in Figure 6.9. The logic of the model is as follows. Stage 1 in the model requires the assessment of resource availability. That is, the help provider determines if there are sufficient resources to help all claimants. If there are, then the model specifies that all claimants will be aided (however, as will soon be discussed, there are qualifications to this decision rule dependent on the political ideology of the allocator).

If there are insufficient resources, which normally is the case, then further information is necessary, and the potential helper advances to Stage 2 of the model. At this stage, the allocator asks why the claimants need help. If the causes are internal and controllable—that is, if the needy are responsible for their condition(s)—then help is not provided. Skitka and Tetlock (1992, 1993a) accept that responsibility relates to the affects of sympathy and anger and, hence, apply the mediational model that has been

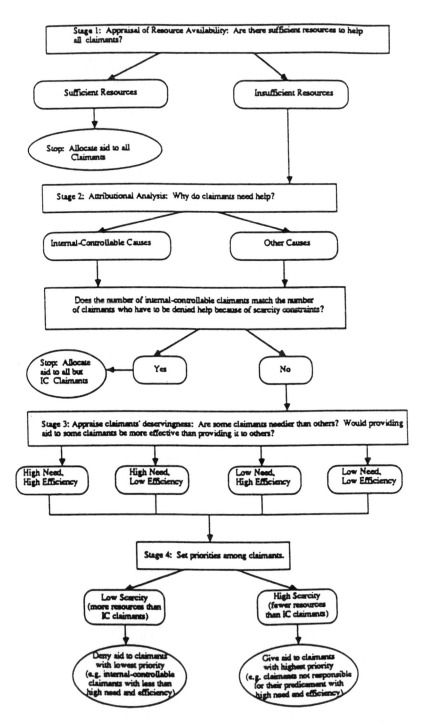

**FIGURE 6.9.** Temporal sequence model of the determinants of support of claimants who are seeking financial aid. From Stitka and Tetlock (1992, p. 494). Copyright 1992 by Academic Press. Reprinted by permission.

advocated here; however, they do not separate these two elements but treat them instead as a unit. This makes it impossible to examine whether thoughts or affects are contributing to the judgments about helping (but this is not of particular concern for them).

The attributional analysis eliminates some of the demands for resources, but this does not presume that all of those not responsible for their needs will be helped. Whether all persons not responsible are aided depends on whether the number of those in need because of internal controllable reasons matches the number of claimants who have to be denied help because of scarcity constraints. If there is a match, that is, if the shortage of funds can be entirely overcome by not providing aid to those who are responsible, then help will be provided to all of the nonresponsible needy. However, often there still are not enough funds to satisfy all of the "worthy" claimants. In this situation, the decision process continues to Stage 3.

In Stage 3, other determinants of help are considered, particularly the severity of the need and the extent to which the needy will in fact be improved by the help. These might be considered among the nonattributional determinants of help that are incorporated by a path from the stimulus situation to helping, as shown in Models 5 and 6 presented earlier. Then, advancing to Stage 4, the help provider sets priorities among the needy as a joint function of all the factors, including deservingness (responsibility), need, and efficiency. In summary, Skitka and Tetlock (1993a) write:

> When there are sufficient resources to help almost everyone (low scarcity), allocators will deny aid only to those claimants with the lowest overall priority: internal–controllable claimants whose needs are not urgent and whose chances of being effectively helped are slim. When there are insufficient resources (high scarcity), allocators will initially respond by denying aid to all personally responsible claimants. However, if even this step is not sufficient to bring resources and needs into balance, allocators will also deny aid to claimants who are not responsible for needing assistance, in particular to those whose needs are not urgent and whose chances of help are slim. (p. 208)

In addition to these predictions, Skitka et al. (1991) reason that political ideology also influences the willingness to provide aid. As documented in the earlier chapters, conservatives believe more than liberals that individuals are responsible for their plights. Conservatives therefore are expected to withhold more resources from those in need when the causes are personally controllable. Indeed, even in times of resource abundance, conservatives may withhold funds from the needy who are responsible for their plight. Hence, as previously noted, there are qualifications to the assumption of Stage 1, which states that if funds are available, all will be helped.

The most thorough test of this model was reported by Skitka and Tetlock (1992). In this research, allocation preferences under conditions of high, low, or no scarcity were examined across three domains: medicine for AIDS patients, organs for people needing transplants, and low-income housing for the poor. For each scarcity, information about the needy was varied on factors of locus (internal or external cause of the need), control (controllable or uncontrollable), severity of need (high or low), and efficiency (high or low), thus yielding 16 types of claimants. For example, in one condition it was read that a person with a genetically defective organ (internal, uncontrollable cause) required this transplant to survive (high need) and would be saved by the procedure (high efficiency).

In the high-scarcity condition, subjects could select only 3 of the 16 persons to be the recipients of aid; for low scarcity, 13 of the 16 were eligible for assistance; and given no scarcity, the respondents could select as many of the needy as they wished to receive help. In addition to these helping judgments, political ideology and other variables were assessed.

Table 6.12 shows the average number of times that the 16 types of claimants were selected to receive aid in the high (top half of the table) and low (bottom half of the table) scarcity conditions. Considering high scarcity, assistance was for the most part denied to all individuals responsible for their plights. Among claimants not personally responsible, assistance was received if the need was urgent and if there was a high likelihood that help would be effective. On the other hand, given low scarcity, allocators recommended help to all claimants not responsible for their needs. Further, those personally responsible were aided if the need was severe and if the help would be effective.

Finally, even assuming no scarcity, conservatives continued to withhold assistance from some claimants responsible for their predicaments, whereas liberals endorsed the position that all should be helped. Skitka and Tetlock (1992, 1993a) suggest that conservatives withhold resources as a punishment. This seems analogous to punishing those who do not try (as discussed in Chapter 2), with the goals of rehabilitation, providing others with a moral education, and extracting retributive justice, perhaps because of the "ultimate" reason that irresponsibility decreases the survival fitness of others in the society. However, in subsequent research Skitka and Tetlock (1993b) report that if a person overcomes a prior stigma (e.g., a recovered alcoholic), then conservatives are particularly open to offer aid!

In sum, this study provides strong support for the model proposed by Skitka and Tetlock. Their approach incorporates the mediators that I have proposed, but expands in a new direction by considering the consequences of resource scarcity and by explicitly identifying other influences on help

**TABLE 6.12.** Average Number of Times Claimants Were Chosen to Receive Available Aid under High versus Low Scarcity as a Function of Locus, Control, Need, and Efficiency

| Locus of responsibility | Need/efficiency | | | |
|---|---|---|---|---|
| | High need-<br>High<br>efficiency | High need-<br>Low<br>efficiency | Low need-<br>High<br>efficiency | Low need-<br>Low<br>efficiency |
| | *High scarcity* | | | |
| Internal–controllable | 0.16 | 0.01 | 0.03 | 0.01 |
| Internal–uncontrollable | **1.97** | 0.23 | 0.56 | 0.19 |
| External–controllable | **2.07** | 0.15 | 0.58 | 0.06 |
| External–uncontrollable | **2.22** | 0.12 | 0.53 | 0.05 |
| | *Low scarcity* | | | |
| Internal–controllable | 2.20 | <u>0.89</u> | <u>1.51</u> | <u>0.42</u> |
| Internal–uncontrollable | 2.97 | 2.72 | 2.95 | 2.78 |
| External–controllable | 2.95 | 2.76 | 2.94 | 2.54 |
| External–uncontrollable | 3.00 | 2.86 | 2.91 | 2.66 |

*Note.* From Skitka and Tetlock (1992, p. 510). Copyright 1992 by Academic Press. Reprinted by permission. Bold-faced numbers highlight claimants predicted to have highest priority under high scarcity, and underlined numbers highlight claimants predicted to have lowest priority under low scarcity.

giving when resources are insufficient to help all. In addition, the process of making a decision to offer aid is more fully explored. This research, therefore, points out both the limitations of the narrow path I have taken as well as the amenability of a responsibility–emotion approach to incorporation within larger and more complex theoretical frameworks (although affects are not explicitly explored in this approach).

## EMPIRICAL SUMMARY AND
## THEORETICAL CONCLUSIONS

Prior to this chapter, it was quite evident that responsibility inferences and/or their affective consequences played important roles in the dispensing of rewards and punishments in achievement contexts (Chapter 2) and in judgments regarding the stigmatized, particularly alcoholics, the obese, the impoverished (Chapter 3), homosexuals and those with AIDS (Chapter

4), as well as depressed individuals and those with a schizophrenic disorder (Chapter 5). But in none of these areas of investigation was there a sufficiently in-depth attempt at building psychological structure; in none was there a sufficient number of investigations to promote theoretical change; and in none was there a systematic examination of key theoretical issues. The unsolved conceptual questions include: (1) Are there direct as well as indirect linkages between thinking and doing? (2) Do the path structures or motivational sequences change as a function of conditions such as the emotion-arousing properties of the situation? and (3) what are some of the conditions that limit the generality of the theory?

This chapter on helping behavior diverged from the prior discussions because a large number of similar investigations have been conducted, guided by the same theoretical framework and using sophisticated statistical techniques to tease apart the temporal sequence of a motivational episode. In contrast to the studies examined in the prior chapters, these characteristics of the literature on helping have promoted theory building, theoretical change, and an examination of central conceptual issues.

The many studies of helping lead to the conclusion that there is a thinking (controllability to responsibility) → feeling → acting order to motivation and that emotions are the proximal determinants of action, with thoughts giving rise to these emotions (and at times linking directly to action). In addition, factors within the situation directly affect decisions about helping, without attributional mediation. However, it also is the case that contextual variables including resource scarcity and lack of personal involvement alter whether specific instances will result in help giving and/or positive intentions to help.

It is evident that the dispensing of rewards and punishments in achievement contexts, reactions to the stigmatized, and helping behavior are subject to the identical theoretical analysis, which is no small accomplishment in the field of motivation, an area of study that has become increasingly loath to search for general laws of behavior. All these domains are subject to a common conceptual analysis because judgments of sin and sickness—that is, being responsible or not responsible for a state, outcome, or condition—and the affects that this generates, mediate between some external stimulus and the behavioral reactions to that stimulus. In traditional terms, this can be represented as an S–O–R (stimulus–organism–response) process.

The search for generality does not end in this chapter, for aggression (Chapter 7) and impression management (confession as well as giving excuses, Chapter 8) remain to be examined. However, it is useful to remind the reader of the general goals for this book introduced in Chapter 1: namely, to document the extensity of judgments of responsibility in everyday life and to build a general psychological system with judgments of responsibility as the key component or foundation. Judgments about helping and helping behavior are determined by inferences of deservingness (responsibility), and this incontrovertible fact fostered the systematic theory building evident in this chapter.

# 7

## Aggression

Speak roughly to your little boy
and beat him when he sneezes.
He only does it to annoy,
because he knows it teases.
—Lewis Carroll,
*Alice in Wonderland*

The psychological study of aggression has had a very different history and focus than the study of helping behavior. Among the issues of most concern to those studying aggression has been the identification of an aggressive trait that makes a person prone to commit antisocial acts. This has lead to the search for genetic determinants of hostile conduct and specific chromosomal anomalies, as well as to the recognition of the dysfunctional child-rearing practices of those with aggressive offspring. Attention also has been given to the demographic variables and social conditions that are associated with and/or generate antisocial conduct, including poverty, youth, living in urban ghettos, and the like (see Berkowitz, 1993). In addition, many investigators have made use of subhuman populations to discover the stimulus conditions that give rise to hostile actions, including particular colors or smells and the onset of aversive stimulation such as shock.

Such extensive research efforts have not been targeted toward an understanding of help giving. There has not been a serious quest to identify an "altruistic" personality, to find the conditions within the family that give rise to subsequent generosity, or to study help giving among infrahumans. Hence, helping behavior and aggression typically are not examined by the same researchers, nor are they often embraced within the same conceptual framework (biological approaches like sociobiology are an exception to this statement).

In contrast to this history, I will argue in this chapter that aggression is subject to the same theoretical analysis and psychological laws as have been applied to achievement evaluation, reactions to the stigmatized, and help giving. Indeed, you might recall that in the very first pages of Chapter 1, a situation was described in which there was a car crash and the party who was hit followed with a hostile retaliation. Thus, aggressive behavior is a focus of this conceptual approach.

The basic argument that will be made is that if a person is the victim of a harmful act, then that person seeks to determine the cause of the infraction. If the act was committed by another person, if the act is perceived as subject to volitional control, and if there were no mitigating circumstances, then the perpetrator of the misdeed is inferred to be responsible for his or her conduct. This gives rise to anger and the tendency to engage in hostile retaliation. This sequence can be represented in the following way:

Event (personal harm) → Attributional search → Personal agency, controllable causality, no mitigating circumstances → Inference of responsibility → Anger → Tendency to retaliate

On the other hand, if the offender is not perceived as responsible for the damage, then anger will not be experienced and the tendency to respond aggressively that is evoked by that emotion will not be aroused. This sequence can be represented in the following way:

Event (personal harm) → Attributional search → No personal agency, uncontrollable causality, or mitigating circumstances → Inference of nonresponsibility → No anger → No tendency to retaliate

Of course, much aggressive behavior is not subject to an attributional explanation or analysis, just as one might help one's mother without considering her responsibility for the need of aid. When a bully takes the toy of another, when a robber threatens to harm others during a criminal act, and when a rapist attacks an unsuspecting target, it is unlikely that the perpetrator of these deeds has engaged in an attributional search and infers victim responsibility for some prior conduct. The aggression considered in the current discussion, therefore, is retaliatory or reactive rather than proactive (as will be discussed in more detail later in the chapter) and typically is directed toward a specific, preselected target.

Hence, a theory of aggression is not being proposed. As was indicated in a prior chapter regarding depression, I am neither smart enough nor foolhardy enough to suggest that. In fact, I do not believe that there can be a "complete" theory of aggression (or achievement, affiliation, or any other broad category of behavior), given that these actions can have disparate, sufficient antecedents. Rather, what is being offered is a mechanism or process that can in part account for some types of aggressive conduct on some occasions, as well as some types of helping on some occasions. It does not invalidate the conception if there are situations that elicit aggression without intervening attributional thoughts or if affects other than anger cause one to behave with hostility. As noted by Averill (1979), "Not all aggression can be characterized as 'angry,' and anger does not always involve aggression. But this does not mean that one can ignore anger when studying aggression" (p. 3).

## AN EXPERIMENTAL DEMONSTRATION

It is once again time for an experimental demonstration, although this one does seem even more self-evident than those in the prior chapters. Perhaps this is because the role of responsibility and anger in aggressive acts is so prevalent and so much part of common sense and everyday psychology. However, obviousness does not minimize the importance or significance of a demonstration. Quite the contrary. It is known, for example, that objects typically fall toward the earth. But this does not minimize the importance of this observation, and it is of fundamental significance in the establishment of the laws of physics.

This experiment is given on the following pages. It will be seen that there are two vignettes describing an act of damage (taken from Betancourt & Blair, 1992). In both, a rock is thrown that breaks a car window. Questions about intentionality and responsibility, as well as anger, sympathy, and action, are asked. Please do this experiment now. I will return to consider the data later in the chapter.

## EXAMINING THE THEORETICAL LINKAGES

Throughout this book, the interconnections between thoughts about holding others responsible or not, the affects of anger and sympathy, and antisocial and prosocial conduct have been discussed and documented. Nonetheless, there is a huge psychological literature about these associations generated in studies of aggression that thus far has been ignored. In the next few pages, some of the literature linking responsibility with anger

## EXPERIMENT 7.1

## Determinants of Aggressive Retaliation

A number of students at a local school drive to an empty lot one evening to have stone-throwing contest. During the course of the competition, it becomes evident that one of them is the best thrower, and a second student becomes increasingly frustrated about this. In his frustration, this second person throws the rock as hard as possible at the target, but it goes astray, accidentally hitting the car of the first student, breaking a window. There is no doubt that this was accidental. Please answer the following questions.

1. Did the second (losing) student intend to break the window of the first (winning) student?

| 1 | 2 | 3 | 4 | 5 | 6 | 7 | 8 | 9 |
|---|---|---|---|---|---|---|---|---|
| Definitely not | | | | | | | | Definitely yes |

2. How responsible would you hold the student for this damage?

| 1 | 2 | 3 | 4 | 5 | 6 | 7 | 8 | 9 |
|---|---|---|---|---|---|---|---|---|
| Not at all | | | | | | | | Totally |

3. If you were this first student, how angry would you be at the second student because of the damage done to the window?

| 1 | 2 | 3 | 4 | 5 | 6 | 7 | 8 | 9 |
|---|---|---|---|---|---|---|---|---|
| Not at all | | | | | | | | Very |

4. If you were this first student, how much sympathy would you feel toward the second student?

| 1 | 2 | 3 | 4 | 5 | 6 | 7 | 8 | 9 |
|---|---|---|---|---|---|---|---|---|
| None at all | | | | | | | | A great deal |

5. If you were this first student, would you retaliate with some aggressive act, such as throwing a stone at the second person's car, or engaging in some other action?

| 1 | 2 | 3 | 4 | 5 | 6 | 7 | 8 | 9 |
|---|---|---|---|---|---|---|---|---|
| Definitely not | | | | | | | | Definitely yes |

Now consider this second situation.

A number of students at a local school drive to an empty lot one evening to have a stone-throwing contest. During the course of the competition, it becomes evident that one of them is the best thrower, and a second student becomes increasingly frustrated about this. In frustration, this second person throws the rock as hard as possible toward the car of the first person, breaking a window. There is no doubt that the throw was on purpose. Please answer the following questions.

1. Did the second (losing) student intend to break the window of the first (winning) student?

| 1 | 2 | 3 | 4 | 5 | 6 | 7 | 8 | 9 |
|---|---|---|---|---|---|---|---|---|

Definitely not                                                                    Definitely yes

2. How responsible would you hold the student for this damage?

| 1 | 2 | 3 | 4 | 5 | 6 | 7 | 8 | 9 |
|---|---|---|---|---|---|---|---|---|

Not at all                                                                              Totally

3. If you were this first student, how angry would you be at the second student because of the damage done to the window?

| 1 | 2 | 3 | 4 | 5 | 6 | 7 | 8 | 9 |
|---|---|---|---|---|---|---|---|---|

Not at all                                                                                 Very

4. If you were this first student, how much sympathy would you feel toward the second student?

| 1 | 2 | 3 | 4 | 5 | 6 | 7 | 8 | 9 |
|---|---|---|---|---|---|---|---|---|

None at all                                                                        A great deal

5. If you were this first student, would you retaliate with some aggressive act, such as throwing a stone at the second student's car or engaging in some other action?

| 1 | 2 | 3 | 4 | 5 | 6 | 7 | 8 | 9 |
|---|---|---|---|---|---|---|---|---|

Definitely not                                                                    Definitely yes

and linking anger and sympathy with aggression is briefly reviewed. Then I turn to an experiment that examined the relations between responsibility, anger, sympathy, and aggressive conduct. The first section of this chapter ends with a consideration of individual differences in aggressive tendencies among children. In the second part of the chapter, child and spousal abuse and international conflict are discussed from a responsibility → anger → aggression theoretical viewpoint.

## Inferences of Responsibility as Precursors to Anger

There have been numerous studies that have examined the relations between anger and concepts that imply responsibility (e.g., controllability, foreseeability, intentionality, volitional control, etc.; see Averill, 1983; Ferguson & Rule, 1983). Consider, for example, the research of Averill (1983). Averill asked persons to report about recent events that made them angry. More than 50% of the events reported were considered "voluntary," that is, the offender was considered to be fully aware of the consequences of the action and the act was perceived to be unjustified. The next largest category of situations that gave rise to anger (30%) was associated with an avoidable harm that was not necessarily intended, such as harm resulting from negligence or carelessness. Hence, nearly 80% of the contexts that elicited anger involved ascriptions to negative prior actions that were under the volitional control of the transgressor, so that an individual was held personally responsible for these instigating actions (see Weiner et al., 1982, for a replication of these results).

In Chapter 1, it was revealed that an intentionally completed action will more likely promote inferences of responsibility than one occurring because of negligence, although both are considered controllable. If this is the case, then intentional actions should elicit greater anger than untoward acts of negligence. In accord with this analysis, Ferguson and Rule (1983) concluded that:

> malevolently intended harm most facilitates anger and aggression. When people receive information that another person deliberately intended harm, they become angrier than if the other person did not intend harm but could have foreseen the harmful consequences. (p. 65)

In contrast to the self-report research undertaken by Averill (1983) and Weiner et al. (1982), many other of the investigations that have examined the relation between responsibility and anger have been conducted in laboratory settings, which enable one to experimentally manipulate perceptions of intent. Of particular relevance here are studies by, for example, Epstein and Taylor (1967), Nickel (1974), and Dyck and Rule (1978), which adhered to a very similar deception paradigm. In these experiments, a subject received an aversive stimulus (e.g., shock, a loud noise) from an experimental partner (who may have been an experimental confederate or did not "actually" exist but was thought to be in an adjoining room). Information was then conveyed that the partner did or did not know of the effects of his or her action, was aware or was not aware of the level of the noxious stimulation that had been administered, and the like. That is, knowledge was transmitted that resulted in the inference that the other person was or was not fully responsible for the pain that had been inflicted.

After undergoing this negative experience, in conjunction with the additional responsibility-related information, the subject was provided with the opportunity to report his or her anger and/or respond aggressively toward this person. In this manner, experimentally manipulated inferences of responsibility have been related to anger and/or behavioral aggression (see also Rule & Duker, 1973; Shantz & Voydanoff, 1973). These experiments primarily were conducted during the 1970s, when research on aggression was particularly popular and laboratory deception studies that involved aggression were more acceptable than they are today.

Consider, more specifically, a study performed by Nickel (1974). To manipulate aggressive intents, Nickel had subjects work in pairs. The experimental context included the administration of shock for incorrect answers at a task, with the shock given by one member of the pair to the other. After delivery of this stimulation, the experimenter made it known that he "noticed" that a switch had been improperly set on the shock apparatus, so that if high shock had been administered it really signified that the partner intended to deliver low shock, while subjects receiving low shock were led to believe that high shock had been intended.

The partners then changed roles as givers and receivers of shock. During the course of the opportunity to retaliate, a self-report measure was administered that included the assessment of anger-related feelings (e.g., mad, furious, enraged). The data revealed that subjects who perceived that the partner intended to give them a high shock reported a great deal of anger (although actually receiving low shock), whereas subjects actually receiving high shock (hence, there was low intended shock) reported low anger. Similar findings characterized the magnitude of shock that was delivered in retaliation. In sum, subjects' level of anger and overt aggression matched the intensity of punishment that they believed the partner intended, rather than the level of aggression that they experienced. Thus, cognitive factors (i.e. inferences of responsibility) were identified as mediating between an aversive event and the hostility of the reactions to that event.

Virtually all cognitive theorists who espouse an appraisal approach to emotion believe that volitional harm by another is included among the antecedents of anger (Roseman, 1984; Smith & Ellsworth, 1985). The evidence regarding this association is incontrovertible.

## Experienced Anger and the Elicitation of Aggression

Charles Darwin first called attention to the facial configuration that accompanies the apparent emotions of anger and rage in infrahumans. This expression includes the baring of teeth toward the threatening other. Baring one's teeth is a communication gesture, warning that an act of retaliation will follow if the transgressor continues the unacceptable behavior. A universally identified expression that accompanies anger that has similar facial characteristics also has been found among humans.

In addition to indicators of anger that serve to warn others, there is abundant evidence that anger is a precursor to overt aggression (see Rule & Nesdale, 1976). As intimated previously, anger need not be followed by overt aggression (although it could be argued that anger must be followed by a tendency toward aggression) and emotions other than anger may serve as elicitors or magnifiers of aggressive tendencies. Nonetheless, anger may be the most prevalent and significant of the emotions that give rise to hostility.

One of the earliest systematic accounts of hostile behavior was the so-called frustration–aggression hypothesis. In its strongest form, this hypothesis stated that, given a frustrating event (the blocking of a goal), aggression would follow, and given an aggressive action, one should be alerted to find prior frustration. Subsequently, Berkowitz (1962) introduced the position that anger intervenes between frustration and aggression. That is, anger is evoked by frustration and increases the likelihood of aggressive behavior (although Berkowitz specified that for anger to enhance aggression, there also must be appropriate cues or releasers in the environment).

The pertinent research investigations did not truly test the position that anger intervenes between frustration and aggression, although they did examine related hypotheses such as the necessity of frustration in producing aggression, particularly in conjunction with such antecedents as intentional hostility that would generate anger. Consider, for example, a study by Epstein and Taylor (1967). These investigators had subjects engage in a competitive task (with a "nonexistent" partner) in which the winner could administer shock to the loser following each victory. The percentage of losses was manipulated, as was the intensity of administered shock. The "true" subject had a chance to retaliate with aggressive shock for the trials that he or she won.

Epstein and Taylor (1967) reported that the percentage of losing experiences, which they considered to be a source of frustration, had no influence on the magnitude of shock retaliation. However, the greater the intentional and freely chosen shock that was received following a loss, the greater was the magnitude of hostile retaliation. Other measures also revealed that the intensity of the shock that was received related to self-reports of experienced anger. Hence, it was argued that intended aggression from the other (which was known to influence anger), rather than frustration, was the determinant of reactive aggression.

Many similar studies, including some already introduced, have been published in the experimental aggression literature, although they typically are unrelated to the frustration–aggression hypothesis. In another prototypical investigation, Baron (1971) again had subjects receive shock from another "apparent" subject in response to errors in a learning task. The "real" subject then had the opportunity to retaliate as the "partner" was put in the role of the learner. It was quite evident from the data that anger was significantly greater when the received shock was high rather than low. In addition, the greater the inflicted pain, the greater the magnitude of hostile retaliation. (These data certainly remind one of the principle of retributive justice that governs many legal decisions.)

In sum, prior research strongly suggests that intentional harm generates greater anger than does unintentional harm and that anger gives rise to aggression. Because there are alternative interpretations of the data, which soon are discussed, these results are not definitive. However, as Rule and Nesdale (1976) conclude:

> Considered together, the results of these studies are consistent with the view that when a person's arousal state is anger, the anger acts as a determinant of aggression, which is directed primarily toward the goal of injuring the source of the anger state. Furthermore, these findings suggest that a person's anger and subsequent aggression can be increased or decreased depending upon that person's attribution. (p. 852)

## Sympathy and Aggressive Inhibition

Thus far, the role of sympathy as a possible inhibitor of antisocial actions has not been examined (recall from the prior chapter that this emotion augments prosocial and helping behaviors). The cause of this neglect is that in the majority of investigations of aggression, sympathy has not been a pertinent emotion.

There is, however, a systematic literature that has considered the effects of empathy (which relates to sympathy) on the doing of harm, as well as studies examining the aggressive–inhibiting effects of the overt suffering of the receiver of a pain-inflicting action. For example, when pain cues are made very salient to the person engaging in an aggressive response, then the intensity of that response decreases (see Berger, 1962). In a study already discussed that was conducted by Baron (1971), as the subject retaliated with aggression, the magnitude of pain believed to be experienced by the paired subject was manipulated from low to high. Figure 7.1 shows the duration of the shock retaliation. As discussed previously, high anger (determined by the magnitude of shock received) increased the duration of shock retaliation relative to low anger. In addition, high pain cues decreased the duration of inflicted shock relative to the presence of low pain cues.

Note that in this research the inferred sympathy is unrelated to perceived responsibility for the initial negative act. Rather, sympathy is elicited

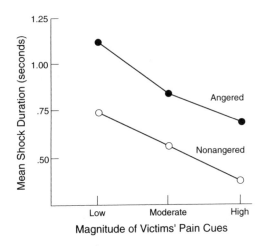

FIGURE 7.1. Mean duration of shock delivered to the learner by subjects in the angered and nonangered conditions as a function of the magnitude of the victim's displayed pain. From Baron (1971, p. 241). Copyright 1971 by the American Psychological Association. Reprinted by permission.

by the salience of perceived pain. Hence, the analysis of aggression from a responsibility perspective is not entirely correspondent with the theoretical interpretation of help giving, wherein the needy person is or is not responsible for the need and this inference consequently gives rise to anger or sympathy. In the study of aggression, anger is believed to be related to another's personal responsibility for the administration of an aversive stimulus, whereas sympathy might be experienced during the "payback," but is unrelated to the inference of responsibility for having been shocked.

## TESTING THE THEORY

As previously intimated, there are shortcomings of the experimental aggression research, and alternative interpretations of the data are possible. From the perspective of this book, among the most significant problems is that the motivational sequence—and, hence, the presumed role of anger in determining aggression—has neither been clearly stated nor documented. To return, for example, to the experiment by Nickel (1974), recall that in this investigation the intention of the aggressive action was varied, and anger as well as shock retaliation were assessed. Intention was related to both of these variables. Hence, one representation of the data is the following:

$$\text{Intentional aggression} \rightarrow \begin{cases} \text{Anger} \\ \text{Aggressive retaliation} \end{cases}$$

That is, intentional aggression gives rise to both anger and aggression. However, these reactions are not causally related to one another (although they are correlated). Another possible representation of the findings is:

$$\text{Intentional aggression} \rightarrow \text{Anger}$$
$$\downarrow$$
$$\text{Intentional aggression} \rightarrow \text{Aggressive retaliation}$$

That is, intentional aggression generates both anger and aggression, and inferences of responsibility along with anger enhance overt aggression (see Graham, Hudley, & Williams, 1992). Finally, the motivational process may be as follows:

$$\text{Intentional aggression} \rightarrow \text{Anger} \rightarrow \text{Aggressive retaliation}$$

In this case, an inference of responsibility gives rise to anger, which then elicits aggression. Of course, still other sequences may be hypothesized (see Figure 6.1), including the possibility that overt aggression precedes feelings of anger.

Unfortunately, in contrast to the experimental analysis of helping, few studies in the aggression area have addressed the goal of discovering the motivational sequence, thereby distinguishing between the distal versus the proximal determinants of aggression (although this desire is implicit in many of the writings). I will next report an investigation by Betancourt and Blair (1992) that was undertaken to answer questions about the mediational role of anger, as well as sympathy, as determinants of overt hostility. Later in the chapter, when discussing individual differences in aggressive tendencies, another investigation (Graham et al., 1992) is introduced that also examines the sequence issue.

Betancourt and Blair (1992) had subjects respond to virtually the same questionnaire that was provided in Experiment 7.1. The research participants read the two scenarios and completed scales assessing the controllability and the intentionality of the act of breaking the window; their feelings of anger, pity, and sympathy at the rock-thrower; and the likelihood that they would retaliate with an act of violence.

The mean responses on these measures are given in Table 7.1. It is evident that when the window was broken "on purpose," the action was rated as more controllable and intentional, there were greater reports of anger and less feelings of pity and sympathy, and a more violent reaction

TABLE 7.1. Mean Ratings of Perceived Controllability,
Perceived Intentionality, and Subjects' Reported Emotions
and Reactions toward the Instigator for Each Condition

|                        | Accidental | Purposeful |
|------------------------|------------|------------|
| Controllability        | 3.22       | 4.89       |
| Intentionality         | 1.77       | 5.34       |
| Anger                  | 2.78       | 4.82       |
| Sympathy               | 4.62       | 2.83       |
| Pity                   | 4.65       | 3.64       |
| Violence of reaction   | 1.82       | 3.18       |

*Note.* From Betancourt and Blair (1992, p. 347). Copyright 1992 by
Sage Publications, Inc. Reprinted by permission. Ratings were made on
scales from 1 to 7; higher numbers indicate greater perceived controllability and intentionality, more intense emotions, and more violent
reactions.

was planned than when the breakage was accidental. The readers should
now compare their responses (not all of these variables were assessed) with
the data in Table 7.1. I am fairly confident that there will be a close
correspondence with the pattern that has been reported.

Next, the correlations between the variables were determined (this is
not possible for the readers to compute without including the data of other
respondents). These correlations are given in Table 7.2. It is apparent from
Table 7.2 that controllability and intentionality, two factors that contribute

TABLE 7.2. Correlations between Attribution Situations, Perceived Attributional
Properties, Emotions toward the Instigator, and Reactions ($N = 154$)

|                          | Situation | Controllability | Intentionality | Anger   | Sympathy | Pity   |
|--------------------------|-----------|-----------------|----------------|---------|----------|--------|
| Attribution situation    |           |                 |                |         |          |        |
| Controllability          | .46*      |                 |                |         |          |        |
| Intentionality           | .79**     | .50**           |                |         |          |        |
| Anger                    | .55**     | .27**           | .54**          |         |          |        |
| Sympathy                 | −.48**    | −.33**          | −.55**         | −.35**  |          |        |
| Pity                     | −.26*     | −.25*           | −.37**         | −.12    | .69**    |        |
| Violence of reaction     | .55**     | .32**           | .53**          | .47**   | −.44**   | −.29*  |

*Note.* From Betancourt and Blair (1992, p. 347). Copyright 1992 by Sage Publications, Inc. Reprinted by permission.
$*p < .01.$  $**p < .001.$

to responsibility, relate positively with anger and negatively with sympathy and pity. In addition, controllability and intentionality, as well as anger, are positively associated with reports of hostile actions, whereas sympathy and pity are related negatively to stated reactive aggression.

Finally, Betancourt and Blair (1992) analyzed these data with path techniques that were able to isolate the relations between the variables, holding all other associations constant. A simplified version of the path best representing the data is shown in Figure 7.2, which reveals that responsibility (determined by the scores of controllability and intentionality) relates positively to anger and negatively to the "empathic" emotions of pity and sympathy. Inferences of responsibility then directly influence aggressive retaliation and also indirectly affect hostility through the more proximal emotional reactions. This supports the sequence depicted in Model 2 in Figure 6.1.

Note, therefore, that in this research the best representation of the motivational sequence is not a linear ordering of thinking, feeling, and action, for both thinking and feeling directly relate to behavior, with thinking (beliefs about responsibility) the more dominant influence. Recall that in the prior chapter it was suggested that the more removed the respondent is from an action, the greater the contribution of "cold" thoughts relative to "hot" emotions as determinants of conduct. In this study, the respondent was relatively removed from the vignettes (the respondent was not even asked to imagine him- or herself as the damaged party). This may account for the fact that emotions played a reduced (albeit significant) role in guiding conduct.

In sum, Betancourt and Blair (1992) addressed the issue of motivational sequence and ascertained the proximal versus the distal antecedents of aggressive action. Of course, this was a hypothetical or role enactment context, with all of the shortcomings (as well as all of the benefits) of this procedure. We know that one swallow doth not a summer make; much more research, some presented later in the chapter, is needed to resolve these complex issues regarding temporal order. But Betancourt and Blair (1992) have contributed to this goal.

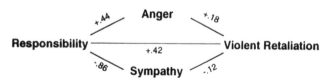

FIGURE 7.2. Structural equation analysis of the determinants of violent reactions. Data from Betancourt and Blair (1992, pp. 343–350).

## INDIVIDUAL DIFFERENCES IN
## AGGRESSIVE TENDENCIES

As indicated at the start of this chapter, one of the most popular research pursuits in the area of aggression is to examine individuals who differ in aggressive tendencies. Geneticists, trait theorists, and developmental psychologists have been equally involved in this endeavor. Geneticists have looked within the organism to identify specific carriers of an "aggressive" gene; trait theorists have constructed instruments to assess the stability and generality of aggressive tendencies; and developmentalists have considered the child-rearing practices that produce an aggressive personality and have searched for the cognitive and affective correlates (or causes) of aggression among children.

Among the developmental psychologists, the conception of responsibility advocated here has been incorporated within a broader theoretical framework. This is known as the social–cognitive or social–informational approach to aggression. As clarified by Dodge and Crick (1990):

> This theory of aggressive events considers the cognitive processes involved in an individual's response to a provocative social stimulus ... [and] relies heavily on an understanding of how individuals perceive cues, make attributions and inferences about those cues, generate solutions to interpersonal cues and problems, and make behavioral decisions about how to respond to those problems (including the decision to aggress). ... The social–cognitive theory maintains that an aggressive response is not inevitable but, rather, is contingent on specific thoughts and patterns of processing information. (p. 9)

This perspective has been supported by an array of empirical evidence. For example, relations have been reported between aggression and favorable self-evaluations for aggressive behavior (Asarnow & Callan, 1985), the anticipation of positive interpersonal outcomes from behaving aggressively (Perry, Perry, & Rasmussen, 1986), and failure to generate alternative solutions (other than aggression) to interpersonal difficulties (Slaby & Guerra, 1988). Recent elaborations of this framework have extended the range of cognitive variables and cognitive deficits that bear upon aggressive behavior in children (see review in Dodge & Crick, 1990).

Taken as a whole, theoretical reasoning and empirical research lend credulity to the belief that dysfunctional cognitive interpretations of the social world provide clues to the understanding of some types of hostile responding. In addition, these characteristic ways of thinking become resistant to change (Huesmann, 1988) and thereby provide the mechanisms for the establishment of individual differences in aggressive tendencies.

Given the focus of this book, what is of prime interest is to determine if aggressive and nonaggressive individuals differ systematically in their inferences about the responsibility of others for untoward events. That is, does the meaning of an event differ between persons who are aggressive and those who are nonaggressive? If so, then this would be a plausible mechanism that could give rise to hostility among the aggressive children.

## Biases in Perceptions of Hostile Intent

Perhaps the main focus of the social–cognitive approach to aggression is on biased inferences regarding the intentionality of others to act aggressively. Knowing that attributions of hostile intent relate to aggressive behavioral reactions (as just reviewed), researchers have hypothesized that individual differences in the tendency to behave aggressively are related to the inclination to ascribe hostile intentions to peers following an action that appears to have a hostile goal (the role of anger in the intention–aggression linkage has not been widely addressed, with the exception of Graham et al., 1992).

Dodge and his colleagues (see Dodge & Crick, 1990) particularly have been associated with this position. In one of the earlier investigations testing the biased inference hypothesis, Dodge (1980) first identified aggressive and nonaggressive boys based on teacher and peer ratings. The children, who were tested individually, were given a puzzle assembly task to complete with the possibility of winning a prize. During the middle of the task, they were interrupted and taken into an adjoining room where they could view a puzzle supposedly being worked on by another child. At this time, they "overheard" a bogus intercom system conveying that this child also was examining their partially completed puzzle. The child was then heard destroying the puzzle. Two experimental conditions conveyed that the damage was done purposefully ("I don't want him to win") or accidentally ("Oh, no, I didn't mean to drop it"). In a third condition, the cause of the damage was unknown. After receiving this information, the child was left alone in the adjoining room and was videotaped to observe his behavioral reactions, particularly to note if there was aggressive retaliation by damaging the other child's puzzle.

Both aggressive and nonaggressive children reacted to the hostile intent condition with retaliatory aggression, whereas given the accidental damage they acted with aggressive restraint. Of most importance, in the ambiguous condition the aggressive children behaved more aggressively than did the nonaggressive ones. Indeed, their aggression in this condition did not significantly differ from the condition in which the damage was intentional, thus suggesting a similar interpretation of these two scenarios. On the other hand, among the nonaggressive boys hostility was significantly lower in the ambiguous than in the intentional condition.

In a follow-up to this study, these same children were presented with vignettes in which a peer either spilled some milk on them or hit them when throwing a ball. The stories were worded ambiguously with regard to intention. Again, only the children identified as aggressive were more likely to see this act as intentional rather than accidental. These children also expected that the other child would continue to behave aggressively and revealed greater distrust of this person than did the children identified as nonaggressive.

Dodge (1980) therefore concluded that aggressive children do not suffer deficits in their ability to integrate information about intention as a behavioral determinant, as some had suggested. Rather, they engage in cue distortion, exhibiting what has been labeled a hostile attributional bias (Nasby, Hayden, & dePaulo, 1980).

In a sequel to this research, Dodge and Frame (1982) again presented ambiguous aggressive-intent stories to aggressive and nonaggressive children. In these vignettes, the negative outcomes were directed either toward another peer or toward the subject. In this manner, it could be determined if the attributional bias uncovered in earlier studies "represented an expectation that peers will act with hostile intent toward all others (a cynical view of their peers) or an expectation that peers will act with hostile intent only toward the subject (a paranoid view of their peers)" (Dodge & Frame, 1982, p. 621). The intent inferences, shown in Figure 7.3, reveal that when

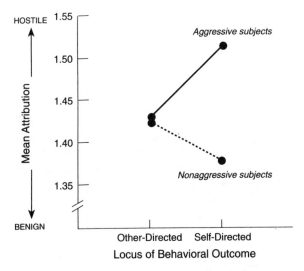

FIGURE 7.3. Subject's attributions of peers' intentions as a function of the subject's aggressive status and the locus of the behavioral outcome. From Dodge and Frame (1982, p. 623). Copyright 1982 by the American Psychological Association. Reprinted by permission.

aggression is directed toward others, there are no differences in ascriptions of intent between the aggressive and the nonaggressive children. However, aggressive subjects infer greater intentionality than do the nonaggressive ones when they are the targets of the hostility. Thus, this information-processing bias is uniquely self-related. In addition, the data revealed that there was reported aggressive retaliation only when a hostile intent was ascribed to the peer.

Earlier in this chapter, it was stated that the responsibility approach advocated here is not applicable to situations in which the aggression is not retaliatory. Inferences of responsibility are not readily amenable to the explanation of unprovoked murder, rape, and the like. Dodge and Coie (1987) also incorporate this position and suggest that the "tendency to over-attribute hostile intent to others is more closely linked to reactive aggression than to proactive aggression" (p. 1146).

To examine this hypothesis, Dodge and Coie (1987) developed a teacher-rating instrument to distinguish between "reactive" and "proactive" aggressive behaviors in children. One of the "proactive" items on the scale was, "The child uses physical force in order to dominate other kids," whereas one of the reactive-aggression statements was, "When this child is teased or threatened, he or she gets angry easily and strikes back." Scores on these two scales were highly intercorrelated ($r = .76$), although there nonetheless was suggestive evidence for maintaining the distinction between the two types of aggressive tendencies. Subsequent studies found that children who were identified as "proactive" aggressive were rated by their peers as bothersome and disruptive but that they were also viewed as leaders and having other positive attributes. These favorable characteristics were not expressed about children who were "reactive" aggressive.

The studies by Dodge and others thus tell a systematic and understandable story (although it must be acknowledged that the data are not as straightforward as have been presented here and that the investigations are not without ambiguity). The simplest story (one that overlooks any empirical inconsistencies) is that there is a subgroup of identifiable children who are inclined to attribute intent following an ambiguously caused event that has an adverse effect on them. Retaliation follows from the biased ascription that the other acted "on purpose." Thus, the manner in which a child attends to and interprets an adverse incident appears to be an enduring structure and provides a mechanism to account for persistent aggressive retaliation (see Graham & Hudley, 1992; Graham, Hudley, & Williams, 1992).

## Utilizing the Full Theory

Although Dodge and his colleagues have related biased ascriptions regarding intent (perceptions of responsibility) to subsequent aggression, they have generally ignored the possible role of anger as a mediator between thinking and action. Further, they have not attempted to determine if inferences of responsibility directly or indirectly result in aggressive retaliation (as have Betancourt & Blair, 1992). As elaborated by Graham and Hudley (1992):

> Although this research [of Dodge] capitalizes on an implicit attribution–behavior linkage, the processes relating intentionality perceptions to peer-directed aggression have yet to be fully explored. Why, for example, does perceiving a classmate as responsible for a negative event lead to hostile reactions? That is, what intervening thoughts and feelings might account for the cognition-to-action sequence suggested by Dodge's work? Dodge and others studying childhood aggression from a social cognitive perspective have not yet addressed this question. (p. 78)

To test the full responsibility conception presented here, Graham et al. (1992) first identified aggressive and nonaggressive young adolescents through the usual peer-nomination and teacher-rating techniques. Then these children were administered an attributional questionnaire in which they read short scenarios that included a negative experience and were asked to imagine themselves in these stories.

The negative experience was accompanied by information that this incident, which involved a hypothetical peer, was accompanied by prosocial, accidental, ambiguous, or hostile intent. For example, one theme that involved a homework assignment and ambiguous intent read as follows:

> Imagine that you are on your way to school one morning. You are walking onto the school grounds. At that moment, you happen to look down and notice that your shoelace is untied. You put the notebook that you are carrying down on the ground to tie your shoelace. An important homework paper that you worked on for a long time falls out of your notebook. Just then, another kid you know walks by and steps on the paper, leaving a muddy footprint right across the middle. The other kid looks down at your homework paper and then up at you. (Graham et al., 1992, pp. 733–734)

Prosocial intent was communicated by the peer's indicating that he did this to keep the paper from blowing away, accidental intent was conveyed by the peer's apology that he did not see the homework paper, and hostile intent was depicted by the peer's laughing as he stepped on the paper.

The subjects then indicated attributions about intent (i.e., Did the peer do this on purpose?), how angry they would feel if this had happened to them, and they judged the likelihood that they would engage in behaviors that differed in the degree of hostile retaliation. Thus, data to more fully test the responsibility conception were gathered.

It was found that aggressive children were more likely than the nonaggressive ones to believe that the peer acted with hostile intention. Furthermore, this was especially the case when the situation was ambiguous. In addition, the aggressive children also expressed greater anger, and more of the aggressive than nonaggressive children endorsed hostile retaliation.

To explore the applicability of the responsibility → anger → aggression conception, path coefficients were reported between these variables for both groups of children (see Figure 7.4). Figure 7.4 reveals that the best model for both nonaggressive and aggressive children is from thinking to feeling to action, that is, from aggressive intent to anger to aggressive retaliation. Graham et al. (1992) also tested models that start with intent but do not include anger as a mediator or that start with anger and have intent as the more proximal determinant of aggression. Neither of these fit the data.

One great advantage of a motivational process with multiple paths is that there may be many points of intervention to change the final behavioral reaction. Given the findings by Graham et al. (1992), aggression theoretically could be reduced if ascriptions of intent were lessened, if emotions other than anger could be elicited in spite of perceptions of responsibility, and if reactions could be modified even with the experience of anger. Hudley and Graham (1993) set out to reduce the overt hostility of aggressive African American boys by creating a program that attempted to influence perceptions of intentionality and inferences of responsibility.

Among the components of Hudley and Graham's 6-week program were procedures to augment aggressive children's ability to accurately detect intention. This was accomplished by means of role-playing and discussion of personal experiences. Videotaped scenarios helped discriminate intentional from ambiguously caused or accidentally caused negative incidents.

To assess the effectiveness of their program, pre- and postmeasures of intentions, affects, and endorsed behaviors regarding an ambiguously caused hostile event were assessed. These ratings are displayed in Figure 7.5. Figure 7.5 includes the data of two control groups. One group, labeled "control," received no intervening treatment; the group labeled "at-

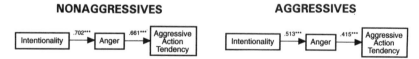

**NONAGGRESSIVES**          **AGGRESSIVES**

FIGURE 7.4. Path models for nonaggressive and aggressive children relating intent to anger to aggressive tendency. Data from Graham et al. (1992).

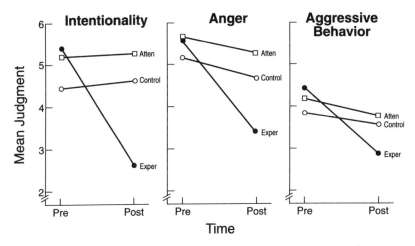

FIGURE 7.5. Pre- and postexperimental intent attributions, anger, and aggressive action as a function of the treatment condition. From Graham and Hudley (1992, p. 88). Copyright 1992 by Lawrence Erlbaum Associates, Inc. Reprinted by permission.

ten(tion)" was given irrelevant training to improve their attention span and focus. Figure 7.5 shows that only in the experimental (intention) intervention group were there decreases in judgments of intent, anger, and aggressive behavior regarding the hypothetical hostile event.

Furthermore, at the end of the training period the subjects were placed in an experimental setting where they communicated with an unseen peer. These two had to cooperate to reach a goal; but, unbeknownst to the pairs, they received contradictory information from the experimenter that impeded their performance and elicited mutual frustration.

The experimenters measured the perceived intentionality of the misbehavior of the peer, reports of anger, and actual behavioral aggression expressed during the task. Table 7.3 shows that aggressive children in the experimental intervention group inferred less intent, reported less anger, and actually exhibited less aggressive behavior (insults, criticisms, and complaints) than the aggressive children placed in the control group or receiving attention training. On the bases of these data, Graham and Hudley (1992) concluded:

> Peer-directed aggression by young Black males is, to at least a modest degree, predictable by these children's causal thoughts and consequent emotions. Furthermore, it is possible to reduce their tendency to respond with hostility by changing the way they causally construe a social dilemma. (p. 90)

**TABLE 7.3.** Attributions to Intent, Reported Anger, and Verbal Behavior in the Analogue Task by Treatment Group

| | Treatment group | | |
| --- | --- | --- | --- |
| Variable | Experimental ($n = 20$) | Attention training ($n = 24$) | Control ($n = 24$) |
| Intentionality | 2.3 | 4.5 | 4.7 |
| Anger | 1.7 | 2.5 | 2.6 |
| Behavior (% total) | | | |
|    Neutral | 61% | 29 | 31 |
|    Complaining | 20 | 25 | 31 |
|    Criticizing | 19 | 29 | 23 |
|    Insulting | 0 | 17 | 15 |

*Note.* From Graham and Hudley (1992, p. 89). Copyright 1992 by Lawrence Erlbaum Associates, Inc. Reprinted by permission. Rating scales for intentionality and anger range from 1 to 7. High numbers indicate greater perceived intent and more intense anger.

# CHILD ABUSE

Prior to an examination of child abuse from a perceived responsibility or "sin" perspective, let me repeat a position that needs restating throughout this book. Behaviors such as help giving, aggression, and even the more specific aggression of child abuse are overdetermined—many factors contribute to these actions. In addition, quite different antecedent conditions may result in the same behavior. As intimated earlier, one may help one's mother because social norms dictate such behavior, because help is given to ingroup members, because it will lead to a large inheritance, or because the mother is perceived as not responsible for her plight, which elicits sympathy and prosocial responses. Only the latter motivational process has been of central concern in this book. In a similar manner, one may aggress toward another and take his or her money because of frustration caused by job loss or as retribution for an unjustified, intentional act that the other committed. This elicits anger and antisocial reactions. Only the latter source of motivation has been of importance in this book. And in the following analysis of child abuse, it is acknowledged that abuse has diverse origins and many determinants. There will not be only one "abusive" psychological configuration of antecedents such that if, and only if, these conditions are met abuse will follow. As a recent review by Belsky (1993) concluded: "All too sadly, there are many pathways to child abuse" (p. 413). There is, however, a particular confluence of factors that I suggest will increase the likelihood of child abuse, and this aggressive response is understandable and interpretable from a responsibility framework. This analysis also generates suggestions of how to intervene and decrease the likelihood of parental aggression. I will present this conceptual framework in the following pages, guided by the empirical literature in the abuse area.

I begin with the assumption that aggression (in this case, child abuse) is retaliatory (even though the punishment far exceeds the crime). That is, an event has happened. For this event to have psychological significance, the parents (I will use this label to represent any adult caretaker) must be aware of the incident. Awareness will increase if the parents and the children are in close proximity. This is more likely if the child is an infant; if there are crowded living conditions; if the parents are unemployed and, therefore, at home; if there are other children, which could increase the likelihood of parental presence; and so on. So important are these demographic predictors of abuse that Light (1973) concluded that unemployment was the single factor most frequently differentiating abusive from nonabusive families (see also Belsky, 1980, 1993; however, I do not believe that it remains the *most* differentiating factor). Of course, unemployment is associated with many other antecedents and consequences, including greater personal instability among the antecedents and increased frustration, stress, and need among the consequences. In this context, however, what is emphasized is that it increases the likelihood that a child's behavior will have a psychological reality to the parent.

Given that the parent(s) are present to observe the behavior of the child, another necessary antecedent of subsequent abuse already intimated is that the behavior must be perceived as negative. There is a great deal of evidence that particular characteristics of the child result in "bad" behavior. Children who are particularly active or are temperamentally disposed toward having a colicky disposition are more likely to be associated with negative outcomes and to be abused (see Belsky, 1993).

In addition to the eliciting actions of these children, it also is the case that abusive parents have less tolerance for the typical negative behavior of children than nonabusive parents do. For example, abusive parents are more annoyed by crying (Frodi & Lamb, 1980). Finally, the demographic factors mentioned earlier, such as living space, increase the occurrence of annoying incidents including, for example, interfering with the movements of others, breakage, and so on. It has been reported, for example, that hyperactive children are "bottlenecks" in the home.

To summarize the discussion thus far, it has been suggested that an act of abuse is initiated when a caretaker perceives an event and when that event is psychologically bothersome. The next step in the abusive sequence relates to the parent's interpretation of the cause of this incident. In the prior section of this chapter, it was contended that the cause (act) must be perceived as controllable and that the person must be held responsible in order for there to be an aggressive retaliation. At one time in the history of the study of child abuse, it was believed that a key antecedent of abuse was unrealistic parental expectations regarding the development of the child "and a corresponding disregard for the infant's or child's own needs, limited abilities, and helplessness" (Spinetta & Rigler, 1972, p. 299). Hence, abusive parents were characterized as lacking child-rearing knowledge; it was their false expectations and inferences of controllability that differentiated these individuals from others who did not abuse their children (see Steele & Pollack, 1968). This hypothesis is still regarded as plausible, although there are published reports that abusive parents in fact do not differ from nonabusive parents in child-related expectations (see, for example, Altemeier, O'Connor, Vietze, Sandler, & Sherrod, 1982; Twentyman & Plotkin, 1982).

Related to this point is the position that abusive parents tend to perceive that an adverse act was committed intentionally by the child and/or that the child was in relative control over this behavior. Bugenthal and her colleagues have espoused this position (see, e.g., Bugenthal, 1987; Bugenthal, Blue, & Cruzcosa, 1989). In one pertinent research investigation, Bugenthal et al. (1989) had parents assign importance ratings to the causes of caregiving success and failure. These investigators concluded:

> Abusive mothers were found to be more likely than nonabusive mothers to believe that they can do little to prevent negative caregiving outcomes; at the same time, they were more likely to believe that children can control such outcomes. . . . When [children who are more likely to be targeted for abuse] are paired with adults with low perceived control, a dysfunctional match is created. The annoyance that such caregivers experience can be thought of as reflecting a combined frustration with their own [in]ability to change the child's behavior and an irritation with the child for "deliberately" acting to create an aversive situation. (pp. 538–539)

MacKinnon-Lewis and her colleagues (1992) reached somewhat similar conclusions regarding biased interpretations of intent by abusive mothers. These experimenters first had their parent–child subject pairs make attributions about intentions in a series of hypothetical vignettes that were ambiguous regarding intent. For example, one story told to the mothers was the following: "Pretend you and your child are playing a board game. You are almost to the finish line and you are winning. Your child knocks the pieces off the board onto the floor" (p. 406). Responses to the inquiry, "Why do you think your child would do this?" were then coded for hostile intent (as opposed to accidental behavior).

In addition, the mother and child were observed while participating in two gamelike tasks. As predicted, it was found that negative perceptions of the other's general intent were related to the likelihood that the individuals would initiate a negative or coercive interchange during the game. This was true for both children and their mothers. The experimenters concluded that "the associations between mother's and children's attributions and behavior underscore the importance of studying the effects of social cognitive biases on coercive and aggressive parent–child interaction" (MacKinnon-Lewis et al., 1992, p. 413).

In yet another study consistent with the conceptual analysis suggested here, Golub (1984) asked parents to discuss any recent positive and negative incidents associated with something that their children did. Golub found that parents of abused children were more likely to infer that the child was intentionally misbehaving (see also Bauer & Twentyman, 1985; Larrance & Twentyman, 1983). They also rated this incident as more serious than the nonabusive parents did.

An abusive adult, then, is more likely to be aware of a negative event, is more likely to label it as adverse, and is more likely than nonabusive parents to infer that it was intentionally caused by the child. The next step in this motivational sequence is to proceed from intention to anger, a linkage documented throughout this book, and to ask as well if sympathetic reactions elicited by the incident or by the parental response to it are relatively absent among abusive caretakers.

The affective descriptions of high anger, negative emotional states, and lack of sympathy frequently are reported in the pertinent abuse literature (see Belsky, 1993). Concerning parental anger, Engfer and Schneewind (1982), for example, found that parental "anger-proneness" was related to harsher child-rearing punishment (see also Golub, 1984). Indeed, some intervention programs created to lessen child abuse primarily are targeted at anger management and are based on the assumptions that abusive parents are easily angered and that anger gives rise to harsh reactions (see Ambrose, Hazzard, & Haworth, 1980).

Emotional reactions of sympathy also are pertinent to nonabuse. Regarding the absence of sympathy among abusive parents, a summary by Belsky (1980) is informative:

> One question that must be raised in this connection is why the victim's pain and suffering does not function to inhibit abusive behavior [as documented in the prior section of this chapter in the research by Baron, 1971]. Consideration of the abuser's own rearing as a child may shed light on this issue. Feshbach and Feshbach (1974) have demonstrated that the inhibitory effect of pain feedback may be dependent on the development of empathy. If this social skill develops through a warm, caring parent–child relationship, as has been sug-

gested . . . then the emotional deprivation that has frequently been noted by clinicians as characteristic of child abusers . . . may very well be responsible for their apparent insensitivity to the pain they cause in their victims. (pp. 325–326)

Finally, the presence of anger and absence of sympathy to their inflicted pain promote antisocial conduct, including harsh physical punishment. Thus, the following sequence or process is suggested as describing the antecedent course of an act of abuse:

Unemployed parent in small living quarters observes incident →
Incident is perceived as aversive → Parent infers controllability
and intentionality (i.e., that the child is responsible) →
Anger → Punishment (without sympathy as an inhibitor)

In addition to being consistent with the prior discussion of aggression, this analysis emphasizes the effects not only of parents on children but also of children on parents. It takes into account the mutual effects of behavior as well as the importance of the way in which events are interpreted or explained.

It is apparent from this line of reasoning that intervention can involve a number of procedures with quite disparate immediate goals in mind. Employment that takes parents from the home or larger living space that makes negative incidents less likely to occur and be observed should result in reduced abuse. Similarly, increasing parental knowledge so that incidents are less likely to be perceived as intentional and controllable, particularly if they are beyond the capabilities of the child, also theoretically will decrease abuse (see Golub, Espinosa, Damon, & Card, 1987). And anger management, as advocated by Ambrose et al. (1980), as well as empathy training, may be effective, even if the antecedents of anger remain unchanged. Indeed, it can safely be stated that if intervening processes and mechanisms include multiple steps and stages, then intervention is possible at any of these steps and theoretically can result in behavioral change.

A similar conclusion was reached in the recent comprehensive review by Belsky (1993). He stated:

There is no single solution to the problem of child maltreatment. A variety of targets of intervention exist, ranging from the specific caregiving behavior of a parent to the social conditions that make it difficult for parents to be emotionally sensitive and psychologically available to their offspring. To be noted, however, is that the research literature . . . does not enable the research community to determine yet which intervention targets are either most likely to prevent or remediate child maltreatment or which are most easily or effectively modified. (p. 413)

## SPOUSAL ABUSE

Abuse in the family certainly is not limited to children. The reported incidents of spousal beating (particularly of husbands battering wives), and even abuse toward parents and grandparents, is increasing. Holtzworth-Munroe and her colleagues (e.g., Holtzworth-Munroe, 1992; Holtzworth-Munroe & Hutchinson, 1993; Holtzworth-Munroe, Jacobson, Fehrenbach, & Fruzetti, 1992) have pursued an attributional interpretation of spousal abuse that is consistent with the prior analysis of child beating. Building on the work of Bradbury and Fincham (1990) (reviewed in Chapter 5) and Dodge and his colleagues, Holtzworth-Munroe and Hutchinson (1993) suggest:

> Violent husbands are more likely than nonviolent husbands to attribute hostile intent to wife behaviors. . . . In situations in which a husband attributes hostile intent to his wife's actions, there is an increased risk of violence because such interpretations ("She was trying to hurt me") may increase the likelihood that the husband will choose a violent response to the situation (e.g., "My violence is a justified retaliation"). (p. 206)

In one test of this hypothesis, husbands in violent, distressed but nonviolent, and normal spousal relationships were identified. A number of hypothetical situations were created, and scales were rated to assess the extent to which the wife acted with negative intent and deserved to be blamed for her actions in these situations. A typical scenario was the following: "You are at a social gathering and you notice that for the past half-hour your wife has been talking and laughing with the same attractive man. He seems to be flirting with her."

The data clearly revealed that violent husbands attributed greater intent to and blamed their wives more than husbands in distressed but nonviolent relationships and husbands in nondistressed relationships. This was particularly the case when the depicted scenarios involved jealousy, rejection from the wife, and potential public embarrassment. Hence, the findings are consistent with the portrayal of abusive parents as overattributing intent. The data therefore support the theme that aggression is instigated by causal beliefs and inferences of responsibility—that is, aggression is a reaction to the sin of another. In this research, as in the majority of studies reviewed in this chapter, anger and sympathy were not assessed, nor was responsibility, and there was no attempt to develop and test a more complete motivational representation of the phenomenon.


## INTERGROUP AND INTERNATIONAL CONFLICT

It is risky to generalize explanations at the individual level to issues that involve groups or nations (see Betancourt, 1990b). The same processes might not be operative at both levels, and for group and national issues molar analyses may prove more fruitful than conceptions that have evolved from the study of the person. Nonetheless, there are reasons to believe that the framework of responsibility presented in the prior pages also is applicable to conflicts involving larger structural entities. An example of a concept that is useful at the personal level and that appears generalizable to larger structures, and that is pertinent to the conception presented in this book, is known as "vicarious personalism" (Cooper & Fazio, 1979). As noted by Betancourt (1990b):

> Cooper and Fazio define "vicarious personalism" as a group's perception of the behavior of another group as intended for them. This phenomenon is supposed to be equivalent to personalism at the interpersonal level. For example, Japanese business people may perceive a U.S. policy to impose a tax on imports as a measure against their economy, intended to harm them, even when the actual motivation may be to increase revenues or something else. (p. 207)

If the interpretation suggested in the above quotation is "correct," and if the conception presented in the prior pages also has some validity, then the Japanese should be angry at the United States and would be goaded to retaliate with some sort of hostile response.

The largest body of group research pertinent to the relation between responsibility and aggression concerns intergroup attributions (see Hewstone, 1989). The typical paradigm in these investigations is to present subjects with hypothetical examples of positive and negative behaviors of their in-group (for instance, others who share, their national, ethnic, and religious identity), as well as examples of positive and negative behaviors of an out-group. For example, Hindu and Muslim respondents might be told that a Hindu (Muslim) person was generous to (or neglected) a stranger in need (note in this case the out-group also is in some conflict with the in-group). Then beliefs regarding the cause of this behavior are examined.

The typical finding in this research is a "hedonic bias," that is, favorable actions by the in-group members are attributed to internal factors (e.g., their dispositions), whereas unfavorable conduct is ascribed to the situation. The reverse pattern of ascriptions characterizes the behavior of the out-group—that is, negative behaviors are attributed to their dispositions or other internal factors, whereas positive actions are attributed to the situation (see reviews in Hewstone, 1989; Weber, 1993). There is some question, however, about the symmetry of these effects. Weber (1993) has contended that there is a greater tendency to externalize the negative behavior of the in-group as well as the positive behavior of the out-group more than there is a bias to internalize in-group positive behavior and out-group negative behavior.

Only recently has this research begun to take into consideration the concepts of controllability and, by implication, responsibility (although these often are implicitly conceived as part of internality). In addition, affective reactions also are just beginning to be incorporated into this research. In an investigation by Islam and Hewstone (1993), Hindu and Muslim respondents were presented with both positive and negative in-group and out-group behaviors. The respondents then indicated the controllability as well as the internality of the cause of the behavior. This study included behavioral examples of nonaggressive as well as aggressive in-group and outgroup behavior, so caution must be exercised when considering this as an investigation concerned solely with aggression. Nonetheless, as anticipated, out-group negative behavior was inferred by the in-group to be more controllable than was out-group positive behavior. In addition, anger was maximized when a negative act was ascribed to something internal to the out-group.

In a recent study of actual international conflict, Bizman and Hoffman (1993) made use of attribution theory to shed light on the Arab–Israeli conflict. Israelis were first classified as politically left (liberal) or center (relatively conservative). They then were asked about the causes of the Arab–Israeli conflict. Among other responses, the Israeli participants indicated whether the conflict was under Arab or Israeli control; they disclosed a number of emotional reactions to the conflict, including anger and guilt; and they also responded to some questions about resolution of the conflict, including the use of force.

It was found that those who were politically conservative, relative to the liberals, perceived greater Arab than Israeli control over the problem, reported greater anger, and were more willing to use force. Furthermore, they revealed greater feelings of anger than guilt. On the other hand, relative to the conservatives, the liberals perceived more Israeli than Arab control over the conflict, reported higher personal guilt, and believed less in the use of force. They also revealed more intense feelings of guilt than anger. In sum, two patterns appeared in the data:

Conservative: Belief that Arab control is relatively greater than Israeli control; low guilt; high anger; hostile action

Liberal: Belief that Israeli control is relatively greater than Arab control; high guilt; low anger; withholding of hostile action

These patterns should remind the reader of the findings presented in prior chapters that conservatives hold others responsible for such stigmas as obesity and poverty. This belief gave rise to high anger, little pity, and the withholding of aid. The opposite pattern was displayed by liberals.

In conclusion, there is reason to believe that the conception that has proved so useful at the individual level also has value as an explanation of some phenomena at the group and national level—that is, the same processes are evident across different types of structures. This is an important extension that opens up many new avenues of research.

## SUMMARY

When a student fails to exert effort, the teacher is angry and is likely to reprimand that student; when a person is in need because he or she failed to help him- or herself, others are angry and withhold aid; and when a person is hit "on purpose," that person becomes angry and there is a tendency to retaliate. Hence, across an array of settings, inferences of responsibility evoke anger, and anger is a goad to action. The type of behavior undertaken may vary greatly; but broadly conceived, the reaction is negative and directed against the transgressor. For the failing student or the needy person, the sin is not sufficient to involve the justice system. However, if an act of aggression is sufficiently severe, then criminal proceedings may be initiated. In this case, the sin against a person is punishable by society.

In the present chapter, I first examined the linkages between inferences of responsibility and anger, and then between anger and aggression. The first of these relations is supported by self-report studies that ask people to describe instances in which they were angry. These reports reveal that anger is elicited primarily by an intended transgression. In addition, experimental studies that manipulate perceptions of the intention of an aggressive action find that intention influences anger (as well as aggressive retaliation). Specifically, investigators have frequently reported that the intended magnitude of an aversive stimulus delivered by another person, rather than the actual magnitude of the delivered stimulation, relates to self-reports of anger. In addition to this, that anger is associated with aggressive retaliation. In contrast to the enhancing effects of intention and anger on aggression, cues that elicit sympathy and empathy such as pain decrease aggressive responding.

Path analytical techniques have been used to determine the motivational ordering or sequence that relates thinking, feeling, and behavior—respectively, inferences of responsibility, anger and sympathy, and aggression. Responsibility directly relates to both the affects and the behavior and indirectly relates to aggression via the mediational effects of emotion. Hence, both thinking and feeling may have proximal influences on aggressive conduct.

I then considered individual differences in aggression in children. It has been reported that aggressive children tend to see ambiguous negative acts as intentionally caused, which then promotes anger and retaliation. Path models in this area of study find that anger is the proximal determinant of retaliation, while inferences of responsibility (intent) are distal determinants. Change programs have been reported that reduce anger and overt aggression by teaching children to be better able to label an unintended aggressive action and to distinguish when the cause of an act was unintentional or unclear.

I then examined child and spousal abuse and international conflict from this theoretical perspective. Regarding child abuse, I argued that demographic variables including unemployment and crowded housing increase the likelihood that a negative action will be perceived by the potential abuser. In addition, this person is more likely to hold the child responsible and, hence, respond with anger. Anger, in turn, contributes to an aggressive reaction.

In a similar manner, in situations of international conflict, opposing countries or groups tend to see the other group as having control over the conflict. This is particularly true for individuals with conservative beliefs; for liberals, there is a greater tendency to maintain beliefs of self-control, which give rise to more guilt than anger.

There are two dominant social motivations: altruism and aggression. Both are amenable to an analysis that highlights the influence of inferences of responsibility and the affects elicited by this construal. Social transgressions can involve a sin of omission (not engaging in expected behavior) or a sin of commission (hurting someone else on purpose). These may elicit actions that involve going away from (neglect) or going against, but the goal in all these instances is antisocial, that is, doing something that the other does not desire. Phenotypically opposing responses can have the same meaning, which are made understandable by a genotypic analysis of the determinants of action.

# 8

---

# Reducing Inferences of Responsibility: Excuses and Confession

There are many kinds of fraud, not all of them criminal.
—ANITA BROOKNER, *Fraud*

He who excuses himself accuses himself.

If we confess our sins, He is faithful and righteous to forgive us.
—1 JOHN 1:9

If there is an unequivocal conclusion that can be reached on the basis of the evidence reviewed in this book, and surely confirmed by experiences in everyday life, it is that being responsible for a negative event has damaging consequences. Failure at an achievement task ascribed to lack of effort generates severe reprimand; stigmatization because of overeating, excessive drinking, sexual permissiveness, lack of financial care, and the like promote adverse reactions from others; unhappy mood states (depression) and withdrawal (schizophrenia) can give rise to criticism even by family members if it is believed that the affected persons are "not trying" to get better; need of class notes from fellow students and requests for financial assistance from the government are neglected if the needy person did not engage in activities to help him- or herself; and an act construed as hostile results in retaliation if it is thought that the conduct was intended.

In sum, humans are held accountable for the violation of social norms or transgressions that break social expectations. The conduct engenders "social predicaments" in that the event "casts undesired aspersions on the lineage, character, conduct, skills, or motives of an actor" (Schlenker, 1980, p. 125). The offense thus results in an account being requested and evaluated. According to Scott and Lyman (1968), an account is defined as "a statement made by a social actor to explain unanticipated or untoward behavior" (p. 46).

An account can be described with the language of commercial exchange. It often is said that we "owe," "give," or "offer" an account, while the reproacher then "receives," "accepts," or "refuses" this explanation. Thus, there is a mutual transaction. The account given often attempts to "neutralize" the negative evaluation or anticipated negative evaluation of the other (Scott & Lyman, 1968). That is, the account is a "conversational move" to prevent reprimand and punishment. Accounts, then, serve social and interpersonal needs and goals (they also may involve only the self, but this aspect of ego enhancement or ego defensiveness is not considered in this context).

Figure 1.1 outlined the (or *a*) responsibility process and provides a foundation for the classification of accounts. Note that in Figure 1.1 (see also Table 8.1) the responsibility process is initiated by a negative occurrence. First, then, one can deny the very event or the meaning of the event for which one is being held accountable. It could be effective to explain to one's parents that, for example, a math test was not yet taken or that it was not failed (when, in fact, it was taken and the test results were poor), that the allowance was saved and not spent foolishly (when indeed the latter was the case), or that the unkempt appearance that characterizes oneself is fashionable in school and is not considered repugnant by others. The strategy often is referred to as denial, which in this case is one type of lie.

Continuing with the responsibility process as shown in Figure 1.1 and Table 8.1, one might admit that the adverse outcome did take place, but that it was caused by an external agent or circumstances rather than by oneself. That is, there was not personal agency. For example, it could be conveyed that teacher bias was the cause of test failure or that a prank in the lunchroom or a malfunctioning juice machine is the reason that one's clothes are dirty. In these instances, the act or state is acknowledged, but the explanation of it is altered from the true cause (the self) to an external source.

Yet another tactic to reduce responsibility perceptions and, by implication, anger is to accept that the cause of a negative event is the self but to convey that this cause was not controllable. For example, exam failure could be said to be due to lack of math aptitude rather than to an absence

**TABLE 8.1.** The Responsibility Process Related to Strategies That Promote Nonresponsibility

| Stage in the responsibility process | Strategy |
| --- | --- |
| Negative outcome occurs | Disavow outcome (denial) |
| Outcome is ascribed by others to the self | Ascribe to external factors (excuse) |
| Outcome is ascribed by others to causes controllable by the self | Ascribe to uncontrollable causes (excuse) |
| No mitigating circumstances are perceived | Indicate mitigating circumstances (excuse and justification) |
| Responsibility inference is made | Apologize and confess |

of effort (see the research by Juvonen and Murdoch in Chapter 2) or that the poor attire is caused not by sloppiness, but by a lack of native ability to have a "good eye" for clothes. The word *excuse* (*ex* = "from," *cuse* = "cause," "i.e., from one cause to another") is often used to refer to any ascription shifted from the true intended and controllable causes to external or internal factors not controllable by the self.

Still further in the responsibility process, it can be accepted that the cause of a negative outcome was due to internal, controllable factors, while the presence of mitigating circumstances are communicated. Telling a teacher that failure to study for a test because of the need (decision) to provide aid to a sick grandmother illustrates the use of one common mitigator. As already discussed, this often is referred to as a justification—a higher moral goal was served. Other mitigators, such as a failure to differentiate right from wrong, can be considered as excuses in that they are not subject to personal alteration.

Finally, even if self-responsibility for an action is admitted, there are still strategic devices used to foster positive impression management. These include apology and confession. Confession represents a paradox in that the individual publicly accepts responsibility for an act, yet this has been shown to *decrease* anger and punishment. Unlike excuses, however, the mollifying effect of confession is not due to lessened responsibility for the transgression. The relations between the responsibility process and the strategies or maneuvers used to "repair the broken and restore the estranged" (Scott & Lyman, 1968, p. 46) are summarized in Table 8.1.

This chapter examines accounts—that is, explanations of or statments about the causes of behavior. Attention primarily is given to excuses, for this tactic has been extensively studied and is the most understood method of decreasing inferences of personal responsibility for a negative act. In addition, there is a detailed examination of confession and the mechanisms that account for its success. As usual, experiments for you to perform are introduced and the discussion is integrated within the larger theoretical framework presented in the prior chapters.

# EXCUSES

Before reading further, you are asked to complete Experiment 8.1. In Experiment 8.1, a number of social transgressions and their causes are given. You are asked to report what the consequences of publicly communicating the reason for the transgression would be. In addition, you are asked to reveal whether this reason would or would not be communicated, that is, would an excuse be provided rather than the real reason. Please complete this experiment now; later in the chapter, these responses will be examined. As usual, you should be as truthful as possible and avoid the desire to either please me or foil my obvious plans.

If you have completed Experiment 8.1, let us turn to the analysis of excuses. An excuse may be defined as a consciously used device, communicated to others who might be reprimanding, to decrease personal responsibility and, in turn, to reduce anger and/or punishment. As considered in this chapter, an excuse is not the truth (although it obviously may be in everyday life). Thus, here we consider incidents when others convey, for example, that their lateness was due to a traffic jam, when in fact this was not the case. Whether the excuse is true or false, the consequences may be the same; but when it is false, the excuse is a strategy, or a device, used only because of its functional value.

Excuses therefore attempt to change perceptions that one has sinned! In so doing, a positive image of the self is maintained and the strength of an interpersonal relationship is not damaged (see Weiner, 1992; Weiner, Figueroa-Munoz, & Kakihara, 1991).

The prevalence of excuses in everyday life is not known. There also is uncertainty about the contexts in which they are elicited (see McLaughlin, Cody, & Rosenstein, 1983), although it is reasonable to assume that they are more likely to be given if the consequences of a transgression are major rather than minor (Schlenker & Darby, 1981; also see McLaughlin et al., 1983). Inasmuch as the majority of social influence attempts are directed toward parents, siblings, roommates and friends, rather than strangers, close interpersonal contexts would be expected to be the dominant settings for giving excuses. Indeed, research has documented that nearly 75% of excuses are furnished in affiliate, as opposed to achievement, contexts (Weiner et al., 1991). Excuses thus primarily involve friendships, personal bonding, and the maintenance of the social fabric.

No doubt the prevalence of excuses is fostered by the fact that they generally go undetected. Inasmuch as the communication delivered by the

## EXPERIMENT 8.1
### Communicating Excuses

Assume that you had made arrangements with an acquaintance to attend a play together. However, you failed to meet him there. In the following, the reasons that you failed to appear are given. Indicate if you would reveal the true cause, if the other would hold you responsible, and how angry the other would be if the cause was revealed.

1. You failed to appear because of sudden illness and could not reach the other.

   a. Would you reveal this cause?

| 1 | 2 | 3 | 4 | 5 | 6 | 7 |
|---|---|---|---|---|---|---|

Definitely yes                                                    Definitely no

   b. How responsible would the other person hold you?

| 1 | 2 | 3 | 4 | 5 | 6 | 7 |
|---|---|---|---|---|---|---|

Not at all                                                           Entirely

   c. How angry would the other person be?

| 1 | 2 | 3 | 4 | 5 | 6 | 7 |
|---|---|---|---|---|---|---|

Very                                                               Not at all

   d. If you would not reveal this cause, write what you would say, and answer the above questions again (using a different marker so that the responses can be distinguished from one another).

2. You failed to appear because you forgot.

   a. Would you reveal this cause?

| 1 | 2 | 3 | 4 | 5 | 6 | 7 |
|---|---|---|---|---|---|---|

Definitely yes                                                    Definitely no

   b. How responsible would the other person hold you?

| 1 | 2 | 3 | 4 | 5 | 6 | 7 |
|---|---|---|---|---|---|---|

Not at all                                                           Entirely

   c. How angry would the other person be?

| 1 | 2 | 3 | 4 | 5 | 6 | 7 |
|---|---|---|---|---|---|---|

Very                                                               Not at all

   d. If you would not reveal this cause, write what you would say, and answer the above questions again (using a different marker so that the responses can be distinguished from one another).

3. You failed to appear because you went to a party instead.

   a. Would you reveal this cause?

| 1 | 2 | 3 | 4 | 5 | 6 | 7 |
|---|---|---|---|---|---|---|
| Definitely yes | | | | | | Definitely no |

   b. How responsible would the other person hold you?

| 1 | 2 | 3 | 4 | 5 | 6 | 7 |
|---|---|---|---|---|---|---|
| Not at all | | | | | | Entirely |

   c. How angry would the other person be?

| 1 | 2 | 3 | 4 | 5 | 6 | 7 |
|---|---|---|---|---|---|---|
| Very | | | | | | Not at all |

   d. If you would not reveal this cause, write what you would say, and answer the above questions again (using a different marker so that the responses can be distinguished from one another).

4. You failed to appear because your boss unexpectedly made you stay overtime at work to finish a project.

   a. Would you reveal this cause?

| 1 | 2 | 3 | 4 | 5 | 6 | 7 |
|---|---|---|---|---|---|---|
| Definitely yes | | | | | | Definitely no |

   b. How responsible would the other person hold you?

| 1 | 2 | 3 | 4 | 5 | 6 | 7 |
|---|---|---|---|---|---|---|
| Not at all | | | | | | Entirely |

   c. How angry would the other person be?

| 1 | 2 | 3 | 4 | 5 | 6 | 7 |
|---|---|---|---|---|---|---|
| Very | | | | | | Not at all |

   d. If you would not reveal this cause, write what you would say, and answer the above questions again (using a different marker so that the responses can be distinguished from one another).

excuse-provider is a lie, a risk is being taken. It is known, however, that individuals are very poor at discriminating false from true communications (Ekman, 1984). It should not be surprising, then, to find that this also is the case regarding excuses. Folkes (1982) reported that when being rejected for a date, the vast majority of the reasons given are accepted as real or true. In contrast, rejecters report that only about half of the reasons are valid. A related study that I conducted with my colleagues (Weiner, Amirkhan, Folkes, & Verette, 1987) found that only about 12% of the communications regarding the reasons for a broken social contract are perceived by the communicator to be disbelieved by the listener. Of these, about half were in fact true, and the other 50% were false! Thus, persons are not able to identify lies; the saying, "He who excuses himself accuses himself," is not empirically substantiated.

Among college students, Weiner et al. (1987) found that when a social transgression such as missing an appointment is said to be due to transportation problems (e.g., one's car could not start), then that was more likely to be a true rather than a false statement. However, when it was reported that an appointment was missed because of requirements at work or at school, then this communication was more likely to be false. Thus, one very imperfect method to infer if the other is providing a false account is to consider the content of the excuse. It also is of interest to note that if a college student pleads lack of responsibility because of illness, then that reason is as likely to describe the true state of affairs as not, and, therefore, does not enable the listener to make any inference regarding "true" responsibility. "Caveat emptor" is the best advice to the recipient regarding communicated causes of a broken social contract.

## Contents of Excuses

Thus far it has been proposed that excuses as defined here are untrue, tactical communications (knowing lies), given primarily to deny responsibility for a social transgression. They are frequent, accepted, and conveyed generally in affiliative contexts, most likely to relatives and friends.

But how specifically does the excuse giver go about this task? What true reasons are withheld and what actually is communicated? One simple research methodology that has been used to investigate this question is to ask research participants to recall a time when they gave an excuse and to report the real (withheld) cause of the transgression as well as the cause that was falsely communicated (the excuse).

Table 8.2 gives the results of one representative study reported by Weiner et al. (1991). Eight categories were sufficient to describe virtually all of the communications. Considering first the withheld or true causes, Table 8.2 reveals that more than 80% of the reasons that are withheld are forgetting/negligence (e.g., "I forgot we had a meeting") or intention ("I did not want to go to the party"). Recall from Chapter I that, given these causes, persons are held responsible because the causes are perceived as subject to volitional control. This is true for forgetting as well as for an intentional transgression, inasmuch as it is presumed that a "reasonable" person would have remembered to keep the appointment. However, one

**TABLE 8.2.** Content of True (Withheld) and False Causes (Excuses)

| Content categories | True | Excuse |
|---|---|---|
| Parents | 1% | 7 |
| Friends | 4 | 7 |
| Illness | 0 | 21 |
| Other commitment | 2 | 24 |
| Transportation | 0 | 2 |
| Work/study | 2 | 15 |
| Forget/negligence | 12 | 2 |
| Intent | 70 | 2 |
| Miscellaneous | 9 | 24 |

*Note.* Data from Weiner, Figuera-Munoz, and Kakihara (1991).

is held more responsible for an intended rather than a negligent act (as represented in the distinction between murder and manslaughter)—and, accordingly, more intentional causes are withheld.

Table 8.2 also reveals the causes that are communicated by the excuse giver. They fall within six general categories: parents ("My parents would not let me go"), friends ("I had to help Mary"), illness ("I had the flu"), other commitments ("I had to take my mother to the airport"), transportation ("The bus came late"), and work/study ("My boss made me work overtime"). Other commitments, illness, and work/study requirements are most frequent among college students. The excuses given are normative and rather mundane and prosaic, most likely out of fear that any unusual explanations will not be believed (also see Riordan, Marlin, & Kellogg, 1983).

In a procedure that did not make use of recollection of past events but involved an experimental manipulation, Weiner et al. (1987) had pairs of subjects participate in an experiment. The two subjects reported to different rooms. One of the subjects was delayed for 15 minutes, while the second subject was led to believe that his or her partner was late.

The delayed subject was then told to join the partner and was asked to communicate a "bad excuse" (which would evoke anger), a "good excuse," or just "any excuse." Table 8.3 shows the reports of the delayed subjects. In the "bad excuse" condition, they said that they were negligent (e.g., "I forgot") or that they came late by free choice (e.g., "I saw some friends and stopped to talk"). On the other hand, in the "good excuse" condition, the subjects reported a sudden obligation (e.g. "I had to take my mother to the hospital"), transportation or arrival problems (e.g., "I could not find the experimental room"), or school demands (e.g., "My midterm

TABLE 8.3. Categories of Explanations and Frequencies as a Function of the
Experimental Condition

| | Experimental condition | | |
|---|---|---|---|
| Categories of explanation | Bad (n = 17) | Good (n = 18) | Any (n = 19) |
| Sudden obligation | 1 | 6 | 3 |
| Transportation, distance, space | 1 | 5 | 3 |
| School demand | 0 | 4 | 5 |
| Negligence | 7 | 0 | 2 |
| Free choice | 6 | 0 | 0 |
| Something missing | 1 | 2 | 2 |
| Miscellaneous/multiple categories | 1 | 1 | 4 |

*Note.* From Weiner, Amirkhan, Folkes, and Verette (1987, p. 321). Copyright 1987 by the
American Psychological Association. Reprinted by permission.

took longer than expected."). The reports in the "any excuse" condition
were similar to those in the "good excuse" condition. Hence, when asked
to give "any excuse," the subjects gave one that would be considered
"good" in that it would absolve them of personal responsibility for coming
late.

Let us now return to Experiment 8.1 and determine if your responses
match those of the experimental results that have been reported. Two of
the reasons provided for the lateness in Experiment 8.1 are "good" in that
you apparently would not be held responsible (illness and work requirements). Hence, little anger is anticipated. I therefore expect these causes to
be revealed. On the other hand, the remaining two causes were "bad" in
that you would be held responsible for the transgression (forgetting and
intentionally deciding to go to a party). A great deal of anger should be
elicited by these reasons. In these instances, it is predicted that there will
be a tendency to withhold the truth and substitute a different cause, such
as illness, other commitments, transportation problems, work demands,
and the like. These causes will reduce inferred responsibility and anger
responses. Comparisons between the responses in the four conditions
provide the opportunity to test the hypotheses.

I feel quite confident that you will conform to the predicted pattern.
Of course, some individuals may hold a "never lie" rule of social relationships, and perhaps others might believe that forgetting is an explanation
that should not be punished or withheld for there was not a "guilty mind"
that accompanied an intentional transgression. Nonetheless, I suspect that
these belief systems will characterize very few people, who are knowl-

edgeable about the rules of social obligation and the consequences of a social transgression for which they are held responsible.

## Excuse Effectiveness

But do excuses work? That is, is this "fraud" successful? It has been implied that they do accomplish their goals inasmuch as excuses are not readily detected and are widespread in everyday life. This is prima facie evidence of their influence. But thus far experimental data have not been provided to support the belief that excuses indeed reduce personal responsibility, elicited anger, and/or unpleasant retaliations.

To be successful, Figure 1.1 and Table 8.1 indicate that the true cause of an event must be controllable by the person and that there must be no mitigating circumstances, whereas the accepted substitute must be considered uncontrollable by the individual (here I exclude the conveyance of justification rather than an excuse, as well as the possibility of forgiveness following a confession). Table 8.2 intimates that the true causes of excuse-instigating events indeed are perceived as controllable by the person (forgetting and intent), whereas the substituted causes (e.g., parents, friends, illness) are perceived as uncontrollable.

To more systematically test this position, when subjects were asked by Weiner et al. (1991) to report incidents in which excuses were given, the true (withheld) and false (excuse) causes were classified by raters as controllable or uncontrollable. Weiner et al. (1991) report that 96% of withheld causes were rated as controllable by the excuse-giver, whereas this was the case for only 10% of the communicated causes. Hence, excuses (if accepted) do shift causality from controllable to uncontrollable—and therefore, by implication, decrease inferences of personal responsibility. This is a necessary condition if excuse goals are to be met.

But an answer to the question of whether the ultimate aims of the communicator are reached still has not been fully addressed. In one study pertinent to the question of whether excuses "work," reported by Weiner et al. (1987), excuse givers were asked to reveal how much their relationship suffered, the degree to which their personal image decreased, their inferred responsibility, and the anger of the other after hearing the excuse for a social transgression. In addition, the subjects were asked to imagine what the other would think and feel if the withheld reasons for the transgression actually had been given. These responses are shown in Table 8.4, where it is shown that respondents benefit on all these indicators from the excuse, as opposed to what they thought would happen if the real (withheld) reason were made known. In addition, Table 8.4 reveals the subjects' beliefs when the communicated excuse was not accepted. It is evident from

JUDGMENTS OF RESPONSIBILITY

TABLE 8.4. Perceived Consequences of Excuse Giving as a Function of Excuse Classification

|  | Type of reason | | |
| Dependent variable | Believed false ($n = 88$) | Not believed false ($n = 15$) | Withheld ($n = 88$) |
| --- | --- | --- | --- |
| Relationship suffer | 1.87 | 3.46 | 3.72 |
| Image suffer | 1.23 | 3.26 | 4.27 |
| Responsibility | 2.33 | 4.06 | 4.72 |
| Anger | 2.26 | 4.26 | 4.39 |

Note. Adapted from Weiner, Amirkhan, Folkes, and Verette (1987). Copyright 1987 by the American Psychological Association. Reprinted by permission.

the table that disbelief has adverse consequences for the response giver, although the excuse giver still benefits.

But again this does not provide definitive evidence for the effectiveness of an excuse, as opposed to its imagined effectiveness. To yet more directly examine whether excuses "work," recall an experiment from Weiner et al. (1987) in which subjects were detained and had to provide a bad excuse, a good excuse, or say anything to their waiting partners. In that study, the partners also were asked for their impressions of the tardy subject following the manipulated communication. This was indexed by ratings of emotional reactions, traits, and possible future social behaviors. These data, given in Table 8.5, show that positive feelings, perceived character, and favorable interpersonal behaviors were lower following a "bad excuse," as opposed to the deliverance of a "good excuse" or "any excuse" (which was, in fact, "good."). Thus, that excuses are functional is not just a fantasy of the excuse giver. Rather, excuses result in a successful

TABLE 8.5. Mean Judgments as a Function of the Experimental Condition among Excuse Receivers

|  | Experimental condition | | |
|  | Good | Any | Bad |
| --- | --- | --- | --- |
| Emotions | 6.15 | 5.92 | 5.32 |
| Traits | 5.37 | 5.29 | 4.71 |
| Behaviors | 5.76 | 5.84 | 5.18 |

Note. Adapted from Weiner, Amirkhan, Folkes, and Verette (1987, p. 322). Copyright 1987 by the American Psychological Association. Reprinted by permission. High numbers indicate positive emotions, positive traits, and approach behavior.

"fraud" in which the communicator avoids being "sentenced" (although the sentence in this case is not one carried out in a court of law; see also Riordan et al., 1983).

## The Excuse Process

It is evident, then, that the naive psychology of the layperson, or beliefs of the "person on the street" regarding the determinants of responsibility, correspond to the scientific or philosophical analysis. Science and philosophy assert that for responsibility to be inferred there must be freedom of choice—that is, controllable causality. Consistent with this, persons communicate uncontrollable causes in order to decrease perceptions of responsibility. This correspondence should not be entirely surprising, for individuals could not function adaptively in society without this knowledge. They can function, however, without knowledge about the process that is activated to call forth and communicate an excuse.

What might this process be? When a social contract is broken, a transgressor may consider the real explanation ("I did not want to go"), analyze this explanation regarding its implications for personal responsibility (the cause is controllable and the act intentional), anticipate the negative consequences of communicating the cause (anger and rejection), and then make a decision about what to communicate (deny the act, withhold the true cause and furnish an excuse, supply a justification, or confess and ask for forgiveness). This captures a controlled or effortful process in which the "sinner," (i.e., the person who has committed a social transgression) logically considers all the alternatives and their likely consequences and selects the "best" tactic.

However, the demands of the situation—for example, a sudden confrontation accusing the transgressor and seeking an explanation—may not permit the luxury of such calculation. In these instances, a more automatic process may be activated and the person's usual or habitual mode of responding (e.g., do not admit the act; say you were ill; etc.) may spontaneously be activated.

The same analysis may be applied to the decision about which excuse to substitute, given that it is decided to furnish an excuse. The communicator could have a schema or a model for a "good excuse" (uncontrollable), consider various excuses and select one having this uncontrollable property ("My car broke down"), and then deliver that explanation. But again, time constraints may not permit this amount of cognitive work. Hence, it is quite possible that we already have a set of good excuses, or a "best" one from which to draw, without going through a complex comparison process.

Even this sequence, however, does not capture the full complexity of the decision-making process, for some excuses that reduce responsibility are unlikely to be communicated in certain contexts (e.g., a student might not want to tell her parents that she did not come home during Christmas because of illness—an uncontrollable and, therefore, a good excuse). Thus, what excuse is presented cannot be divorced from the context in which it is elicited.

One surely can hypothesize many account-giving processes, from the most simple habit of always denying to extremely complex chains of reasoning that might characterize the pleas of a psychopathic criminal. At present, there has been very little experimental work related to the process that accompanies the giving of accounts.

## Developmental Considerations

Throughout this book, I have avoided developmental issues. It surely can be asked at what point children come to understand responsibility–anger and lack of responsibility–sympathy linkages; what determines an understanding of controllable and uncontrollable causality; and the like. These are fascinating questions that remain to be fully explored.

There have been some developmental investigations related to the understanding of the function of excuse giving that are appropriate to at least briefly acknowledge here. In one study that I conducted with a colleague (Weiner & Handel, 1985), children varying in age from 5 to 12 were given scenarios that involved a broken social engagement. The reasons for not appearing at an appointment to play with a friend were varied so that they would be perceived as controllable or uncontrollable, in a manner quite similar to Experiment 8.1 that you completed. The controllable causes included such reasons as "You decided to play with another friend," while uncontrollable causes included such reasons as, "Just that day your mother made you stay home." The children were asked if they would tell this cause to their friend and how angry the friend would be if that reason were communicated.

Table 8.6 shows that the expected anger and the likelihood of revealing the cause as a function of its controllability and the age of the children. It is evident that even among the 5 to 7 year-olds, more anger is anticipated for controllable causes and that the uncontrollable causes are more likely to be revealed. Thus, from a very early age children understand social rules regarding transgressions and how to avoid being held responsible by employing a "conversational move." However, anticipated anger and the likelihood of withholding the truth do grow over time between the ages of 5 and 12.

It also is of interest to report the correlations between anticipated anger and the withholding of responses. If anger, or anticipated anger, is

**TABLE 8.6.** Anticipated Anger and Reported Likelihood of
Revealing Cause as a Function of Causal Controllability and Age

| Cause | Age | | |
|---|---|---|---|
| | 5–7 | 8–9 | 10–12 |
| | Expected anger[a] | | |
| Controllable | 3.96 | 4.21 | 4.32 |
| Uncontrollable | 2.06 | 2.01 | 2.07 |
| | Likelihood of revealing | | |
| Controllable | 3.65 | 2.49 | 1.98 |
| Uncontrollable | 5.52 | 5.70 | 5.74 |

*Note.* From Weiner and Handel (1985, p. 105). Copyright 1985 by the
American Psychological Association. Reprinted by permission.
[a]The higher the number, the greater the expected anger and the greater the
likelihood of revealing causes.

the proximal determinant of behavior, then one would expect high correlations between these two variables. Among the 5 to 7-year-olds, this correlation is $r = .40$; the correlation increases to $r = .78$ for the 8 to 9-year-olds and to $r = .83$ for the 10 to 12-year-olds. Again, then, for all age groups there is a strong association between anticipated emotion and conduct, but this relation does display a developmental increment.

There are many possible explanations for the developmental trend, ranging from very young children's adherence to communicating the truth to their lesser concern about arousing negative feelings in others. In this context, what is of primary importance is not this trend, but rather that the function of the withholding of responses is learned very early in life, thus attesting to the significance of the giving of accounts in everyday functioning. Young children might not have a concept of "sin," but they do understand the role of personal responsibility in judgments of inappropriate social behavior and the consequences of such a transgression. From the perspective of this book, they do comprehend what is meant by a social sin!

## Excuses for Aggression

It would be reasonable to anticipate that excuses are particularly prevalent in the case of aggressive actions. After all, criminal proceedings are not initiated if one is obese because of overeating, if one is poor because of a failure to save money, or if one needs class notes because one went to the beach. But an intentional hostile action can result in a legally sanctioned response that could have dire consequences for the offender.

There have been some empirical studies of the explanations given by those who have engaged in harmful actions. In criminal trials, most offenders contend that their conduct was justified, in the service of self-protection (Felson & Ribner, 1981).

There also has been an examination of the statements of child molesters regarding the cause of their misconduct. Pollock and Hashmall (1991) examined the clinical records of persons referred for psychiatric assessment following a charge of sexual assault on a child. All were convicted, with the victims ranging in age from 2 to 13 (see also Stermac & Segal, 1989).

These molesters gave multiple accounts for their action. Pollock and Hashmall (1991) report that 21% of the molesters denied the act (stating that "nothing happened" or that the victim was "lying"), 35% contended that the incident was nonsexual (and that they were "just being affectionate"), and 36% stated that sex with children is not wrong and/or that the victim consented. Within Figure 1.1 and Table 8.1, these explanations would be considered denial of the act in that either the act itself or the negative aspects of the conduct are not accepted. (It is not known from the data if these reports are tactics or strategies that are conscious lies to reduce responsibility or whether they are truly believed by the wrongdoers).

In addition, 22% of the molesters stated that the action was victim initiated, that is, the behavior occurred but causality was external to the self. This would be construed as an excuse within the framework of Table 8.1 (if this were a conscious manipulation ploy). Finally, 48% of the molesters cited situational mitigators (e.g., "I was intoxicated," "There was family stress"), while 35% made reference to psychological mitigators ("I was sexually abused as a child").

The structure of explanations of child molesters proposed by Pollock and Hashmall (1991) is shown in Figure 8.1. There is some correspondence between this analysis and the structure of responsibility outlined in Figure 1.1 and Table 8.1. As already suggested, I would combine "Nothing happened," "It wasn't sexual," and "It wasn't wrong" into one category of act denial; "It was not my idea" appears to be external causality; and the final stage introduces uncontrollable causality. The explanations in this very real context (as opposed to the simulational studies that I often conduct) are consistent with the line of reasoning that has been presented.

## Excuses of Aggressive Children

Recall that in the prior chapter it was reported that aggressive children are more likely than nonaggressive children to perceive ambiguous harmful

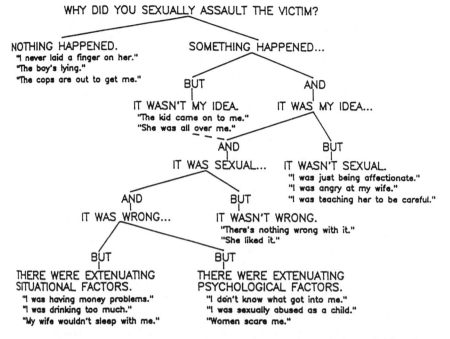

**FIGURE 8.1.** Schematic diagram of excuses for sexual assault from child molesters. From Pollock and Hashmall (1991, p. 57). Copyright 1991 by John Wiley Sons, Ltd. Reprinted by permission.

conduct as intentionally caused. Misperceptions, in turn, arouse the anger of aggressive children as well as a tendency to retaliate. This analysis of the determinants of aggression is part of what has been called a social–cognitive approach, which seeks the causes of aggression, not in the personality traits of the aggressor, but rather in the manner in which these individuals perceive their social world, make decisions, solve problems, and the like.

This position guided an investigation conducted by Graham, Weiner, and Benesh-Weiner (in press) that examined the excuse giving of aggressive children. The prior section of this chapter examined excuses in average, normally adjusted children. It also is worthwhile to consider excuse-giving skills among children known to have adjustment problems, particularly in the domain of aggression. Considering excuse giving, a number of findings in the peer-aggression literature suggest that there might be differences between aggressive and nonaggressive children in their adaptive use of excuses. As indicated, one goal of excuses is to maintain the social bond. However, aggressive children are less likely than nonaggressive children to pursue social goals in their relations with others (see, for example, Crick & Ladd, 1990; Rabiner & Gordon, 1993). Even when aggressive children do report social goals, they have difficulty in translating these goals into effective social problem-solving strategies (Rabiner & Gordon, 1992). Hence, a common theme and finding is that aggressive children, compared to their nonaggressive counterparts, are less motivated by relationship-enhancing goals with peers and/or lack the necessary social skills to foster positive relationships.

It therefore was reasoned by Graham et al. (in press) that among the social–cognitive shortcomings of aggressive children might be a failure to engage in "conversational moves" that mask their responsibility for social transgression. Adherence to the truth and honesty are considered fundamental to society. However, as indicated throughout this chapter, social competence also entails the realization that maintaining the social fabric often depends on intentional miscommunication. If indeed aggressive children do communicate in a maladaptive manner (e.g., relatively withhold uncontrollable causes and reveal controllable causes of a transgression), then following a transgression anger would tend to be evoked in others and there would be a tendency to engage in some form of hostile retaliation. Hence, an aggressive cycle could be set in motion.

To examine excuse giving among aggressive children, Graham et al. (in press) created scenarios similar to those in Experiment 8.1. Younger (ages 7 to 11) and older (ages 12 to 13) aggressive and nonaggressive children, classified from peer nominations and teacher ratings, were told to imagine that they did not show up at an expected time either to meet their mother or a friend. Again, uncontrollable and controllable reasons were provided (e.g., "I had to stay after school," "I decided to play instead"). The two groups of children rated how responsible they would be perceived if they communicated the true cause, how angry the other person (mother or peer) would be, and whether they would reveal this cause or withhold it and disclose something else (tell a lie).

Table 8.7 shows the relations among the dependent variables of perceived responsibility, anticipated anger, and communication strategy (i.e., whether the truth was told). Table 8.7 indicates that all children realize that responsibility results in anger and that the greater the inferred responsibility and anticipated anger the less the likelihood that they would reveal the cause. It also is evident from Table 8.7 that there is a developmental trend—namely, that older children perceive these associations to a greater extent than younger children do. And, of most importance in this context, there is a difference between the aggressive and the nonaggressive children that grows over time (see Figure 8.2). In Figure 8.2, this difference is represented by combining the correlations in each column of Table 8.7 into

TABLE 8.7. Correlations between Responsibility, Anticipated Anger, and Revealing the Truth among Younger and Older Aggressive and Nonaggressive Children

| | Status group | | | |
|---|---|---|---|---|
| | Aggressive | | Nonaggressive | |
| Correlation | Younger ($n$ = 32) | Older ($n$ = 28) | Younger ($n$ = 22) | Older ($n$ = 24) |
| Respons. × anger | .41* | .60* | .47* | .80*** |
| Respons. × reveal | −.20 | −.45* | −.30 | −.69*** |
| Anger × reveal | −.23 | −.48** | −.34 | −.74*** |

*$p$ < .05. **$p$ < .01. ***$p$ < .001.

one index. This summary index might be considered one of "social awareness" regarding the components of excuse giving. Considering simultaneously all three correlations, there is relatively little difference in their strengths among the younger aggressive versus nonaggressive children. On the other hand, the overall difference in association strengths is quite pronounced among the older children. It is unknown what gives rise to this developmental disparity, and this issue is beyond the scope of the chapter. Rather, what is of most interest here is that older aggressive children indeed appear to be deficient either in their social understanding of the function of excuse giving or in the adaptiveness of their social behavior (see also Caprara, Pastorelli, & Weiner, 1994).

## Summary of Excuse Giving

In the criminal justice system, the sentence for manslaughter is less than that for murder because only in the latter was there an intention to kill. It thus is in the interest of the criminal to "prove" that the intention to kill was absent during the act. In a similar manner, in everyday transgressions such as not showing up for an appointment, arriving late, not doing something that was expected, or doing an act that "should not" have been completed, it is in the self-interest of the transgressor to convince others that controllability was absent. This would free the individual from responsibility and its consequences, which include anger and social punishment.

Excuses provide a ready vehicle for attaining the goal of convincing

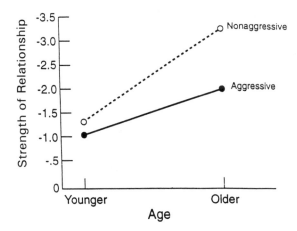

**FIGURE 8.2.** Combined strengths of the associations between perceived controllability of a transgression and response withholding, perceived controllability of a transgression and anticipated anger, and anticipated anger and response withholding. Strengths of relations are added standard scores. From Graham, Weiner, and Benesh-Weiner (in press). Copyright by the American Psychological Association. Reprinted by permission.

others of the uncontrollability of one's social transgression. This miscommunication, or excuse giving, is common and effective and develops quite early in life. The absence of this strategy is more prevalent among aggressive youths, which could contribute to their interpersonal difficulties and hostile activities.

Finally, the use of excuses in everyday life provides evidence that the determinants of inferences of responsibility are understood by all. That is, there is a correspondence between naive psychology and the laws of psychology as formulated by professional psychologists. Currently, this knowledge is particularly dramatic in the courtroom. Those who harm others with intent, with crimes including the killing of parents, the beating of others, and even male castration, are arguing that these acts were fostered by an abused childhood, an abusing spouse, or a society that does not permit attainment of personal goals. That is, they have a "good" excuse (the so-called abuse excuse) for their conduct. And indeed, courtroom juries appear prone to accept these excuses that, in turn, reduce responsibility, anger, and punishment. Perhaps, then, "crimes of passion" are re-entering into the legal arena, with passion more broadly defined as the "absence of freedom of choice," which indeed is an acceptable excuse.

## CONFESSION

Unlike denial, in confession an untoward act is admitted; unlike excuses, given a confession the transgressor accepts personal responsibility; and unlike justification, mitigating circumstances are not used to convince another that the untoward act really served a higher moral goal. In a "complete" confession the individual admits doing the act, accepts full responsibility, includes an apology and self-castigation, and offers some restitution. Why, then, would this tactic be used as a "conversational move?"

The assumption first must be made that the confessor is consciously seeking to be exonerated and to be perceived more positively. It certainly is possible that confession is not used as a conscious ploy but, rather, springs from overriding guilt. Jung (1933), for example, once stated that: "every personal secret has the effect of sin or guilt" (p. 34). Guilt, in turn, has been postulated to be a goad that moves the individual to admit fault and to comply with social rules (Carlsmith & Gross, 1969). Presumptions of a "compulsion to confess" have been noted in the psychoanalytic literature and, like slips of the tongue and dreams, is considered beyond volitional control and a product of unconscious forces acting on the individual (see Belgum, 1963). This determinant of confession is not pertinent in the present context, which focuses only upon the conscious use of confession as a tactic or maneuver to influence the impressions of others. That is, just like an excuse, confession as considered here is a form of impression management.

When used as a method of impression management, what might be the perceived function of a "conversational move" that accepts responsibility? There is a naive or commonsense association between confession and forgiveness. This relation even is found in aphorisms, as in the saying: "A fault confessed is half forgiven." Perhaps this linkage can be traced to religious writings, for in the Scriptures confession gives rise to forgiveness. There it is clearly stated that confession is the sine qua non for divine pardon. In the Saint John affirmation of the divine, it is written: "If we confess our sins, He is faithful and righteous to forgive us" (1 John 1:9). Prayers also are based on this belief: Witness the supplication, "I have sinned, O Lord, forgive me."

There is reason, then, for individuals to believe that confession, just as denial, excuses, and justifications, will "work." But prior to pursuing this question further, it is time to present you, the reader, with another experiment so that you may provide your own data. Again, all that is asked of you is to be as honest as possible. It is not readily feasible to disguise the purpose of these experiments, which are quite transparent. Thus, the only recourse I have is to ask for openness and for you to truthfully reveal your thoughts and beliefs.

The experiment you are asked to perform is quite simple, yet not far removed from an experience that may have been encountered in everyday life. A short vignette is to be read in which a senator (correctly) accuses another senator of wrongdoing. After reading this story, you are asked to respond to seven questions: two regarding the traits of the accused senator, two concerned with your emotional reactions of anger and sympathy, one assessing forgiveness, and two behavioral judgments about recommended punishment and voting behavior.

There are two conditions or experimentally created situations: (1) a control condition in which nothing further is added and (2) a confession. The reader is asked to rate the same variables in the two conditions. Please go ahead and complete the experiment now.

## The Effectiveness of Confessions

Prior to examining the results of this experiment, let us determine if confession actually results in forgiveness from others. There is some real-world evidence that confession does have this consequence. For example, in the late 1980s two television evangelists, Jimmy Swaggart and Jim Bakker, were accused of immoral sexual activities. Swaggart immediately confessed, admitting that the charges were true and acknowledging wrongdoing. He stated: "I do not call it a mistake . . . I call it a sin . . . I have no one to blame but myself" (see Osting, 1988, p. 46). Bakker, on the other hand, did not ever accept full responsibility. He accused others of blackmail, his wife of lack of caring, and his accuser (Jessica Hahn) of lying. He subsequently did offer a public apology, but not one of strong repentance (see Hackett, 1987). Later opinion polls revealed less condemnation for Swaggart following his confession than for Bakker, who received a severe punishment for his misdeed (see "Public Opinion Poll," 1987).

Perhaps the most infamous modern example of lack of confession given public perception of a misdeed involves former President Richard Nixon and what is known as the Watergate scandal. Nixon never acknowledged personal guilt, although there was compelling evidence of his involvement in this affair, which included an illegal entry into the headquarters of the Democratic Party. In a popular autobiography, Senator Barry Goldwater (1988), a prominent Republican, expressed the following: "I wanted the President . . . to tell . . . the truth. If it was bad, he could ask for help and forgiveness. He could say he made a mistake and explicitly say he was sorry" (p. 269). Senator Goldwater obviously believed in the power of confession.

A similar analysis of the Nixon episode was offered by Larry Speakes, Press Secretary for Ronald Reagan. Speakes stated: "We attempted to convince the President to say, 'I take full responsibility.' " This was in

## EXPERIMENT 8.2

## Confession and Forgiveness

Please read the following two vignettes and answer the questions related to them.

1. Senator Joe McNally has accused Senator James Dunn of misusing his senatorial expense account. Senator McNally stated: "Senator Dunn has used his expense account, which is funded by taxpayers, to print up and mail out advertisements for his own benefit and reelection. He knows that current expense account regulations prohibit the use of such expenses for elections and other self-related purposes." When informed of this charge, Senator Dunn refused to comment. The charge was subsequently substantiated.

Please answer the following questions about Senator Dunn.

1. How honest is Senator Dunn?

| 1 | 2 | 3 | 4 | 5 | 6 | 7 | 8 | 9 | 10 |
|---|---|---|---|---|---|---|---|---|---|
| Totally honest | | | | | | | | | Totally dishonest |

2. How trustworthy is Senator Dunn?

| 1 | 2 | 3 | 4 | 5 | 6 | 7 | 8 | 9 | 10 |
|---|---|---|---|---|---|---|---|---|---|
| Totally trustworthy | | | | | | | | | Totally untrustworthy |

3. How much sympathy do you feel toward Senator Dunn?

| 1 | 2 | 3 | 4 | 5 | 6 | 7 | 8 | 9 | 10 |
|---|---|---|---|---|---|---|---|---|---|
| A great deal | | | | | | | | | None at all |

4. How angry would you be at Senator Dunn?

| 1 | 2 | 3 | 4 | 5 | 6 | 7 | 8 | 9 | 10 |
|---|---|---|---|---|---|---|---|---|---|
| Very | | | | | | | | | Not at all |

5. Would you forgive Senator Dunn?

| 1 | 2 | 3 | 4 | 5 | 6 | 7 | 8 | 9 | 10 |
|---|---|---|---|---|---|---|---|---|---|
| Definitely yes | | | | | | | | | Definitely not |

6. What kind of punishment should be given to Senator Dunn?

| 1 | 2 | 3 | 4 | 5 | 6 | 7 | 8 | 9 | 10 |
|---|---|---|---|---|---|---|---|---|---|
| None at all | | | | | | | | | The maximum possible |

7. Would you vote for Senator Dunn?

| 1 | 2 | 3 | 4 | 5 | 6 | 7 | 8 | 9 | 10 |
|---|---|---|---|---|---|---|---|---|---|
| Definitely no | | | | | | | | | Definitely yes |

2. Senator William Smith has accused Senator Thomas Case of misusing his senatorial expense account. Senator Smith stated: "Senator Case has used his expense
account, which is funded by taxpayers, to print up and mail out advertisements
for his own benefit and reelection. He knows that current expense account
regulations prohibit the use of such expenses for elections and other self-related
purposes." This charge was subsequently substantiated. When informed of this
charge, Senator Case said: "I apologize; I'm terribly sorry for what has happened.
I feel terribly guilty. It's my fault; I am responsible for this. I have gone through
all the entries to my expense account and have paid back all the expenses that
even have a remote possibility of having been used to fund my campaign."

Please answer the following questions about Senator Case.

1. How honest is Senator Case?

| 1 | 2 | 3 | 4 | 5 | 6 | 7 | 8 | 9 | 10 |
|---|---|---|---|---|---|---|---|---|---|

Totally honest                                                    Totally dishonest

2. How trustworthy is Senator Case?

| 1 | 2 | 3 | 4 | 5 | 6 | 7 | 8 | 9 | 10 |
|---|---|---|---|---|---|---|---|---|---|

Totally trustworthy                                              Totally untrustworthy

3. How much sympathy do you feel toward Senator Case?

| 1 | 2 | 3 | 4 | 5 | 6 | 7 | 8 | 9 | 10 |
|---|---|---|---|---|---|---|---|---|---|

A great deal                                                         None at all

4. How angry would you be at Senator Case?

| 1 | 2 | 3 | 4 | 5 | 6 | 7 | 8 | 9 | 10 |
|---|---|---|---|---|---|---|---|---|---|

Very                                                                  Not at all

5. Would you forgive Senator Case?

| 1 | 2 | 3 | 4 | 5 | 6 | 7 | 8 | 9 | 10 |
|---|---|---|---|---|---|---|---|---|---|

Definitely yes                                                      Definitely not

6. What kind of punishment should be given to Senator Case?

| 1 | 2 | 3 | 4 | 5 | 6 | 7 | 8 | 9 | 10 |
|---|---|---|---|---|---|---|---|---|---|

None at all                                                    The maximum possible

7. Would you vote for Senator Case?

| 1 | 2 | 3 | 4 | 5 | 6 | 7 | 8 | 9 | 10 |
|---|---|---|---|---|---|---|---|---|---|

Definitely no                                                       Definitely yes agreement with the conclusion of former Kennedy advisor, Pierre Salinger, who noted:

> If in the first two or three days of the Watergate story, Richard Nixon had gone on television and said: "I made a stupid mistake" . . . and fired a couple of people, Watergate would have never happened . . . It would have been a thing that would have gone away if he had accepted responsibility for it. (quoted in Hortsman, 1990)

There are observations from real life, then, that lack of confession when others perceive that a transgression was committed results in harsh reactions, that confession does result in forgiveness, and that many individuals believe in the functional value of confessing.

The experimental evidence regarding the positive benefits of confession is sparse but convincing. For example, Holtgraves (1989) described to subjects a variety of social transgressions, followed by various types of communications that might be beneficial to the relationship between the transgressor and the "victim." He also asked his subjects how satisfied the hearer would be with these accounts, how difficult it would be for the speaker to make these statements, and how helpful the communications would be in resolving a conflict. As shown in Table 8.8, a full-blown apology (i.e., a confession) is rated as most satisfying, most difficult to communicate, and most helpful in solving interpersonal conflict (also see Felson & Ribner, 1981; Hale, 1987). Note also in the table that a confession is rated as more effective than an excuse or a justification. However, this obviously will depend on a number of factors. It certainly intuitively appears that, for example, stealing money because one is "forced to" by powerful others, or in order to give it to your sick parent (a justification), will be perceived as a more effective strategy for impression management (if accepted) than a confession!

TABLE 8.8. Mean Ratings of Remedial Moves

| Remedial move | Satisfaction | Difficulty | Helpful |
|---|---|---|---|
| Justification | 1.18 | 2.85 | 1.33 |
| Regret plus justification | 1.68 | 3.0 | 2.03 |
| Excuse | 2.91 | 2.38 | 2.64 |
| Regret plus excuse | 3.95 | 2.09 | 3.96 |
| Regret | 3.53 | 3.18 | 3.54 |
| Apology | 3.91 | 3.59 | 4.12 |
| Full-blown apology (confession) | 5.53 | 4.78 | 5.26 |

*Note.* Adapted from Holtgraves (1989, p. 12). Copyright 1989 by Multilingual Matters, Ltd. Reprinted by permission.

My colleagues and I (Weiner et al., 1991) conducted a series of studies examining the consequences of confession. Some of the studies were similar to the one that you completed in the prior pages. Consider, for example, an investigation in which the senatorial vignette was given. After reading about the transgression, the subjects rated the same variables as you did. The subjects then were informed that the accused senator confessed, denied the accusation, or said nothing. The variables were subsequently rerated.

The results of this investigation are given in Table 8.9. This table shows that there were no differences between the three conditions at Time 1, prior to receiving impression management information. In addition, there were only minor changes in the ratings from Time 1 to Time 2 in the control (no confession) condition. However, compared to Time 1, following a confession the senator was rated as more honest and trustworthy, there was increased sympathy and forgiveness and less anger, and there was less recommended punishment as well as a greater likelihood of voting for this person. In addition, at Time 2 the data show that it was more beneficial to confess than to deny the act, although in this study the vignette did not state that the accused senator was in fact guilty. Hence, if others have reasons to think that you are guilty, although that guilt is not proved, it still may be of personal benefit to confess (even if one is innocent)!

You should now examine your data from Experiment 8.2 and determine if confession resulted in more positive perceptions of the confessor, more favorable emotional reactions, greater forgiveness, and more positive behavioral reactions, as opposed to the condition in which a confession was not delivered. I feel fairly confident that this will indeed be the case.

TABLE 8.9. Mean Judgments in Three Experimental Conditions, before and after a Confession

| Variable | Time 1 (before) | | | Time 2 (after) | | |
|---|---|---|---|---|---|---|
| | Control | Confess | Deny | Control | Confess | Deny |
| Honesty | 1.95 | 1.96 | 2.38 | 1.71 | 4.13 | 2.71 |
| Trustworthiness | 2.12 | 2.25 | 2.62 | 1.75 | 3.16 | 2.62 |
| Sympathy | 2.00 | 2.29 | 2.54 | 2.75 | 3.20 | 2.58 |
| Anger | 5.70 | 5.25 | 4.87 | 6.13 | 4.25 | 4.37 |
| Forgiveness | 2.16 | 2.95 | 3.38 | 1.96 | 4.08 | 2.66 |
| Punishment | 5.79 | 6.04 | 5.66 | 6.33 | 4.38 | 5.38 |
| Vote | 1.96 | 2.29 | 3.00 | 1.75 | 3.29 | 3.29 |

*Note.* Adapted from Weiner, Graham, Peter, and Zmuidinas (1991, p. 297). Copyright 1991 by Duke University Press. Reprinted by permission.

## Why Does Confession Work?

The question to be addressed, then, is why confession is effective in reducing negative trait perceptions, undesirable emotional reactions, and retaliatory punishment? There are a number of answers to this question, none with sufficient empirical evidence to consider the issue settled. It may be that a confession signals that the individual feels guilty and has suffered, so that some of the "sentence" to be imposed already has been served. It also may be that a confession indicates that the person will not engage in the untoward act again. This explanation also would account for a reduction in punishment, which is perceived as an inhibitor of future transgressions.

Perhaps the best current explanation of the effectiveness of a confession can be traced to correspondent inference theory as espoused by Jones and Davis (1965). This theory states that an observer views an action and then, on the basis of the act, reaches inferences about the actor. For example, if a person acts in a dominant way, then we describe that individual as being dominant. Certain conditions, such as the conduct being forced, or information that all have engaged in this behavior, lessen the tendency to move from the act to a dispositional inference.

It has been contended that a confession signals recognition of the basic rule that has been violated and reaffirms that the transgressor values that rule (Darby & Schlenker, 1982). Hence, accepting personal responsibility may alter inferences about the person who violated expectations and social norms and may restore perceptions of that person's moral character. As Blumstein et al. (1974) cogently write:

> An offender may also return to a proper moral position by a display of penitence. By showing respect for the rule he broke, the offender lays claim to the right to reenter the moral graces of the offended party who, by demanding an account, becomes the momentary guardian of responsibility. . . . Showing penitence, like claiming reduced responsibility, splits the identity of the offender. He asserts his own guilt for the act and accepts the momentary blows to his moral character, while at the same time reaffirms his overriding righteousness (awareness of the rules) and acknowledges the offended's rights to demand an account. (p. 552)

According to the prior interpretation, if the offender confesses, there is a loosening of the linkage between the negative act and the correspondent inference of the offender's unfavorable personality characteristics. That is, the behavior and the inferred intention that produced it are less likely to be perceived as corresponding to some underlying dispositional attribute of the person. When viewed from a correspondent inference perspective, confession is thus presumed to have the same severing effect on act-to-disposition correspondence as does information that all others have engaged in the same action (Kremer & Stephens, 1983). This differs from the function of excuses, which reduce responsibility for the particular transgression.

## Why Don't Others Always Confess?

Given that there is such a strong confession–forgiveness relation in naive psychology, a puzzling fact is why individuals such as Bakker and Nixon chose not to confess, when it appeared that they were guilty. Two possible answers to this question come to mind. It may be that these individuals incorrectly miscalculated reactions to their misdeeds and wrongly assumed that public indignation would eventually dissipate. In this case, the absence of confession was guided by impression management concerns and, in hindsight, the wrongdoers selected an incorrect tactic. On the other hand, it may be that lack of public confession is better explained by the dynamics of denial and ego defensiveness, and thus is a topic of concern more for clinical than for social psychologists!

Finally, my discussion has considered "benefit" and "harm" only from the perspective of the confessor. What is beneficial to the confessor ultimately may be harmful to larger society. Forgiving Swaggart and others because they publicly confess could encourage individuals to engage in similar behavior and then ask for forgiveness. The final long-term social consequences of forgiveness and the conditions that promote it are complex issues that have not been addressed here.

## SUMMARY

It is evident that there is a convergence between the law, naive psychology, and theology in the arena of impression management. In a jury trial, defendants who are responsible for a criminal act seek a favorable, or at least a relatively favorable, verdict by either denying the act, offering an excuse or a justification, or confessing when guilt is presumed. In a similar manner, in an interpersonal setting a spouse guilty of a social transgression, such as failing to appear at an appointment, can strive for a reduced "sentence" (e.g., not speaking to the other) by using the same maneuvers. And a parishioner who is facing a priest may endeavor to receive relatively lenient judgments from divine authorities by confessing his or her sins and misdeeds.

What is common in these situations is that there is an attempt to reduce perceptions of either responsibility for the act itself (an excuse) or for the inference that one is an irresponsible person (a confession). Furthermore, there is an understanding of the tactics that will result in this goal. There are shared thoughts and knowledge about the role of responsibility in judgments of others, and there is an overlap of legally defined sin with a more broadly defined social sin.

Excuses and confession, the two strategies considered in this chapter, differ in a number of characteristics. Most importantly, given an excuse, the person does not accept personal responsibility for an untoward act. Rather, causality is shifted to something external to the person or to a cause that is internal to the person but not controllable. At times, mitigators also can be used to excuse an act. Being a victim of abuse now is considered sufficient to reduce responsibility for an intentional act of revenge. On the other hand, in confession the sinning person accepts full responsibility for the past conduct. Given either strategy, there is personal benefit for the communicator; failure to engage in such tactical communications can have dire consequences.

Which strategy a person selects obviously depends on a number of factors, like the following: Is guilt presumed by others? How acceptable are the mitigators? Is the audience the public or an all-knowing God? What is the developmental level of the communicator? What personal goals are sought? Selection of the "best" tactic, therefore, is a complex process. But for most persons, what is communicated will be guided by the ultimate goal of influencing others and creating a favorable impression.

# 9

## On the Construction
## of Psychological Theory
## and Other Issues

If we discover a complete theory, it should in time be understandable
in broad principle by everyone, not just a few scientists. Then we
shall all, philosophers, scientists, and ordinary people, be able to take
part in the discussion . . .
—STEPHEN HAWKING, *A Brief History of Time*

In this final chapter, I reorganize what has been presented and consider the
logical or sequential steps in the construction of a psychological theory.
This discussion is somewhat myopic or self-centered in that the principles
and ordering that I suggest are derived from the development of the theory
that has been offered in this book. However, I do believe that my particular
travels and travails (these have the same linguistic root) may be useful to
others as well. The task of reconstruction also provides the opportunity to
review the substantial material in the previous chapters.

In addition to metatheoretical concerns, a number of issues remain to
be considered. These issues include the relations of popular psychological
phrases and phenomena (e.g., "compassion fatigue," "culture of victimiza-

tion," and "naive psychology") to the analyses already given. In this chapter, I examine these observations and topics as well as a diverse array of pertinent themes that thus far have not been addressed.

## STEPS IN THE CONSTRUCTION OF PSYCHOLOGICAL THEORY

There appear to be several stages or steps in the development of a psychological theory. Of course, there need not be one invariant sequence (just as there was not one ordering in the responsibility process or in the relations between thinking, feeling and action). In addition, the steps or stages that are proposed do overlap.

The theory that has been formulated proceeded in the following manner (these phases will be subject to extended discussion in the remainder of the chapter):

1. The initial step in theory building was *descriptive*, that is, it involved the gathering of empirical facts and evidence. The evidence must be unequivocal if there is to be theoretical progress; it must be replicable; it must have the certainty of the results of mixing two parts of hydrogen with one part oxygen. In my endeavors, the "first fact" upon which all other observations were built relates to the disparate consequences of failure caused by lack of effort versus low ability on achievement evaluation. However, this has been followed by many other indisputable observations, some illustrated in the experiments carried out by you. Providing experiments for you to complete shows my confidence in the replicability of these observations.

2. A specific fact in and of itself is of less interest than what that evidence more broadly represents. For example, it is of great importance that lack of effort is punished more than lack of ability (the "first fact" referred to above). But it is of greater significance to realize that, given a transgression, causal controllability, which is substantiated or materialized by lack of effort, generates greater punishment than does causal uncontrollability, which is embodied within low ability (aptitude). Lack of effort as a cause of achievement failure and promiscuity as a cause of HIV infection are the "same" in that both are controllable determinants of a negative outcome. These determinants elicit greater social reprimand than do lack of ability as a cause of failure to achieve or a blood transfusion as a cause of AIDS—both uncontrollable causes. This step in theory building, which involves the grouping of disparate descriptions, necessitated the creation of a *taxonomy* or a *classification system*. Here, this specifically

incorporated the grouping of causes into more embracing categories. Description therefore was followed by a *structural analysis*, or an identification of the basic properties of phenomenal causality.

3. Description and classification were then followed by explanation, which is a higher level of scientific activity. Two types of explanation require distinction. One involves the *processes and mechanisms* that intervene between an observation (e.g., failure) and the behavior linked with the stimulus (e.g., punishment). The second type of explanation concerns the *function* of a behavioral reaction to a stimulus.

The distinction between a process versus a functional explanation is illustrated in the interpretation of why a stickleback fish attacks other stickleback fish (a topic addressed in most introductory psychology and zoology texts). It is now known that the color red, which is on the belly of the fish, acts as a sign-stimulus that releases an innate attacking response. These mechanisms are involved in the action sequence and, in part, "explain" the aggressive behavior. But a functional interpretation, which often includes evolutionary considerations, embraces the significance, or meaning, or the ultimate consequences of the act. In this case, the attack response chases the fish into another territory. In so doing, there is a greater likelihood of personal reproductive activity as well as spreading of the species. Species spreading enables all the fish to have access to food, thereby abetting their survival.

In the theory championed in this book, the underlying mechanisms and processes include the classification of causes according to causal properties, an inference concerning the responsibility of the person, the emotions elicited by this inference, and the direction or motivational effect of these emotions along with the cognitions of cause and responsibility. For example, failure believed to be caused by lack of effort is construed as controllable; the person may then be held responsible; responsibility for a negative event gives rise to anger; and anger (as well as) beliefs about responsibility are cues or goads to "eliminate" the wrongdoer.

The functional explanation of the associations outlined above examines what goals are fulfilled by the linkages between lack of effort → punishment, on the one hand, and lack of ability → withholding of punishment, on the other, and what the evolutionary gains or advantages of these unions are. The answers to these questions center on the rehabilitation of the wrongdoer, teaching transgressors and others a moral lesson, and the administration of "just deserts." Evolutionary or functional explanations in this context are thus closely related to theories of justice.

4. The search for observations to which a theory can be applied is one of the final steps in the validation of a conception. The theory presented in this book was derived from the study of achievement evaluation. However,

it has proved effective in explaining reactions to the stigmatized, helping behavior, aggression, excuses, and other more circumscribed phenomena.

In addition, seeking to explain new psychological domains, or broadening the range of convenience of a theory, also provides the opportunity for additional theoretical development. For example, when the theory of responsibility was used to interpret reactions to the poor, it was found that the proximal versus the distal determinants of personal help differed from the determinants of attitudes about governmental welfare for the poor. Personal help was particularly influenced by emotions, whereas governmental welfare beliefs were related to political ideology and thoughts about responsibility rather than to the affective reactions of anger and sympathy. This finding can result in further theoretical distinctions that are pertinent to the evaluation of others in achievement contexts. For example, a teacher's appraisal of a student in her classroom might not be the same as evaluations of a similar student located in a different school, with whom she has had no personal contact.

In addition to extending the generality of the theory, another step in the service of theoretical growth is to combine the conception with other existing conceptions, and in so doing situate the theories within a broader framework. This issue was not addressed in the prior chapters, but will be examined in this final chapter.

With this broad overview of theoretical construction in mind, let me now turn to each distinct theoretical phase in more detail, both reviewing the content that already has been presented and examining a number of additional pertinent topics.

## THE INITIAL STEPS: EMPIRICAL FACTS AND DESCRIPTION

As just indicated, the initial stage in the construction of this (and, I assume, most) theories was the discovery of empirical facts and relations. The evidence that provided the foundation for the building of a responsibility-based conception of social motivation was that lack of effort in the event of failure is punished more than lack of ability. Following this, other associations also were detected (although these were not without some theoretical direction).

The observations that formed the heart of the empirical basis of the theory were guided by the metaphor that humans are gods (or godlike). Thus, they judge others and have the "right" to judge others as good or bad (moral or immoral); they react to others with anger and compassion; and they are guided in their behaviors by these thoughts and feelings. Another directing metaphor with similar implications regarding empirical search is that life is a courtroom where the participants judge one another and defend themselves, where sentences are passed and parole is sought, and so on. And still a third related metaphor is that we are moral vigilantes.

Among the facts that provided additional support for theory building, guided by these metaphors, were the following:

1. Adolescent students communicate to parents and teachers that their failure was due to lack of ability, whereas they communicate to peers that failure was caused by the absence of effort (Chapter 2).

2. Stigmas including AIDS, alcoholism, child abuse, drug addiction, and homosexuality elicit anger and little sympathy in comparison to stigmas like Alzheimer's disease, blindness, cancer, heart disease, and paraplegia, which evoke much sympathy and little anger (Chapter 3).

3. Cancer and heart disease caused by unhealthy life styles that include smoking and lack of exercise are reacted to more negatively than the same stigmas are when caused by unknowingly living in a toxic area or a genetic predisposition for this problem (Chapter 3).

4. Obesity caused by overeating and/or lack of exercise gives rise to more intense antisocial reactions than when this stigma is caused by a thyroid dysfunction (Chapter 3).

5. Poverty that is perceived to be caused by laziness, lack of thrift, and/or poor financial planning results in greater social sanctions than when this state is perceived to be caused by lack of educational or job opportunities provided by the government (Chapter 3).

6. HIV infection caused by sexual promiscuity calls forth greater antisocial responses than the same infection caused by a transfusion with contaminated blood (Chapters 3 and 4).

7. When homosexuality is construed as a choice or preference it results in greater negative reactions from others than when it is conceived as a genetic sexual orientation (Chapter 4).

8. Negative mood states, including depression, are believed to be linked with personal causality; depressed people often elicit anger and rejection (Chapter 5).

9. Families that respond to a schizophrenic member with criticism and hostility perceive that schizophrenic behavior is more a free choice than do families that respond to this illness with fewer negative emotions (Chapter 5).

10. Distressed couples are more likely than nondistressed couples to consider that a negative act by a spouse was intentionally caused. This belief weakens the marital bond (Chapter 5).

11. Help is more likely to be extended to those with eye problems, other physical illnesses, or lack of ability than to those who need help because of alcoholism or laziness (Chapter 6).

12. People respond more harshly to intentional aggression than to accidental aggression (Chapter 7).

13. Aggressive children more than nonaggressive children perceive that others have intentionally committed an ambiguously caused negative action (Chapter 7).

14. Abusive parents more than nonabusive parents believe that their children committed a negative act on purpose (Chapter 7).

15. Excuses communicated after a social transgression state that the cause of the transgression was personal illness, transportation problems, other commitments, and work/study requirements. In contrast, reasons for a social transgression that are withheld are primarily intentional decisions to engage or not to engage in the action or negligence or forgetting (Chapter 8).

16. Confession gives rise to forgiveness and alters inferences about the moral character of the offender (Chapter 8).

These are just a few of the documented facts and relations that concern social transgressions and social behavior. The evidence certainly is in accord with our "common sense," or shared knowledge, although the data reviewed above were based on experimental procedures with pertinent variables either manipulated or controlled.

There are a myriad of other responsibility-related facts that concern criminal behavior rather than social transgressions. It is known, for example, that murder results in a harsher sentence than involuntary manslaughter does, and that the former but not the latter involves purposive or intended misconduct. But legal facts were not highlighted in the book.

## The Immutability of Empirical Relations: Phenotypic versus Genotypic Representation

A question that remains to be answered is whether the listing of the empirical findings, which I put forth as "facts," is contradicted by research documenting that scientific announcements to the public and attributional change programs can alter the established relations. Specifically, for example, if it is initially believed that individuals are held responsible for homosexuality, and if later a "homosexual gene" is discovered so that homosexuals are no longer perceived as responsible for their orientation, then the initial empirical reality is indeed altered. However, if this analysis is made at a conceptual (genotypic) level, then there is less change than there appears. For persons to be held responsible, there must be controllable causality or freedom of choice. Thus, if homosexuality is believed to be a preference or choice, then homosexuals are likely to be found responsible for their state; if at a subsequent time homosexuality is construed as a genetic predisposition or sexual orientation, then homosexuals will not be deemed responsible for their state. At this level of genotypic interpretation, the shifting phenotypic beliefs about responsibility are quite consistent with theoretical predictions and do not represent any change or inconsistency. To state this somewhat differently, in the example of change that I presented, there was indeed transformation at the observable level (e.g., homosexuals are no longer inferred to be responsible for their state). But there was compatibility at the theoretical level, i.e., responsibility is in part determined by perceived freedom.

## Empirical Replicability and Cross-Cultural Psychology

The prior discussion also captures my beliefs about the interpretation of cross-cultural research in this domain. Studies regarding the evaluative consequences of ability and effort have been consistent across a wide array of cultures, so that there is little doubt about the generalization that across many cultures (and time) lack of effort is punished more than lack of ability as a cause of failure. In a similar manner, it was documented that reactions to stigmas are relatively the same in the People's Republic of China and in the United States, and that helping among Japanese is amenable to a thinking–feeling–action sequence. I anticipate that these findings also will have wide generality.

   However, it is certainly conceivable that responses to stigmas may be quite disparate in different cultures. For example, one might imagine a "slim" culture in which all obesity is conceived as genetic or hormonal in origin. In this society, people should respond to obesity in the same manner as, say, blindness, i.e., the obese person will not be held responsible and the reactions to the obese will be sympathy rather than anger. Note, therefore, that there again may be disparities in phenotypical relations across cultures, while genotypic constancy is found.

## FROM DESCRIPTION TO TAXONOMY (STRUCTURE)

The importance of the advancement from description to taxonomy already has been disclosed. Phenotypic analysis may reveal differences, but genotypic interpretation, which includes taxonomic placement, points out similarities. Classification may take many forms, from the grouping of external stimuli to the categorization of internal mechanisms and behavioral expressions.

In the present book, two classifications have proved essential. The first involved the creation of a taxonomy of the causes of events. There are as many causes of behavioral outcomes as the imagination can allow. In achievement contexts, failure may be caused by (or be perceived as caused by) lack of effort, an absence of ability, poor strategy, bad luck, the bias of teachers, hindrance from others, illness, and so on (see review in Weiner, 1986). In a similar manner, an affiliative rejection might be due to poor social skills; the desired partner's having already made plans; the parents of the desired date, who will not let him or her go out; the other's regarding you as boring; school demands; and so on.

But these diverse and manifestly "different" causes have common characteristics or properties and therefore could be genotypically similar in spite of phenotypic differences. For example, ability, effort, social skills, and being boring all describe (are internal to) the person; whereas teacher bias, hindrance from others, the desired date's being busy, and parents as obstacles all place causality external to the unsatisfied individual. It therefore may be stated that lack of math ability and being a boring person are, in some respects, similar, just as are teacher bias and the desired mate's having already made plans. The property of causal location is the same within each of these pairings but differs between the pairs (internal vs. external).

A second causal property that proved of great importance in this book is controllability, or the degree to which a cause is volitionally alterable. Lack of effort is perceived as controllable and thus may elicit perceptions of personal responsibility. In addition, often traits like being sloppy or boring also are judged by others as controllable—the causal agent can dress better or converse about more interesting topics. Lack of effort as a cause of failure to achieve and the perception that one is boring as a cause of social rejection, therefore, are in some sense identical, as are lack of aptitude as a cause of math failure and greater-than-average height as a cause of social rejection, in that the last two are classified as uncontrollable.

Related to this causal taxonomy is a second classification, which can be construed as a grouping of behaviors, states, and/or conditions. Not trying hard enough in school, overeating, consuming alcohol, and coming late for an appointment because of negligence all can be conceived as sin: The person is held responsible for these acts or states, which elicit anger, rebuke, and retribution. On the other hand, lack of ability, Alzheimer's disease, blindness, and so forth, are "sicknesses" inasmuch as the person is not considered to be responsible for these conditions or states (see Weiner, 1993b).

Clearly, classification of states, conditions, and behaviors as sin corresponds closely with a causal analysis that results in inferences of personal responsibility. This inference, in turn, necessitates personal and controllable causality. Conversely, sickness presumes lack of personal responsibility, which follows from beliefs of impersonal causality, the absence of personal controllability, and/or the presence of mitigating circumstances. The scientific leap from description to classification was absolutely essential for the creation of a theoretical system that embraces a variety of contexts in which beliefs about responsibility determine social conduct.

## FROM TAXONOMY TO EXPLANATION

I now come to the next highest stage of theoretical advancement, that of explanation. First I consider mechanisms and processes as explanation, and then I turn to function or purpose.

To first repeat the theoretical sequences that have been documented throughout the prior chapters:

1. Motivationally relevant explanation begins with an event that is interpreted as positive (e.g., success at achievement) or negative (failure).
2. Then the cause of this event is sought (with search most likely given a negative and unexpected outcome; see Weiner, 1986).
3. The cause is classified according to its basic properties. In this context, the causal dimensions of locus and controllability are of foremost importance.
4. If there is personal causality, controllability, and no mitigating circumstances, then the person is held responsible. External causality, lack of controllability and/or mitigating circumstances result in the absence of a judgment of responsibility. Thus, the process goes from causal understanding to an inference about the person.
5. The responsibility of others for an adverse event gives rise to anger; lack of responsibility for an adverse state or condition in others gives rise to sympathy.
6. Anger acts as a goad to eliminate or to act against others, displayed behaviorally as reprimand, withholding of help, and aggression. Sympathy, on the other hand, causes the person who experiences this emotion to go toward the other and not to reprimand but to help.

Two sequences that capture social conduct from a responsibility perspective therefore are:

Failure → Cause (e.g., lack of effort) → Internal and personal controllability → Responsibility → Anger → Reprimand

Failure → Cause (e.g., lack of ability) → Internal but no personal controllability → No responsibility → Sympathy → No reprimand

(These sequences do not include direct linkages between thinking and doing.)

This theory of social conduct may be broken down and shown to be composed of three sub- or minitheories:

1. A theory of how responsibility inferences are reached
2. A cognitive theory of emotion that assumes that thoughts (appraisals) are the necessary and sufficient determinants of feelings
3. A theory of social conduct presuming that thoughts and/or affects are the determinants of action (In the two sequences outlined above, it was assumed that thinking gives rise to feelings which, in turn, promote action.)

Let me, then, consider the responsibility, affective, and motivational processes incorporated within the broader conceptual picture.

## The Responsibility Process

Recall that the hypothesized responsibility process includes the assumption that an event has occurred and then the person to whom that event happened, as well as others, search for the cause. The first step in the responsibility process after the perception of the event involves a determination of whether there was personal or situational causality; only with personal causality can another be construed as responsible.

Given that responsibility inferences are so prevalent, it follows that beliefs of person causality also are widespread. This may be accounted for by a number of facts. First, there is abundant evidence that perceivers tend to minimize the causal effect of the situation and overestimate the causal contribution or importance of an individual in that situation. The underestimation of situational constraints is so well documented that it has the title of the "fundamental attribution error" (see Ross & Nisbett, 1991). This "error" may be traced to perceptual tendencies, including the focus of attention on the individual rather on the situation or context.

Motivational factors, including the belief that if causality is located within the person, then it is more controllable, also can account for the prevalence of perceiving the other as responsible. In addition, in today's society, finding causality within another person can result in great financial benefit. For example, if a banana peel is believed to have been left intentionally or carelessly in front of a door, then a personal accident is more likely to lead to financial remuneration than if the perceived cause was a strong wind that scattered garbage throughout the neighborhood.

Finally, finding another person or even a larger entity responsible for a negative event can protect an individual from an inference of self-responsibility. For example, ascribing school failure to an unfair teacher or to a biased school system may be more hedonically positive than attributing that failure to lack of personal effort. Finding others responsible thus is entangled with thoughts about the self. The movie character who "blamed society" in the film *Repo Man* can feel justified about his social anger and maintain his self-esteem—consequences that would not follow if the self is inferred to be responsible for negative life events.

Indeed, it has been said that contemporary America can be described as a "culture of victimization," where others are blamed for personal problems, instead of accepting self-responsibility. These "others" range from parents who are held responsible by their children for poor child-rearing practices to larger bureaucratic structures that then become the target for responsibility judgments. Acts of violence against governmental officials, as witnessed recently when an unemployed person shot and killed a number of individuals working in a government-operated welfare and employment agency, then become somewhat more "understandable" in that frustration for a negative state (unemployment) is accompanied by inferences of responsibility and anger.

Of course, there often is actual responsibility of the other for victimization, and the appropriate allocation of responsibility then becomes a salient issue. A number of years ago it was reported that African Americans who were classified as external on locus of control engaged in more social activism than did those who were considered as internal on this trait. This finding follows inasmuch as African Americans placed responsibility for their problems on external forces in the society and then acted according to this belief (Lao, 1970; see also the discussion of feminist beliefs in Chapter 3).

One might argue that there are negative as well as positive benefits to holding others responsible for one's plight in that it breeds paranoia and lack of self-responsibility. These complex issues go beyond the scope of this book and the abilities of this writer. Rather, here I merely want to point out the everyday importance of judgments of responsibility and the interactiveness of judgments of the responsibility of the self with judgments of the responsibility of the other.

## Speculations about Inferences of Responsibility among Infrahumans

It is of interest to consider whether humans are unique in judging others as responsible or not, basing their social behavior on this inference. Behavior directed by inferences regarding the responsibility of others requires that we understand their mental states, knowing whether they were doing something "on purpose" as opposed to acting "without volitional control," "without knowledge," or "with good intentions."

Even for humans, discriminations between intended versus unintended behavior, or between actions for which the person is or is not responsible, are difficult to make. Did the battered wife kill her husband as an act of cold-blooded and thoughtful revenge, or was this crime committed because "there was no other choice?" Did the husband whose wife was having an affair kill her as an act of uncontrollable passion, or was this a carefully planned murder? Did a friend miss your party "on purpose," or did the car really not start? As the reader well knows, such inferences about others are quite complex.

Seyfarth and Cheny (1992) add a very mundane yet revealing example to this list regarding the dilemma of interpreting whether the behavior of another was or was not intentional and controllable:

> During the Wimbledon tennis championship in 1981, officials were confronted with an unusual problem. Some male players, notably Jimmy Connors, were regularly grunting loudly as they hit the ball. Their opponents protested, demanding that this practice be stopped. These quieter players claimed that the noises were distracting and were emitted deliberately to throw off their timing.
>
> When officials confronted Connors and other "vocal" players, they received a slightly different explanation. Connors said that some players do grunt on purpose—but not him. He explained that he had no control over his grunting; it just happened when he hit the ball hard.
>
> The Wimbledon officials then observed the different players, trying to discern which grunts were intentional and which were not. They found the distinction virtually impossible to make. (p. 122)

Grunting is an appropriate response to consider when examining inferences about intentions in infrahumans, for this is one type of vocalization of monkeys and chimps. Do their vocalizations and behaviors provide evidence regarding intended versus unintended acts, and do they reveal knowledge of the difference between an intentional act and an unintended one when committed by others? That is, do monkeys and chimps have a theory of the mind, and can they infer the mental states of others?

There is anecdotal evidence that animals in the wild do intentionally deceive one another, withholding information "on purpose." For example, there are stories of chimps knowing where there is a supply of food and then walking away from that food to mislead other chimps. They then return to the stash by themselves and consume the bounty (see Seyfarth & Cheny, 1992, for other examples as well). Of course, there are more parsimonious explanations of this behavior that do not involve assumptions that the chimp "knows" what others do and do not know. Nonetheless, intended deception is one possible interpretation of such conduct.

In one experimental study that called into question the mental abilities of macaques monkeys, a mother and her child were placed in separate chambers where they could observe one another. In one experimental condition, only the mother had the opportunity to view a third adjoining room, while in a second experimental condition both the mother and the child could observe this other enclosure. Then the experimenter either placed some food in that room or hid within the room after making threatening gestures. If the mother was able to infer the knowledge of the child, then she might exhibit different behaviors or express different sounds when the child did or did not have knowledge about what had taken place, given that the child now had access to the room. However, differences in the two conditions were not displayed, suggesting that either the monkey mothers did not have a theory of the mind, i.e., could not infer the knowledge of the other, or else they could not vocally make use of this ability (if indeed they had it).

A different variation of these conditions might allow us to determine if monkeys are guided by judgments of responsibility. Assume in the above experiment that a predator was in the area and in one condition a youngster was unaware of this danger, whereas the mother did have such knowledge. In another condition, the young chimp as well as the mother had pertinent information about the predator. If the young chimp now strayed into danger in these two conditions, then would the mother express different reprimands (vocal communications)? That is, would there be evidence for a differentiation between ability and effort attributions for "dangerous" behavior (the reader should assume here, for the sake of the illustration, that the present danger does not mask or overwhelm the possibility of differential expressions). If the mother differentially punished on the basis of the cause of behavior, could it then be contended that humans are not the only species with a concept of "sin," i.e., a differentiation between transgressions based on inferences of responsibility?

I offered this flawed experiment only to point out that there remains much of value and interest regarding the development of a cognitive psychology of infrahumans that relates to issues raised in this book. Based on current evidence, one would be surprised if responsibility inferences are part of the capacity of nonhuman species (this would create havoc for theologians!). However, it does appear that mothers differentiate an "accidental" hit by an infant from a purposive hostility by an enemy, and research on animal knowledge and communication has yielded many unexpected findings. Thus, it is not unreasonable to raise questions regarding these issues.

## The Affective Process

Recall that the theory of social behavior championed in this book can be described as composed of the responsibility process (just discussed), the affective process (to be discussed now) and a motivational process (to be soon introduced). Let me therefore turn to the affective process.

A very central position assumed throughout this book is that cognitive appraisals are necessary and/or sufficient antecedents of certain affective experiences. Specifically, anger follows from the perception that others are responsible for a negative plight, whereas sympathy is generated when others are not responsible for their unfortunate condition. Of course, the more important or personally relevant the context, the greater the affective intensity. We may have relatively little anger toward students who do not study, but this anger increases greatly if we are their teachers or parents. In a similar manner, we have some sympathy for others who are living under a totalitarian regime, but we have greater sympathy if a personal acquaintance is being held in prison by that regime. The evidence regarding these appraisal–emotion linkages is unequivocal.

### On Altering Appraisal–Emotion Linkages

Can the responsibility–anger and the nonresponsibility–sympathy linkages be altered? In one illustration of this possibility, it has been noted that there may be limits on how much sympathy we "give," as if emotional feelings can be represented as a closed system with fixed amounts "available" for use.

The assumption of what is known as "compassion fatigue" has been derived from apparent shifts in attitudes toward homeless people. It has been noted that the government as well as individuals are becoming harsher in their treatment of the poor and of homeless people: these sufferers are no longer being allowed to sleep in the park, while kitchens for homeless people, the availability of volunteer helpers, and charity donations are all relatively decreasing. Because of the number of homeless people, it has been postulated that persons are experiencing "compassion fatigue," i.e., their capacity for the experience of sympathy toward this group is dwindling because of overuse. This presumes that inferences of responsibility have not shifted (they could have), but rather that the affective responses to this ascription have undergone modification and/or habituation (see Blackburn, 1988; Rolland, 1988; and Smyer & Birkel, 1991, for related discussions).

Another issue to be considered is whether anger and sympathy can be aroused in situations where responsibility is not inferred. This is a difficult question, but I believe that the answer is no (see also Chapter 1). We are frustrated and unhappy when our tire is flat, but not angry (or nonspecifically angry) at the tire. We might, however, be angry at the (unknown) person who left a glass bottle in the street, thus causing the flat tire. Sympathetic affects may be more complex. Might we be sympathetic to someone dying of AIDS, even if the cause of the HIV infection that led to AIDS was promiscuous sexual behavior? Intuitively the answer to this is yes, but what is not clear is whether this reaction is elicited because dying is uncontrollable—instrumental actions cannot be undertaken. Would similar feelings of sympathy be elicited, for example, by a person with anorexia who refused to eat and, thus, was literally starving him- or herself to death? Perhaps, but I think not to the same extent as the person dying of AIDS (if starving oneself, or not eating, truly is perceived as controllable). However, these obviously are difficult issues and, as I previously indicated, the fine-grained indicators of disparate emotional experiences are not available to definitively answer the questions that have been raised.

Finally, can there be help without sympathy, and aggression without anger? I am more confident in answering these affirmatively. I may help my irresponsible brother, and robbers have been known to express their apologies following a robbery (an experience I once encountered). It has not been contended that only anger gives rise to aggression or that only sympathy gives rise to prosocial conduct. In addition, it is not the case the anger must generate antisocial behavior or that sympathy must promote displays of prosocial behavior. Rather, the affects give rise to behavioral tendencies; the actual expression of the tendency is quite overdetermined. This reasoning, in part, led me to contend that there will not be a general theory of achievement, or aggression, or altruism. These behaviors may be displayed given any number of antecedents and may not be displayed although there is a known antecedent present.

In sum, I suspect that the proper characterization of the thinking–emotion union is just short of being "strong," i.e., one can reasonably contend that the relation between responsibility for a negative act and anger, as well as between nonresponsibility for a personal plight and sympathy, is both sufficient and perhaps even necessary. On the other hand, the feeling–behavior union is "weak" in that there is neither necessary nor sufficient causality—for example, there may be aggression without anger, and the presence of anger is not sufficient for aggression.

Again this is not the appropriate context to address such complex issues, which themselves require the writing of a book. For now, I wish to make clear the fundamental assumptions in the book and, at the same time, prevent misunderstandings about the proposed linkages between thinking–feeling–acting.

## The Motivational Process

While a thinking–feeling–acting sequence has been featured in this book, it also has been acknowledged that this is not an invariant sequence. Indeed, a note of caution and the likelihood of multiple processes characterizes the position taken in all the previous chapters. The data presented in the prior pages suggest that this ordering is most applicable with actions that reflect on the self and with important goals. Thus, it is predicted that if another intentionally interferes with my academic career, or my spousal relationship, then I will infer responsibility, become angry, and act on those feelings. However, if I am informed that there was intentional interference with the career of someone I barely know, I again infer responsibility, experience modulated anger, and am likely to base my actions on more abstract and distal beliefs rather than (or in addition to) my feelings. This may be because events unimportant to oneself arouse minimal affect, or it could be that the motivational sequence differs as events become less and less personally relevant. I suspect that both mechanisms may be operative, but particularly the latter.

The issue of motivational sequence is of great importance and has far-reaching psychological implications, particularly in regard to what intervention techniques will prove most effective for behavioral change. There are very little data pertinent to this issue.

## THEORETICAL GENERALIZATION AND INTEGRATION

As is well accepted, the broader the generality of a theory, the more its power and contribution to the scientific goal of creating order in the universe in the simplest manner possible. Throughout this book, I have attempted to document that the theoretical principles first derived from the study of achievement evaluation generalize to explain some aspects of reactions to the stigmatized, helping behavior, aggression, and impression management techniques. The usefulness of the basic principles across this diversity of situations is indeed impressive. This generality is fostered by the unmistakable observation that inferences of responsibility and/or their linked affects are central in guiding behaviors in all of these contexts. The prior discussion regarding achievement evaluation, reactions to those who are stigmatized, helping behavior, and aggression are summarized in Table 9.1.

I therefore believe that what has been proposed in the previous chapters are some of the basic principles that guide human conduct, across cultures and over time. Stated with still more bravado, a few of the underlying rules of the social universe have been presented. I do not believe that this is an outrageous statement. Indeed, you, the reader, may have concluded that you knew all these rules or principles already and that nothing really "new" has been discussed. I will return to briefly address this issue later in the chapter, when examining the overlap between the contents of the book and naive psychology.

## Theoretical Integration with Personal Motivation

There is another aspect of theoretical generality that has not yet been discussed, namely, theoretical integration. This perhaps is the highest stage of conceptual development (recall that the prior steps were description, taxonomy, explanation, and generalization). By integration, I mean the unification of this theory with another theory or theories, thereby embracing the data that support each of the conceptions. If this is possible, then

TABLE 9.1. A Foundation for a Theory of Social Conduct

| Event | Cause/type | Responsibility antecedent | | Behavioral reaction |
|---|---|---|---|---|
| Failure to achieve | Lack of effort | Causal controllability | | Reprimand |
| Stigmatizing condition | Behavioral/ mental type | Causal controllability | Responsibility ⟶ Anger | Condemnation |
| Need for help | Drinking, lack of effort | Causal controllability | | Neglect |
| Aggressive act of another | | Intentionality | | Retaliation |
| Failure to achieve | Lack of aptitude | Causal uncontrollability | | Withholding of reprimand |
| Stigmatizing condition | Somatic type | Causal uncontrollability | No responsibility ⟶ Sympathy | No condemnation |
| Need for help | Illness, low ability | Causal uncontrollability | | Help |
| Aggressive act of another | | Unintentionality | | No retaliation |

an overarching framework with even greater power would have been created.

Social motivation was the focus of this book—evaluation and appraisal of others, helping and aggression, interpersonal communications, and so on—that is, motivation in an interpersonal context. Personal motivations explained by intrapsychic processes and mechanisms have not been addressed. Can, then, a responsibility-based theory of social motivation be integrated with a theory of personal motivation, thereby increasing theoretical generality and power? I turn now to this topic, starting with an examination of a theory of achievement striving.

## An Attributional Analysis of Achievement Behavior

An attributional approach to behavior, which is one description of the present theory of social motivation, has been most prominent and useful in the achievement domain. There is a "main" finding related to achievement performance that corresponds in importance to the observation that lack of effort more than lack of ability is punished by others when it is a cause of failure. This finding is that if personal failure is ascribed to insufficient effort, then performance on the next occasion or opportunity to attain this same goal will be better than if the prior failure is attributed to lack of ability (see review in Weiner, 1986). That is, performance is relatively enhanced if it is accepted that prior failure was due to the lack of "try" rather than to the absence of "can" (or personal efficacy). This finding does not have the certainty of the difference in reprimand for failure caused by low effort versus low ability, but it begins to approximate that status (see, for example, Bandura, 1986, for a discussion of the detrimental effects of a belief that "I cannot").

In the 1980s, along with many colleagues and students, I developed a theory to account for this observation (see Weiner, 1985, 1986). Classification of causes into underlying dimensions (as already discussed), identification of affective consequences of causal beliefs that are self directed (i.e., emotions that are directed toward oneself) and associations between attributions for prior performance and future expectancy of success were found to be the main processes and mechanisms aroused in achievement performance (see Figure 9.1). This theory regarding personal performance therefore, shares much with the conception of social motivation put forth in this book.

Figure 9.1 (which does not include all of the components in the theory as described in Weiner, 1985, 1986) indicates that the motivational sequence pertinent to achievement motivation is initiated with an outcome that is interpreted as a success or a failure. Based on information including past personal history of success and failure, the number of others who are

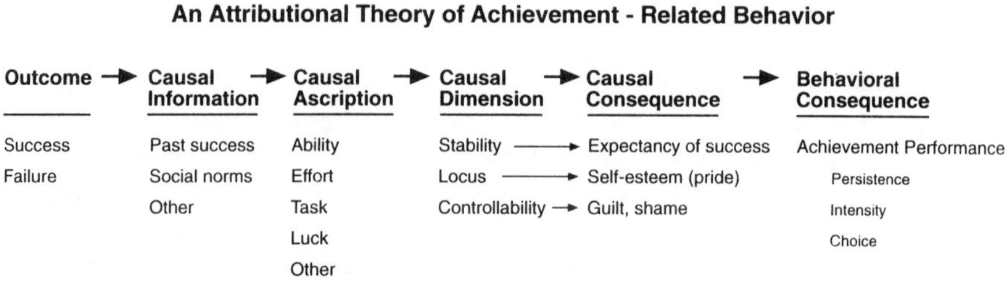

**An Attributional Theory of Achievement - Related Behavior**

| Outcome ➡ | Causal<br>Information | ➡ Causal<br>Ascription | ➡ Causal<br>Dimension | ➡ Causal<br>Consequence | ➡ Behavioral<br>Consequence |
|---|---|---|---|---|---|
| Success | Past success | Ability | Stability ────➤ | Expectancy of success | Achievement Performance |
| Failure | Social norms | Effort | Locus ────➤ | Self-esteem (pride) | Persistence |
| | Other | Task | Controllability ➤ | Guilt, shame | Intensity |
| | | Luck | | | Choice |
| | | Other | | | |

FIGURE 9.1. Simplified model of the determinants of achievement-related behavior. Data from Weiner (1986, p. 240).

succeeding and failing (social norms) and other antecedents not in need of mentioning here, an attribution for that outcome is reached. The attributions are quite varied and include such things as ability, effort, task characteristics, and luck. The specific attribution is then classified according to its dimensional properties. These properties include one that was not previously considered and two that were focused upon in this book. The newly introduced causal property is stability, which refers to the relative duration of a cause. Causes can be constant over time (stable), such as aptitude, or variable over time (unstable), such as luck. The two remaining properties of causes, already known to you, are locus (internal versus external to the actor) and controllability (controllable versus uncontrollable).

Causal stability influences the subjective probability of future success and failure. If an outcome (e.g., failure) is ascribed to a stable cause such as low aptitude, then that outcome will be anticipated again in the future. On the other hand, if the ascription for failure is to an unstable cause such as bad luck, then future failure may not be anticipated. Hence, an attribution of failure to low ability or aptitude results in a lower expectancy of future success than does an ascription of failure to lack of effort or bad luck, for aptitude is unchangeable, whereas effort and luck can vary over time.

In this theory of personal motivation, the locus of causality and causal controllability influence self-directed affective reactions. Causal locus is linked with pride in accomplishment and self-esteem. If an outcome (e.g., success) is ascribed to the self, then greater pride is experienced than if the outcome is attributed to external factors. Hence, for example, success caused by ability or effort results in greater pride in accomplishment than does success attributed to the ease of the task.

Causal controllability is related to the affects of guilt and shame. If failure is ascribed to an internal controllable cause such as lack of effort, then guilt is experienced. On the other hand, failure ascribed to an internal uncontrollable cause, such as low aptitude, gives rise to shame, humiliation, and embarrassment (see reviews in Weiner, 1986). Guilt, in turn, acts as a motivational goad that activates the person and enhances performance (assuming that its intensity is not too great), whereas shame promotes withdrawal from the task and inhibits subsequent performance (for more detailed discussion and supporting empirical evidence, see Weiner, 1986).

Let us, then, consider two motivational sequences to understand the processes and mechanisms that account for achievement strivings. Consider first the scenario of a student who does poorly on an exam and then drops out of school. Figure 9.1 reveals that following this negative outcome, the student will make use of certain information to reach a causal understanding of the event. Assume that the student has failed in the past and that other students did well on this exam. Given this information, the poor performance is ascribed to low intelligence, or aptitude. Aptitude is a stable cause, so that future failure is anticipated; aptitude is internal, so that there is a loss of self-esteem; and aptitude is uncontrollable, so that there is an experience of shame and humiliation. Low expectancy of success accompanied by low self-esteem and shame will result in dropping out of school.

Conversely, assume that another student who did poorly on the test recalls that she has performed well in the past and that she has not been studying recently. She then attributes the failure to lack of effort. Effort is unstable so that better outcomes are anticipated in the future. There is loss of self-esteem because effort is internal, and inasmuch as it is controllable, there is guilt over the poor performance. Reasonable expectation of success along with the positive motivational consequences of guilt result in performance enhancement.

In sum, ability and effort ascriptions produce differences in subsequent behavioral reactions to failure because they promote disparities in expectation of success (respectively, low vs. high) as well as differences in affective experiences (shame vs. guilt), with the former a motivational inhibitor and the latter a motivational enhancer. What has been outlined, then, are the mechanisms or processes that intervene between an outcome (failure) and the subsequent performance. This describes a theory of personal motivation that was developed prior to the conception of social motivation presented in this book.

## Combining the Theories

Figure 9.2 combines this theory of achievement striving with the theory of social motivation. These theories lend themselves to unification because both self-related and other-oriented motivational sequences are initiated with an outcome, that outcome is ascribed to a specific cause, the cause is classified according to its basic properties, these characteristics have affec-

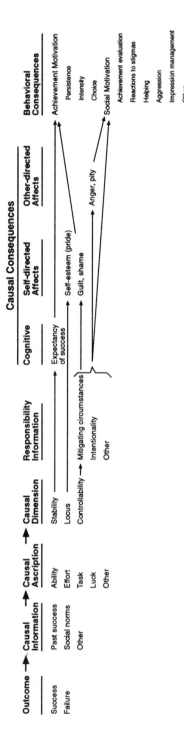

FIGURE 9.2. Combining theories of social motivation and personal motivation within a more embracing conceptual framework.

tive and/or cognitive consequences, and the consequences have motivational implications.

Self-related motivation incorporates expectancy of success (which also is likely to play some role in social motivation, although not discussed in the book), and the specified emotions (guilt and shame) are self-directed. On the other hand, social motivation includes the responsibility process in regard to inferences about others, and the emotions (anger and pity) are other-directed (i.e., directed by the self toward another or others). But the general structure of the two theories is identical.

Self-directed emotions, which are part of personal motivation, and other-directed emotions, which are part of social motivation, are not separate emotional systems, but are highly interactive. Hence, the motivational systems also will be intertwined.

Consider again the student who performs poorly because of lack of aptitude. Inasmuch as this is perceived as an uncontrollable cause, involved observers will communicate sympathy and pity to this person following failure. Introspect, for example, about your own reactions to a mentally handicapped person who is failing at some exam. These communications then add further information to the person that he or she "cannot," which then contributes to his or her feelings of shame and humiliation. That is, if pity and sympathy are "accepted," this contributes to or is an antecedent of a low-ability ascription, which gives rise to shame and humiliation. Little wonder, then, that the teacher of Helen Keller said to her parents, "We do not want your pity," for this "good" emotion is a performance inhibitor.

On the other hand, if the student fails because of lack of effort, the teacher will communicate anger. Anger is a cue that the other is responsible for the failure and that failure is controllable. Hence, if this affect is "accepted," then the student will ascribe his or her personal failure to lack of effort, which increases guilt.

The relations between self-directed and other-directed emotions are depicted in Table 9.2, where the emotions are differentiated according to the causal dimension of controllability and their direction (self vs. other). This theoretical analysis has been supported in an experimental study

TABLE 9.2. The Interaction between Personal and Social Motivation when Examining Affective Reactions

|  | Controllable causality | Uncontrollable causality |
| --- | --- | --- |
| Self-directed emotion | Guilt | Shame |
| Other-directed emotion | Anger | Sympathy |

conducted by Graham (1984). She found that when experimenters communicated sympathy to a subject who was experiencing failure in an experimental setting, that subject tended to ascribe the failure to lack of
ability. On the other hand, communicated anger resulted in a personal
ascription of failure to lack of effort. Self-directed emotions were not
examined in that study, but the relations between self-directed ascriptions
and emotions are well-documented.


## FUNCTIONAL EXPLANATIONS

I previously indicated that two types of scientific explanations of psychological phenomena have been differentiated. One, just discussed in some
detail, establishes the processes and the mechanisms that intervene between
a stimulus and the response to that situation. The second, which I address
now, considers the function of the behavior in that context.

A functional interpretation begins with the assumption that the behavior that has evolved has positive consequences either for the individual,
the species, or the genetic pool of a particular individual, depending on
one's evolutionary stance. Here these differences are not of significance.
What is important is that this approach leads one to ask questions about the
functions of attributions, emotions, and behaviors. What function or purpose might it have to experience guilt or shame, or anger or pity? What is
the significance of the linkages between causal appraisals and feeling states?
What are the positive effects of communicating anger? In addition, what
are the results of punishing lack of effort? Why should we refuse to help
the needy who require aid because they are lazy? Why should intentional,
but not unintended, aggression give rise to retaliation?

Let us consider emotional experiences first. It has been contended that
failure ascribed to lack of effort, a controllable cause, produces guilt, which
is a behavioral motivator. On the other hand, failure caused by lack of
aptitude, an uncontrollable cause, generates shame, which is a behavioral
inhibitor. The positive consequences of these emotions can be understood
if the assumption articulated by Heider (1958) that both "can" and "try"
are necessary for achievement performance, is accepted. If failure is caused
by (or is perceived to be caused by) low aptitude, which is constant over
time and not controllable, then success cannot be attained. It therefore
would be dysfunctional to continue to expend effort. Hence, it could be
argued that an emotion has evolved (shame) that prevents the organism
from persisting in the face of an unattainable goal. Goal persistence is not
invariably positive (see Janoff-Bulman & Brickman, 1982).

On the other hand, effort is modifiable and unstable. Hence, failure caused by lack of effort gives rise to an affect, namely, guilt, which promotes increased effort (see Trivers, 1971). This should then result in a more favorable outcome. Both the affective reactions of shame and guilt, which have opposing motivational consequences, therefore enhance the survival fitness of the person experiencing these emotions (assuming, of course, that the causal assessment is "correct").

Now consider the other-directed emotions of anger and sympathy. Anger is experienced when another has done something that he or she "should not have." Anger communicates that this behavior is unacceptable, and it is interpreted as a threat by the transgressor (see Trivers, 1971). Anger also promotes retaliation, which prevents the other from continuing the untoward behavior. Anger thus teaches the offender a lesson, thereby contributing to behavioral change and rehabilitation. In addition, inferences of personal responsibility for the transgressions of another and their links to anger promote a "tit-for-tat" philosophy, giving in return what is believed to be "just." The evolution of this system of justice is in service of the survival of the individual who has been the target of transgression.

Sympathy, on the other hand, is experienced when another is not responsible for his or her plight. This emotion promotes the giving of help, which increases the survival likelihood of the recipient of this aid. If, for example, the needy person is one's helpless infant, then it is evident that prosocial behavior benefits the survival of the helper's genetic pool.

In sum, it is possible to examine each linkage in the general theory shown in Figure 9.2 from a functional perspective, although posthoc interpretations that give every association a "reason" can be scientifically suspect. Nonetheless, mechanisms and functional analyses are closely intertwined.

## A FEW CONCLUDING REMARKS

I will now close the book with a brief discussion of a few unrelated but nagging topics that I find fascinating and pertinent to theory building related to social conduct.

### On Strong versus Weak Theory

A distinction has been made between strong versus weak theories (see Eysenck, 1993). According to Eysenck (1993):

> For weak theories, positive results are much more important than negative results, because a positive result from testing a deduction from a theory suggests both hypotheses and K [assumptions] are cor-

rect. . . . For strong theories, negative results are much more important, as the role of K has been much reduced. (p. 245)

Given a responsibility analysis of social conduct, relatively little is now
to be learned if lack of effort is punished more than lack of ability as the
cause of failure, if HIV infection caused by promiscuity is reacted to with
less sympathy than HIV infection caused by a blood transfusion, and so on.
The conceptual network supporting these facts is so strong that theoretical
progress will not be made with further confirmation of these hypotheses.
On the other hand, if a culture or group or situation is found in which these
relations do not hold, or are reversed, then this could serve as the spring-
board for much theoretical alteration and great insight into that culture,
group, or situation. It is perhaps now time for the conscious search for
conditions in which theoretically derived hypotheses might not be
confirmed!

## Naive Psychology

Bertrand Russell is said to have asserted that philosophy starts with something so intuitively obvious that no one wants to discuss it and ends with
something so paradoxical that no one believes it. Perhaps this description
characterizes the present book as well. I started with the obvious fact that
students who do not try are admonished. I then documented that people
have little sympathy toward drug users, individuals who overeat, and those
infected with the HIV virus because of homosexual behavior. I also reported that people do not help others who have brought about their own
problems and are likely to aggressively retaliate against others who commit
hostile acts "on purpose." And I documented how excuses and confessions
are used by transgressors to ameliorate their targets. None of these findings
should be surprising to the reader; they are in accord with common sense,
or general knowledge.

But then I attempted to show that all these phenotypically diverse
phenomena can be comprised within the identical theoretical framework,
shown in Table 9.1. This is beyond the creation of the "naive person," who
is not concerned with conscious systematization of knowledge and the
imposition of order. Yet these are precisely the goals of science. Indeed, if
it was stated that helping the blind and revealing that one was late for a date
because of car problems are "similar," this would be met by the naive
person with skepticism (at best)!

There is no reason to believe that the contents of everyday psychology,
as opposed to psychological processes, are beyond the knowledge of the
person on the street (see Kelley, 1992). But this should not create fear that
psychology is obvious. It is just, at times, the study of the obvious. I believe

that social psychologists search for what is not obvious because they are afraid that their investigations are not worthwhile. I do not accept this condition of fear: What is worthwhile is the creation of theoretical or conceptual systems that create order and establish regularity. If Stephen Hawking, as quoted at the start of the chapter, believes that all individuals will be able to understand the laws of physics, then why should we not think the same about psychological laws?

## The Rules of Social Conduct

Many of the rules of social conduct that are related to beliefs about responsibility already have been prescribed. The law describes what is to be and not to be punished and the determinants of the severity of the punishment. In a similar manner, the Bible and other theological writings tell what transgressions are not allowed. Naive psychology borrows from these sources and changes them as well. Thus, for example, as we come to understand the psychological restrictions that burden abused children and battered wives, the laws for their retaliatory crimes are amended. And as society changes, so does the interpretation of theological writings. These two written sources—legal and religious writings, combine with common sense and naive psychology to define the rules of social conduct. I believe that understanding the mutual influences of written and everyday rules on one another lies at the heart of the study of social behavior. This book has addressed that interrelationship.

# References

Aarons, M., Cameron, T., Roizen, J., Roizen, R., Room, R., Schneberk, D., & Wingard, D. (1977). *Alcohol, casualties, and crime.* Berkeley, CA: UCB Alcohol Research Group.

Aguero, J. E., Bloch, L., & Byrne, D. (1984). The relationship among sexual beliefs, attitudes, experience and homophobia. *Journal of Homosexuality, 10,* 95–107.

Allon, N. (1979). Self-perception of the stigma of overweight in relationship to weight-losing patients. *American Journal of Nutrition, 32,* 470–480.

Allon, N. (1982). The stigma of overweight in everyday life. In B. Wolman (Ed.), *Psychological aspects of obesity: A handbook* (pp. 130–147). New York: Van Nostrand Reinhold.

Altemeir, W. A., III, O'Connor, S., Vietze, P. M., Sandler, H. M., & Sherrod, K. B. (1982). Antecedents of child abuse. *Journal of Pediatrics, 100,* 823–829.

Ambrose, S., Hazzard, A., & Haworth, J. (1980). Cognitive-behavioral parenting groups for abusive families. *Child Abuse and Neglect, 4,* 119–125.

Anderson, D. (1991, November 14). Sorry, but Magic Johnson isn't a hero. *New York Times,* p. B-7.

Anderson, V. N. (1992). For whom is this world just? Sexual orientation and AIDS. *Journal of Applied Social Psychology, 22,* 248–259.

Aramburu, B. F., & Leigh, B. C. (1991). For better or worse: Attributions about drunken aggression toward male and female victims. *Violence and Victims, 6,* 31–41.

Archer, D. (1985). Social deviance. In G. Lindzey & E. Aronson (Eds.),

*Handbook of social psychology* (3rd ed., Vol. 2, pp. 743–804). New York: Random House.

Asarnow, J. R., & Callan, J. W. (1985). Boys with peer adjustment problems: Social cognitive processes. *Journal of Consulting and Clinical Psychology, 53*, 500–505.

Attitudes toward homosexuals poll. (1993, March 5). *New York Times*, p. A14.

Averill, J. R. (1979). Anger. In R. A. Dienstbier (Ed.), *Nebraska symposium on motivation* (Vol. 26, pp. 1–80). Lincoln: University of Nebraska Press.

Averill, J. R. (1982). *Anger and aggression: An essay on emotion.* New York: Springer-Verlag.

Averill, J. R. (1983). Studies on anger and aggression. *American Psychologist, 38*, 1145–1160.

Bandura, A. (1986). *Social foundations of thought and action: A social cognitive theory.* Englewood Cliffs, NJ: Prentice-Hall.

Barnes, R. D., Ickes, W., & Kidd, R. F. (1979). Effects of the perceived intentionality and stability of another's dependency on helping behavior. *Personality and Social Psychology Bulletin, 5*, 367–372.

Baron, R. A. (1971). Magnitude of victim's pain cues and level of prior arousal as determinants of adult aggressive behavior. *Journal of Personality and Social Psychology, 17*, 236–243.

Barrowclough, C., Johnston, M., & Tarrier, N. (1994). Attributions, expressed emotion, and patient relapse: An attributional model of relatives' response to schizophrenic illness. *Behavior Therapy, 25*, 67–88.

Batson, C. D., Duncan, B., Ackerman, P., Buckley, T., & Birch, K. (1981). Is empathic emotion a source of altruistic motivation? *Journal of Personality and Social Psychology, 40*, 290–302.

Bauer, W. D., & Twentyman, C. T. (1985). Abusing, neglectful, and comparison mothers' responses to child-related and non-child-related stressors. *Journal of Abnormal Psychology, 53*, 335–343.

Beckman, L. (1979). Beliefs about the causes of alcohol-related problems among alcoholic and non-alcoholic women. *Journal of Clinical Psychology, 35*, 663–670.

Belgum, D. (1963). *Guilt: Where psychology and religion meet.* Englewood Cliffs, NJ: Prentice-Hall.

Belsky, J. (1980). Child maltreatment: An ecological integration. *American Psychologist, 35*, 320–335.

Belsky, J. (1993). Etiology of child maltreatment: A developmental–ecological analysis. *Psychological Bulletin, 114*, 413–434.

Bennett, W., & Gurin, J. (1982). *The dieter's dilemma.* New York: Basic Books.

Berger, S. M. (1962). Conditioning through vicarious instigation. *Psychological Review, 69,* 450–466.

Berkowitz, L. (1962). *Aggression: A social psychological analysis.* New York: McGraw-Hill.

Berkowitz, L. (1969). Resistance to improper dependency relationships. *Journal of Experimental Social Psychology, 5,* 283–294.

Berkowitz, L. (1993). *Aggression.* New York: McGraw-Hill.

Betancourt, H. (1990a). An attribution–empathy model of helping behavior. *Personality and Social Psychology Bulletin, 16,* 573–591.

Betancourt, H. (1990b). Intergroup and international conflict. In S. Graham & V. S. Folkes (Eds.), *Attribution theory: Applications to achievement, mental health, and interpersonal conflict* (pp. 205–220). Hillsdale, NJ: Erlbaum.

Betancourt, H., & Blair, I. (1992). A cognition (attribution)–emotion model of violence in conflict situations. *Personality and Social Psychology Bulletin, 18,* 343–350.

Bishop, G. D. (1987). Lay conceptions of physical symptoms. *Journal of Applied Social Psychology, 17,* 127–146.

Bishop, G. D., Alva, A. L., Cantu, L., & Rittman, T. K. (1991). Responses to persons with AIDS: Fear of contagion or stigma? *Journal of Applied Social Psychology, 21,* 1877–1888.

Bizman, A., & Hoffman, M. (1993). Expectations, emotions, and preferred responses regarding the Arab–Israeli conflict: An attributional analysis. *Journal of Conflict Resolution, 37,* 139–159.

Blackburn, J. (1988). Chronic health problems of the elderly. In C. S. Chilman, E. W. Nunnally, & F. M. Cox (Eds.), *Chronic illness and disability: Families in trouble series* (Vol. 2, pp. 108–122). Newbury Park: Sage.

Blum, T. C., Roman, P. M., & Bennett, N. (1989). Public images of alcoholism: Data from a Georgia survey. *Journal of Studies on Alcoholism, 50,* 5–14.

Blumstein, P. W., Carssow, K. G., Hall, J., Hawkins, B., Hoffman, R., Ishem, E., Maurer, C. P., Spens, D., Taylor, J., & Zimmerman, D. L. (1974). The honoring of accounts. *American Sociological Review, 39,* 551–566.

Bradbury, T. N., & Fincham, F. D. (1988). Assessing spontaneous attributions in marital interaction: Methodological and conceptual considerations. *Journal of Social and Clinical Psychology, 7,* 122–130.

Bradbury, T. N., & Fincham, F. D. (1989). Behavior and satisfaction in marriage: Prospective mediating processes. *Review of Personality and Social Psychology, 10,* 119–143.

Bradbury, T. N., & Fincham, F. D. (1990). Attributions in marriage: Review and critique. *Psychological Bulletin, 107*, 3–33.

Bradbury, T. N., & Fincham, F. D. (1992). Attributions and behavior in marital interaction. *Journal of Personality and Social Psychology, 63*, 613–628.

Brewer, M. B. (1977). An information processing approach to attribution of responsibility. *Journal of Experimental Social Psychology, 13*, 58–69.

Brewin, C. R. (1984). Perceived controllability of life-events and willingness to prescribe psychotropic drugs. *British Journal of Social Psychology, 23*, 285–287.

Brewin, C. R., MacCarthy, B., Duda, K., & Vaughn, C. E. (1991). Attribution and expressed emotion in the relatives of patients with schizophrenia. *Journal of Abnormal Psychology, 100*, 546–554.

Brickman, P., Rabinowitz, V. C., Karuza, J., Coates, D., Cohn, E., & Kidder, L. (1982). Models of helping and coping. *American Psychologist, 37*, 368–384.

Brown, J., & Weiner, B. (1984). Affective consequences of ability versus effort ascriptions: Controversies, resolutions, and quandaries. *Journal of Educational Psychology, 76*, 146–158.

Bugenthal, D. B. (1987). Attributions as moderator variables within social interaction systems. *Journal of Social and Clinical Psychology, 5*, 469–484.

Bugenthal, D. B., Blue, J., & Cruzcosa, M. (1989). Perceived control over caregiving outcomes: Implications for child abuse. *Developmental Psychology, 25*, 532–539.

Caprara, G. V., Pastorelli, C., & Weiner, B. (1994). At-risk children's causal inferences given emotional feedback and their understanding of excuse-giving processes. *European Journal of Personality, 8*, 31–43.

Carlsmith, J. M., & Gross, S. E. (1969). Some effects of guilt on compliance. *Journal of Personality and Social Psychology, 11*, 232–239.

Carlson, M., & Miller, N. (1987). Explanation of the relation between negative mood and helping. *Psychological Bulletin, 102*, 72–90.

Chapman, D. P., & Levin, I. P. (1989). *Attribution in AIDS victimization: Experimental paradigm and theoretical model.* Paper presented at the 97th annual convention of the American Psychological Association, New Orleans, LA.

Chlouverakis, C. S. (1975). Controversies in medicine (II): Nature and nurture in human obesity. In B. Q. Hafen (Ed.), *Overweight and obesity: Causes, fallacies, treatment* (pp. 36–39). Provo, UT: Brigham Young University Press.

Coates, D., & Wortman, C. (1980). Depression maintenance and interpersonal control. In A. Baum & J. Singer (Eds.), *Advances in environmental psychology* (Vol. 2, pp. 149–182). Hillsdale, NJ: Erlbaum.

Collins, R. L. (in press). Social support provision to HIV-infected gay men. *Journal of Applied Social Psychology.*

Cooper, J. (1976). Deception and role playing: On telling the good guys from the bad guys. *American Psychologist, 31,* 605–610.

Cooper, J., & Fazio, R. (1979). The formation and persistence of attitudes that support intergroup conflict. In W. G. Austin & S. Worchel (Eds.), *The social psychology of intergroup relations* (pp. 183–195). Monterey, CA: Brooks/Cole.

Covington, M. V., & Omelich, C. L. (1979a). Effort: The double-edged sword in school achievement. *Journal of Educational Psychology, 71,* 169–182.

Covington, M. V., & Omelich, C. L. (1979b). It's best to be able and virtuous too: Student and teacher evaluative responses to successful effort. *Journal of Educational Psychology, 71,* 688–700.

Coyne, J. C. (1976a). Depression and the responses of others. *Journal of Abnormal Psychology, 85,* 186–193.

Coyne, J. C. (1976b). Towards an interactional description of depression. *Psychiatry, 39,* 28–40.

Coyne, J. C., Kahn, J., & Gotlib, I. H. (1987). Depression. In T. Jacob (Ed.), *Family interaction in psychopathology* (pp. 509–533). New York: Plenum Press.

Crandall, C. S. (1994). Prejudice against fat people: Ideology and self-interest. *Journal of Personality and Social Psychology, 66,* 882–894.

Crandall, C. S. (in press). Do parents discriminate against their heavyweight daughters? *Personality and Social Psychology Bulletin.*

Crandall, C. S., & Biernat, M. R. (1990). The ideology of anti-fat attitudes. *Journal of Applied Social Psychology, 20,* 227–243.

Crandall, C. S., & Martinez, R. (1993). *Culture, ideology, and anti-fat attitudes.* Unpublished manuscript, University of Kansas, Lawrence.

Crandall, C. S., & Moriarty, D. (in press). The dimensions of stigma: Physical illness and social rejection. *Personality and Social Psychology Bulletin.*

Crick, N., & Ladd, G. (1990). Children's perceptions of the outcomes of social strategies: Do the ends justify the means? *Developmental Psychology, 26,* 612–620.

Critchlow, B. (1986). The powers of John Barlecorn. *American Psychologist, 41,* 751–764.

D'Andrade, R. G., Quinn, N. R., Nerlove, S. B., & Romney, A. K. (1972). Categories of disease in American–English and Mexican–Spanish. In

A. K. Romney, R. N. Shepard, & S. B. Nerlove (Eds.), *Multidimensional scaling: Theory and applications in the behavioral sciences* (Vol. 2, pp. 9–54). New York: Seminar Press.

Darby, B. W., & Schlenker, B. R. (1982). Children's reactions to apologies. *Journal of Personality and Social Psychology, 43,* 742–753.

Davitz, J. R. (1969). *The language of emotion.* New York: Academic.

deJong, W. (1980). The stigma of obesity: The consequences of naive assumptions concerning the causes of physical deviance. *Journal of Health and Social Behavior, 21,* 75–87.

Dionne, E. J., Jr. (1991). *Why Americans hate politics.* New York: Simon & Schuster.

Dodge, K. A. (1980). Social cognition and children's aggressive behavior. *Child Development, 51,* 162–170.

Dodge, K. A., & Coie, J. (1987). Social information processing factors in reactive and proactive aggression in children's peer groups. *Journal of Personality and Social Psychology, 53,* 1146–1158.

Dodge, K. A., & Crick, N. (1990). Social information-processing bases of aggressive behavior in children. *Personality and Social Psychology Bulletin, 16,* 8–22.

Dodge, K. A., & Frame, C. L. (1982). Social cognitive biases and deficits in aggressive boys. *Child Development, 53,* 620–635.

Dooley, P. A. (in press). Perceptions of the onset controllability of AIDS and helping judgments: An attributional analysis. *Journal of Applied Social Psychology.*

Downey, M. (1991, November 17). His lifestyle can't blunt the pain of loss. *Los Angeles Times,* p. C-1.

Dyck, R. J., & Rule, B. G. (1978). Effect of retaliation of causal attributions concerning attack. *Journal of Personality and Social Psychology, 36,* 521–529.

Eisenberg, L. (1977). Disease and illness: Distinction between professional and popular ideas of sickness. *Culture, Medicine, and Psychiatry, 1,* 9–23.

Ekman, P. (1984). *Telling lies.* New York: Norton.

Engfer, A., & Schneewind, K. A. (1982). Causes and consequences of harsh parental punishment: An empirical investigation in a representative sample of 570 German families. *Child Abuse and Neglect, 6,* 129–139.

Epstein, S., & Taylor, S. P. (1967). Instigation to aggression as a function of degree of defeat and perceived aggressive intent of the opponent. *Journal of Personality, 35,* 265–289.

Eswara, H. S. (1972). Administration of reward and punishment in relation to ability, effort, and performance. *Journal of Social Psychology, 87,* 139–140.

Eysenck, H. (1993). Creativity and personality: An attempt to bridge divergent traditions. *Psychological Inquiry, 4,* 238–246.

Farwell, L., & Weiner, B. (1993). *On perceptions of the "fairness" of others in achievement evaluation.* Unpublished manuscript, University of California, Los Angeles.

Feagin, J. R. (1972). Poverty: We still believe that God helps those who help themselves. *Psychology Today, 6,* 101–110.

Feather, N. T. (1974). Explanations of poverty in Australian and American samples: The person, society, or fate? *Australian Journal of Psychology, 26,* 199–216.

Feather, N. T. (1992). An attributional and value analysis of deservingness in success and failure situations. *British Journal of Social Psychology, 31,* 125–145.

Feather, N. T., Volkmer, R. E., & McKee, I. R. (1991). Attitudes towards high achievers in public life: Attributions, deservingness, personality, and affect. *Australian Journal of Psychology, 43,* 85–91.

Felson, R. B., & Ribner, S. A. (1981). An attributional approach to accounts and sanctions for violence. *Social Psychology Quarterly, 44,* 137–142.

Ferguson, T., & Rule, B. (1983). An attributional perspective on anger and aggression. In R. Geen & E. Donnerstein (Eds.), *Aggression: Theoretical and empirical reviews: Vol. 1. Theoretical and methodological issues* (pp. 41–74). Orlando, FL: Academic Press.

Feshbach, N., & Feshbach, S. (1974). The relationship between empathy and aggression in two age groups. *Developmental Psychology, 7,* 306–313.

Fincham, F. D. (1985). Attribution processes in distressed and nondistressed couples: 2. Responsibility for marital problems. *Journal of Abnormal Psychology, 94,* 183–190.

Fincham, F. D., & Beach, S. R. (1988). Attribution processes in distressed and nondistressed couples: 5. Real versus hypothetical events. *Cognitive Therapy and Research, 12,* 505–514.

Fincham, F. D., & Bradbury, T. N. (1987). The impact of attributions in marriage: A longitudinal analysis. *Journal of Personality and Social Psychology, 53,* 510–517.

Fincham, F. D., & Bradbury, T. N. (1992). Assessing attributions in marriage: The Relationship Attribution Measure. *Journal of Personality and Social Psychology, 62,* 457–468.

Fincham, F. D., & Bradbury, T. N. (1993). Marital satisfaction, depression, and attributions: A longitudinal analysis. *Journal of Personality and Social Psychology, 64,* 442–452.

Fincham, F. D., & Roberts, C. (1985). Intervening causation and the mitigation of responsibility for harm doing. *Journal of Experimental Social Psychology, 21,* 178–194.

Fincham, F. D., & Shultz, T. R. (1981). Intervening causation and the mitigation of responsibility for harm. *British Journal of Social Psychology, 20,* 113–120.

Folkes, V. S. (1982). Communicating the causes of social rejection. *Journal of Experimental Social Psychology, 18,* 235–252.

Folkes, V. S. (1985). Mindlessness or mindfulness: A partial replication and extension of Langer, Blank, and Chanowitz. *Journal of Personality and Social Psychology, 48,* 600–604.

Fox, R. (1992). Prejudice and the unfinished mind: A new look at an old failing. *Psychological Inquiry, 3,* 137–152.

Frijda, N. (1986). *The emotions.* New York: Cambridge University Press.

Frodi, A. M., & Lamb, M. E. (1980). Child abusers' responses to infant smiles and cries. *Child Development, 51,* 238–241.

Fuller, L. (1969). *The morality of law* (2nd ed.). New Haven: Yale University Press.

Fuller, T. (1642). *The holy state.* Cambridge, England: Cambridge University Press.

Funk, C. E. (1950). *Thereby hang a tale.* New York: Harper & Row.

Furnham, A. (1982). Why are the poor always with us? Explanations for poverty in Britain. *British Journal of Social Psychology, 21,* 311–322.

Furnham, A., & Lowick, V. (1984). Lay theories of the causes of alcoholism. *British Journal of Medical Psychology, 57,* 319–332.

Furnham, A., & Rees, J. (1988). Lay theories of schizophrenia. *The International Journal of Social Psychiatry, 34,* 212–220.

Gilbert, D. T., Pelham, B. W., & Krull, D. S. (1988). Inference and interaction: The person perceiver meets the person perceived. *Journal of Personality and Social Psychology, 54,* 733–740.

Goethals, G. R. (1986). Fabricating and ignoring social reality: Self-serving estimates of consensus. In J. M. Olson, C. P. Herman, & M. P. Zanna (Eds.), *Relative deprivation and social comparison: The Ontario Symposium* (Vol. 4, pp. 135–157). Hillsdale, NJ: Erlbaum.

Goffman, E. (1963). *Stigma: Notes on the management of spoiled identity.* New York: Simon & Schuster.

Goldwater, B. M. (1988). *Goldwater.* New York: Doubleday.

Golub, J. S. (1984). *Abusive and nonabusive parents' perceptions of their children's behavior: An attributional analysis.* Unpublished doctoral dissertation, University of California, Los Angeles.

Golub, J. S., Espinosa, M., Damon, L., & Card, J. (1987). A videotape parent education program for abusive parents. *Child Abuse and Neglect, 11,* 255–265.

Graham, S. (1984). Communicated sympathy and anger to black and white children: The cognitive (attributional) consequences of affective cues. *Journal of Personality and Social Psychology, 47,* 40–54.

Graham, S. (1991). A review of attribution theory in achievement contexts. *Educational Psychology Review, 3,* 5–39.

Graham, S., & Hudley, C. (1992). An attributional approach to aggression in African-American children. In D. Schunk & J. Meece (Eds.), *Social perceptions in the classroom: Causes and consequences* (pp. 75–94). Hillsdale, NJ: Erlbaum.

Graham, S., Hudley, C., & Williams, E. (1992). Attributional and emotional determinants of aggression among African-American and Latino young adolescents. *Developmental Psychology, 28,* 731–740.

Graham, S., Weiner, B., & Benesh-Weiner, M. (in press). An attributional analysis of the development of excuse giving in aggressive and non-aggressive African-American boys. *Developmental Psychology.*

Graham, S., Weiner, B., Giuliano, T., & Williams, E. (1993). An attributional analysis of reactions to Magic Johnson. *Journal of Applied Social Psychology, 23*(12), 996–1010.

Gurtman, M. B. (1986). Depression and the responses of others: Reevaluating the reevaluation. *Journal of Abnormal Psychology, 95,* 99–101.

Hackett, G. (1987, March 30). Paying the wages of sin. *Newsweek,* p. 28.

Hale, C. L. (1987). A comparison of accounts: When is a failure not a failure? *Journal of Language and Social Psychology, 6,* 117–132.

Hamilton, V. L., Blumenfeld, P. C., & Kushler, R. H. (1988). A question of standards: Attributions of blame and credit for classroom acts. *Journal of Personality and Social Psychology, 54,* 34–48.

Hart, H. L. A. (1968). *Punishment and responsibility.* Oxford: Clarendon Press.

Hart, H. L. A., & Honoré, A. M. (1959). *Causation in the law.* Oxford: Clarendon Press.

Heider, F. (1958). *The psychology of interpersonal relations.* New York: Wiley.

Helman, C. G. (1978). "Feed a cold, starve a fever": Folk models of infection in an English suburban community and their relation to medical treatment. *Culture, Medicine, and Psychiatry, 2,* 107–137.

Herek, G. M. (1987). Can functions be measured? A new perspective on the functional approach to attitudes. *Social Psychology Quarterly, 50,* 285–303.

Hewstone, M. (1989). *Causal attributions: From cognitive processes to collective beliefs.* Oxford, England: Basil Blackwell.

Holtgraves, T. (1989). The form and function of remedial moves: Reported use, psychological reality and perceived effectiveness. *Journal of Language and Social Psychology, 8,* 1–16.

Holtzworth-Munroe, A. (1992). Attributions and maritally violent men: The role of cognitions in marital violence. In J. Harvey, T. Orbush, & A. L. Weber (Eds.), *Attributions, accounts, and close relationships* (pp. 165–175). New York: Springer-Verlag.

Holtzworth-Munroe, A., & Hutchinson, G. (1993). Attributing negative intent to wife behavior: The attributions of maritally violent versus nonviolent men. *Journal of Abnormal Psychology, 102,* 206–211.

Holtzworth-Munroe, A., Jacobson, N. S., Fehrenbach, P. A., & Fruzetti, A. (1992). Violent married couples' attributions for violent and nonviolent self and partner behaviors. *Behavioral Assessment, 14,* 53–64.

Hooley, J. M. (1987). The nature and origins of expressed emotion. In K. Hahlweg & M. Goldstein (Eds.), *Understanding major mental disorder: The contribution of family interaction research* (pp. 176–194). New York: Family Process.

Hortsman, B. (1990, January 8). Bay of Pigs press strategy ruled out for Reagan. *Los Angeles Times,* p. A3.

Hudley, C., & Graham, S. (1993). An attributional intervention to reduce peer-directed aggression among African-American boys. *Child Development, 64,* 124–138.

Huesmann, L. R. (1988). An information-processing model for the development of aggression. *Aggressive Behavior, 14,* 13–24.

Humphreys, K., & Rappaport, J. (1993). From the community mental health movement to the war on drugs. *American Psychologist, 48,* 892–901.

Ickes, W., & Kidd, R. (1976). An attributional analysis of helping behavior. In J. Harvey, W. Ickes, & R. Kidd (Eds.), *New directions in attribution research* (Vol. 1, pp. 311–334). Hillsdale, NJ: Erlbaum.

Islam, M. R., & Hewstone, M. (1993). Intergroup attributions and affective consequences in majority and minority groups. *Journal of Personality and Social Psychology, 64,* 936–950.

Jagacinski, C. M., & Nicholls, J. G. (1990). Reducing effort to protect ability: "They'd do it but I wouldn't." *Journal of Educational Psychology, 82,* 15–21.

Janoff-Bulman, R. (1979). Characterological versus behavioral self-blame: Inquiries into depression and rape. *Journal of Personality and Social Psychology, 37,* 1798–1809.

Janoff-Bulman, R., & Brickman, P. (1982). Expectations and what people learn from failure. In N. T. Feather (Ed.), *Expectations and actions* (pp. 207–240). Hillsdale, NJ: Erlbaum.

Jenkins, J. H., & Karno, M. (1992). The meaning of expressed emotion: Theoretical issues raised by cross-cultural research. *American Journal of Psychiatry, 149,* 9–21.

Johnson, M. (1991, November 18). I'll deal with it. *Sports Illustrated*, pp. 18–26.

Jones, E. E., & Berglas, S. (1978). Control of attributions about the self through self-handicapping strategies: The appeal of alcohol and the role of underachievement. *Personality and Social Psychology Bulletin*, 4, 200–206.

Jones, E. E., & Davis, K. E. (1965). From acts to dispositions: The attribution process in person perception. In L. Berkowitz (Ed.), *Advances in experimental social psychology* (Vol. 2, pp. 219–266). New York: Academic.

Jones, E. E., Farina, A., Hastorf, A. H., Markus, H., Miller, D. T., & Scott, R. A. (1984). *Social stigma*. San Francisco: Freeman.

Jung, C. G. (1933). *Modern man in search of a soul*. New York: Harvest Books.

Juvonen, J., & Murdock, T. B. (1993). How to promote social approval: The effect of audience and outcome on publicly communicated attributions. *Journal of Educational Psychology, 85*, 365–376.

Karasawa, K. (1991). The effects of onset and offset responsibility and affects on helping judgments. *Journal of Applied Social Psychology, 21*, 482–499.

Karasawa, K. (in press). An attributional analysis of reaction to negative emotions. *Personality and Social Psychology Bulletin*.

Katz, I., Hass, R. G., Parisi, N., Astone, J., McEvaddy, D., & Lucido, D. J. (1987). Lay people's and health care personnel's perceptions of cancer, AIDS, cardiac, and diabetic patients. *Psychological Reports, 60*, 615–629.

Katz, M. B. (1986). *In the shadow of the poorhouse: A social history of welfare in America*. New York: Basic Books.

Kelley, H. H. (1967). Attribution theory in social psychology. In D. Levine (Ed.), *Nebraska symposium on motivation* (Vol. 15, pp. 192–238). Lincoln: University of Nebraska Press.

Kelley, H. H. (1972). Causal schemata and the attribution process. In E. E. Jones, D. E. Kanouse, H. H. Kelley, R. E. Nisbett, S. Valins, & B. Weiner (Eds.), *Attribution: Perceiving the causes of behavior* (pp. 151–174). Morristown, NJ: General Learning.

Kelley, H. H. (1992). Common sense psychology and scientific psychology. *Annual Review of Psychology, 43*, 1–23.

Kerrick, J. S. (1969). Dimensions in the judgment of illness. *Genetic Psychology Monographs, 79*, 191–209.

Kidder, L. H., & Cohn, E. S. (1979). Public views of crime and crime prevention. In I. H. Frieze, D. Bar-Tal, & J. S. Carroll (Eds.), *New approaches to social problems* (pp. 237–264). San Francisco: Jossey-Bass.

Kinder, D. R., & Sears, D. O. (1981). Prejudice and politics: Symbolic racism versus racial threats to the good life. *Journal of Personality and Social Psychology, 40,* 414–431.

Kleinke, C. L., & Baldwin, M. R. (1993). Responsibility attributions for men and women giving sane versus crazy explanations for good and bad deeds. *The Journal of Psychology, 127,* 37–50.

Kluegel, J., & Smith, E. R. (1986). *Beliefs about inequality.* New York: Aldine.

Kojima, M. (1992). An analysis of attributional processes in helping behavior. *Bulletin of the Tamagawa Guken Junior College for Women, 17,* 57–83.

Kremer, J. E., & Stephens, L. (1983). Attributions and arousal as mediators of mitigation's effects on retaliation. *Journal of Personality and Social Psychology, 45,* 335–343.

Krull, D. S. (1993). Does the grist change the mill? The effect of perceiver's inferential goal on the process of social inferences. *Personality and Social Psychology Bulletin, 19,* 340–348.

Lam, D. H. (1991). Psychosocial family intervention in schizophrenia: A review of empirical studies. *Psychological Medicine, 21,* 423–441.

Lane, R. (1962). *Political ideology: Why the American common man believes what he does.* New York: Macmillan.

Langer, E., Blank, A., & Chanowitz, B. (1978). The mindlessness of ostensibly thoughtful action. *Journal of Personality and Social Psychology, 36,* 635–642.

Lao, R. C. (1970). Internal–external control and competent and innovative behavior among Negro college students. *Journal of Personality and Social Psychology, 14,* 263–270.

Larrance, D. T., & Twentyman, C. T. (1983). Maternal attributions and child abuse. *Journal of Abnormal Psychology, 92,* 449–457.

Lear, M. W. (1991, November 5). Shades of loneliness. *Family Circle,* pp. 70–73.

Leff, J., & Vaughn, C. (1985). *Expressed emotion in families: Its significance for mental illness.* New York: Guilford Press.

Levin, I. P., & Chapman, D. P. (1990). Risk taking, fame of reference, and characterization of victim groups in AIDS treatment decisions. *Journal of Experimental Social Psychology, 26,* 421–434.

Liebrand, W. B. G., Messick, D. M., & Wolters, F. J. M. (1986). Why are we fairer than others? A cross-cultural replication and extension. *Journal of Experimental Social Psychology, 22,* 590–604.

Light, R. (1973). Abuse and neglected children in America: A study of alternative policies. *Harvard Educational Review, 43,* 556–598.

Lin, Z. (1993). An exploratory study of the social judgments of Chinese college students from the perspective of attributional theory. *Acta Psychologica Sinica, 2,* 155–164.

Liu, J. H., Karasawa, K., & Weiner, B. (1992). Inferences about the causes of positive and negative emotions. *Personality and Social Psychology Bulletin, 18,* 603–615.

Long, A. (1990). *Dimensions of illness.* Unpublished doctoral dissertation, University of California, Los Angeles.

Lopez, S., & Wolkenstein, B. (1990). Attribution, person perception, and clinical issues. In S. Graham & V. Folkes (Eds.), *Attribution theory: Applications to achievement, mental health, and interpersonal conflict* (pp. 103–121). Hillsdale, NJ: Erlbaum.

Lussier, Y., Sabourin, S., & Wright, J. (1993). On causality, responsibility, and blame in marriage: Validity of the entailment model. *Journal of Family Psychology, 2,* 322–332.

MacAndrew, C., & Edgerton, R. B. (1969). *Drunken comportment: A social explanation.* Chicago: Aldine.

Mackenzie, M. (1984). *Fear of fat.* New York: Columbia University Press.

Maddox, G. L., Back, K. W., & Liederman, V. R. (1968). Overweight as social deviance and disability. *Journal of Health and Social Behavior, 9,* 287–298.

Madey, S. F., DePalma, M. T., Bahrt, A. E., & Beirne, J. (1993). The effect of perceived patient responsibility on characterological, behavioral, and quality-of-care assessments. *Basic and Applied Social Psychology, 14,* 193–213.

Mallery, P. (1991). *Attributions and attitudes towards AIDS.* Unpublished manuscript, University of California, Los Angeles.

Margolin, G., & Weiss, R. L. (1978). Comparative evaluation of therapeutic components associated with behavioral marital treatments. *Journal of Consulting and Clinical Psychology, 46,* 1476–1486.

Matsui, T., & Matsuda, Y. (1992). *Testing for the robustness of Weiner's attribution–affect model of helping judgments for exogenous impact.* Unpublished manuscript, Rikkyo University, Tokyo, Japan.

MacKinnon-Lewis, C., Lamb, M. E., Arbuckle, B., Baradaran, L. P., & Volling, B. L. (1992). The relationship between biased maternal and filial attributions and the aggressiveness of their interactions. *Development and Psychopathology, 4,* 403–415.

McClelland, D. C. (1961). *The achieving society.* Princeton, NJ: Van Nostrand.

McLaughlin, M. L., Cody, M. J. & Rosenstein, N. E. (1983). Account sequences in conversations between strangers. *Communications Monographs, 50,* 102–125.

Medvene, L. J., & Krauss, D. H. (1989). Causal attributions and parent–child relationships in a self-help group for families of the mentally ill. *Journal of Applied Social Psychology, 19,* 1413–1430.

Medway, F. J. (1979). Causal attributions for school-related problems: Teacher perceptions and teacher feedback. *Journal of Educational Psychology, 71,* 809–818.

Meehl, P. (1983). The insanity defense. *Minnesota Psychologist, 32*(Summer), 11–17.

Messick, D. M., Bloom, S., Boldizar, J. P., & Samuelson, C. D. (1985). Why are we fairer than others. *Journal of Experimental Social Psychology, 21,* 480–500.

Meyer, J. P., & Mulherin, A. (1980). From attribution to helping: An analysis of the mediating effects of affect and expectancy. *Journal of Personality and Social Psychology, 39,* 201–210.

Millman, M. (1980). *Such a pretty face: Being fat in America.* New York: Norton.

Morse, S. J. (1992). The "guilty mind"; Mens Rea. In D. K. Kagehiro & W. S. Laufer (Eds.), *Handbook of psychology and law* (pp. 207–229). New York: Springer-Verlag.

Murdock, G. P. (1980). *Theories of illness: A world survey.* Pittsburgh: University of Pittsburgh Press.

Nasby, W., Hayden, B., & dePaulo, B. M. (1980). Attributional bias among aggressive boys to interpret ambiguous social stimuli as displays of hostility. *Journal of Abnormal Psychology, 89,* 459–468.

Neff, J. A., & Husaini, B. A. (1985). Lay images of mental health: Social knowledge and tolerance of the mentally ill. *Journal of Community Psychology, 13,* 3–12.

Nicholls, J. G. (1975). Causal attributions and other achievement-related cognitions: Effects of task outcome, attainment value, and sex. *Journal of Personality and Social Psychology, 31,* 379–389.

Nicholls, J. G. (1976). Effort is virtuous, but it's better to have ability: Evaluative responses to perceptions of effort and ability. *Journal of Research in Personality, 10,* 306–315.

Nickel, T. W. (1974). The attribution of intention as a critical factor in the relation between frustration and aggression. *Journal of Personality, 42,* 484–492.

Osting, R. N. (1988, March 7). Now it's Jimmy's turn. *Time,* pp. 46–48.

Pence, E. C., Pendleton, W. C., Dobbins, G. H., & Sgro, J. A. (1982). Effects of causal explanations and sex variables on recommendations for corrective actions following employee failure. *Organizational Behavior and Human Performance, 29,* 227–240.

Perry, D. G., Perry, L. C., & Rasmussen, P. R. (1986). Aggressive children believe that aggression is easy to perform and leads to rewards. *Child Development, 56,* 700–711.

Piliavin, I. M., Rodin, J., & Piliavan, J. A. (1969). Good Samaritanism: An underground phenomenon? *Journal of Personality and Social Psychology, 13*, 289–299.

Pollock, N. L., & Hashmall, J. M. (1991). The excuses of child molesters. *Behavioral Sciences and the Law, 9*, 53–59.

Pryor, J. B., & Reeder, G. D. (1993). Collective and individual representations of HIV/AIDS stigma. In J. B. Pryor & G. D. Reeder (Eds.), *The social psychology of HIV infection* (pp. 263–286). Hillsdale, NJ: Erlbaum.

Pryor, J. B., Reeder, G. D., & McManus, J. A. (1991). Fear and loathing in the workplace: Reactions to AIDS-infected co-workers. *Personality and Social Psychology Bulletin, 17*, 133–139.

Pryor, J. B., Reeder, G. D., Vinacco, R., Jr., & Kott, T. (1989). The instrumental and symbolic functions of attitudes toward persons with AIDS. *Journal of Applied Social Psychology, 19*, 377–404.

Public opinion poll. (1987, July 7). *Newsweek*, p. 52.

Rabiner, D., & Gordon, L. (1992). The coordination of conflicting social goals: Differences between rejected and nonrejected children. *Child Development, 63*, 1344–1350.

Rabiner, D., & Gordon, L. (1993). The relationship between children's social concerns and their social interaction strategies: Differences between rejected and accepted boys. *Social Development, 2*, 83–95.

Reisenzein, R. (1983). The Schachter theory of emotion: Two decades later. *Psychological Bulletin, 94*, 239–264.

Reisenzein, R. (1986). A structural equation analysis of Weiner's attribution–affect model of helping behavior. *Journal of Personality and Social Psychology, 50*, 1123–1133.

Richardson, D. C., & Campbell, J. L. (1980). Alcohol and wife abuse: The effects of alcohol on attributions of blame for wife abuse. *Personality and Social Psychology Bulletin, 8*, 468–476.

Richardson, S. A., Hastorf, A. H., Goodman, N., & Dornbusch, S. M. (1961). Cultural uniformity in reaction to physical disabilities. *American Sociological Review, 26*, 241–247.

Riordan, C. A., Marlin, N. A., & Kellogg, R. T. (1983). The effectiveness of accounts following transgression. *Social Psychology Quarterly, 46*, 213–219.

Rippere, V. (1977). Commonsense beliefs about depression and antidepressive behavior: A study of social consensus. *Behavioral Research and Therapy, 15*, 465–473.

Rivers, P. C., Sarata, B. P. V., Dill, R., & Anagnostopulous, M. (1990). *Alcohol workers, mental health workers, school personnel, and judges' perception of deviant stereotypes: Implications for the caregiver-law interface.* Unpublished manuscript, University of Nebraska, Lincoln.

Roberts, C. F., Golding, S. L., & Fincham, F. D. (1987). Implicit theories of criminal behavior: Decision making and the insanity defense. *Law and Human Behavior, 11*, 207–232.

Rodin, M., Price, J., Sanchez, F., & McElligot, S. (1989). Derogation, exclusion, and unfair treatment of persons with social flaws. *Personality and Social Psychology Bulletin, 15*, 439–451.

Rolland, J. S. (1988). A conceptual model of chronic and life-threatening illness and its impact on families. In C. S. Chilman, E. W. Nunnally, & F. M. Cox (Eds.), *Chronic illness and disability: Families of in trouble series* (Vol. 2, pp. 17–68). Newbury Park, CA: Sage.

Roseman, I. J. (1984). Cognitive determinants of emotion: A structural theory. In P. Shaver (Ed.), *Review of personality and social psychology* (Vol. 5, pp. 11–36). Beverly Hills, CA: Sage.

Roseman, I. J., Spindel, M. S., & Jose, P. E. (1990). Appraisals of emotion-eliciting events: Testing a theory of discrete emotions. *Journal of Personality and Social Psychology, 59*, 899–915.

Rosenthal, N. B. (1984). Consciousness raising: From revolution to re-evaluation. *Psychology of Women Quarterly, 8*, 309–326.

Ross, L., & Nisbett, R. E. (1991). *The person and the situation.* New York: McGraw-Hill.

Rule, B. G., & Duker, P. (1973). Effects of intentions and consequences on children's evaluations of aggressors. *Journal of Personality and Social Psychology, 27*, 184–189.

Rule, B. G., & Nesdale, A. R. (1976). Emotional arousal and aggressive behavior. *Psychological Bulletin, 83*, 851–863.

Sacco, W. P., & Dunn, V. K. (1990). Effect of actor depression and observer attributions: Existence and impact of negative attributions toward the depressed. *Journal of Personality and Social Psychology, 59*, 517–524.

Sarbin, T. R. (1990). Metaphors and unwanted conduct: A historical sketch. In D. E. Leary (Ed.), *Metaphors in the history of psychology* (pp. 300–330). Cambridge, England: Cambridge University Press.

Schachter, S., & Singer, J. E. (1962). Cognitive, social, and physiological determinants of emotional state. *Psychological Review, 69*, 379–399.

Scheer, R. (1987, July 28). AIDS: Is widespread threat an exaggeration? *Los Angeles Times,* Pt.1, p. 9.

Schlenker, B. R. (1980). *Impression management.* New York: Brooks/Cole.

Schlenker, B. R., & Darby, B. W. (1981). The use of apologies in social predicaments. *Social Psychology Quarterly, 44*, 271–278.

Schmelkin, L. P., Wachtel, A. B., Schneiderman, B. E., & Hecht, D. (1988). The dimensional structure of medical students' perceptions of diseases. *Journal of Behavioral Medicine, 11*, 171–183.

Schmidt, G., & Weiner, B. (1988). An attribution–affect–action theory of behavior: Replications of judgments of help giving. *Personality and Social Psychology Bulletin, 14,* 610–621.

Schneider, W., & Lewis, I. A. (1984). The straight story on homosexuality and gay rights. *Public Opinion, 7,* 16–20, 59–60.

Schoeneman, T. J., Sergerstrom, S., Griffin, P., & Gresham, D. (1993). The psychiatric nosology of everyday life: Categories in implicit abnormal psychology. *Journal of Social and Clinical Psychology, 12,* 429–453.

Schopler, J., & Matthews, M. W. (1965). The influence of perceived causal locus of partner's dependence on the use of interpersonal power. *Journal of Personality and Social Psychology, 4,* 609–612.

Scott, M. B., & Lyman, S. M. (1968). Accounts. *American Sociological Review, 5,* 46–62.

Sears, D. O. (1988). Symbolic racism. In P. A. Katz & D. A. Taylor (Eds.), *Eliminating racism: Profiles in controversy* (pp. 53–84). New York: Plenum Press.

Sears, D. O., & Kinder, D. R. (1971). Racial tensions and voting in Los Angeles. In W. Z. Hirsch (Ed.), *Los Angeles: Viability and prospects for metropolitan leadership* (pp. 51–88). New York: Praeger.

Seyfarth, R. M., & Cheney, D. L. (1992, December). Meaning and mind in monkeys. *Scientific American,* pp. 122–128.

Shantz, D. W., & Voydanoff, D. A. (1973). Situational effects on retaliatory aggression at three age levels. *Child Development, 44,* 149–153.

Shaver, K. G. (1985). *The attribution of blame: Causality, responsibility, and blameworthiness.* New York: Springer-Verlag.

Shaver, K. G., & Drown, D. (1986). On causality, responsibility, and self-blame: A theoretical note. *Journal of Personality and Social Psychology, 50,* 697–702.

Shultz, T. R., Schleifer, M., & Altman, I. (1981). Judgments of causation, responsibility, and punishment in cases of harmdoing. *Canadian Journal of the Behavioural Science, 13,* 238–253.

Shultz, T. R., & Wright, K. (1985). Concepts of negligence and intention in the assignment of moral responsibility. *Canadian Journal of Behavioural Science, 17,* 97–108.

Siller, J. (1986). The measurement of attitudes toward physically disabled persons. In C. Herman, M. Zanna, & E. Higgins (Eds.), *Physical appearance, stigma, and social behavior: The Ontario symposium* (pp. 245–288). Hillsdale, NJ: Erlbaum.

Skitka, L. J., McMurray, P. J., & Burroughs, T. E. (1991). Willingness to provide post-war aid to Iraq and Kuwait: An application of the contingency model of distributive justice. *Contemporary Social Psychology, 15,* 179–188.

Skitka, L. J., & Tetlock, P. E. (1992). Allocating scarce resources: A contingency model of distributive justice. *Journal of Experimental Social Psychology, 28,* 491–522.

Skitka, L. J., & Tetlock, P. E. (1993a). Of ants and grasshoppers: The political psychology of allocating public assistance. In B. Mellers & J. Baron (Eds.), *Psychological perspectives on justice* (pp. 205–233). New York: Cambridge University Press.

Skitka, L. J., & Tetlock, P. E. (1993b). Providing public assistance: Cognitive and motivational processes underlying liberal and conservative policy preferences. *Journal of Personality and Social Psychology, 65,* 1205–1223.

Slaby, R. G., & Guerra, N. G. (1988). Cognitive mediators of aggression in adolescent offenders: I. Assessment. *Developmental Psychology, 24,* 580–588.

Slavin, R. E. (1983). *Cooperative learning.* New York: Longman.

Smith, C. A., & Ellsworth, P. C. (1985). Patterns of cognitive appraisal in emotion. *Journal of Personality and Social Psychology, 48,* 813–838.

Smyer, M. A., & Birkel, R. C. (1991). Research focused on intervention with families of the chronically mentally ill elderly. In E. Light & B. D. Lebowitz (Eds.), *The elderly with chronic mental illness* (pp. 111–130). New York: Springer.

Sontag, S. (1978). *Illness as metaphor.* New York: Farrar, Straus, & Giroux.

Spinetta, J. J., & Rigler, D. (1972). The child-abusing parent: A psychological review. *Psychological Bulletin, 77,* 296–304.

St. Lawrence, J. S., Husfeldt, B. A., Kelly, J. A., Hood, H. V., & Smith, S., Jr. (1990). The stigma of AIDS: Fear of disease and prejudice toward gay men. *Journal of Homosexuality, 19,* 85–99.

Staffieri, J. R. (1967). A study of social stereotypes of body image in children. *Journal of Personality and Social Psychology, 7,* 101–104.

Steele, B. F., & Pollack, C. B. (1968). A psychiatric study of parents who abuse infants and small children. In R. Helfer & C. H. Kempe (Eds.), *The battered child* (pp. 103–147). Chicago: University of Chicago Press.

Stermac, L. W., & Segal, Z. V. (1989). Adult sexual contact with children: An examination of cognitive factors. *Behavior Therapy, 20,* 573–584.

Stevenson, M. R. (1988). Promoting tolerance for homosexuality: An evaluation of intervention strategies. *Journal of Sex Research, 25,* 500–511.

Strasser, J. A., & Damrosch, S. (1992). Graduate nursing students' attitudes toward gay and hemophiliac men with AIDS. *Evaluation and the Health Professions, 15,* 115–127.

Stunkard, A. J., Sorenson, T. I. A., Hanis, C., Teasdale, T. W., Chakroaborty, R., Schull, W. H., & Schulsinger, F. (1986). An adoption study of human obesity. *New England Journal of Medicine, 314,* 193–198.

Teltsch, K. (1987, July 18). Foundations increase support for AIDS patients. *New York Times,* Pt.1, p. 9.

Titus, T. G., & Thompson, D. (1991). *The lay person's conceptualization of the causes of alcohol and drug dependency.* Unpublished manuscript, Spalding University, Louisville.

Tringo, J. L. (1970). The hierarchy of preferences toward disability groups. *Journal of Special Education, 4,* 295–306.

Triplet, R. G., & Sugarman, D. B. (1987). Reactions to AIDS victims: Ambiguity breeds contempt. *Personality and Social Psychology Bulletin, 13,* 265–274.

Trivers, R. L. (1971). The evolution of reciprocal altruism. *Quarterly Review of Biology, 46,* 35–57.

Turk, D. C., Rudy, T. E., & Salovey, P. (1986). Implicit models of illness. *Journal of Behavioral Medicine, 9,* 453–474.

Twentyman, C. T., & Plotkin, R. C. (1982). Unrealistic expectations of parents who maltreat their children: An educational deficit that pertains to child development. *Journal of Clinical Psychology, 38,* 497–503.

Van Lange, P. A. M. (1991). Being better but not smarter than others: The Muhammad Ali Effect at work in interpersonal situations. *Personality and Social Psychology Bulletin, 17,* 689–693.

VanderStoep, S. W., & Green, C. W. (1988). Religiosity and homonegativism: A path-analytic study. *Basic and Applied Social Psychology, 2,* 135–147.

Vaughn, C. E., & Leff, J. P. (1976). The influence of family and social factors on the course of psychiatric illness. *British Journal of Psychiatry, 129,* 125–137.

Wallack, J. J. (1989). AIDS anxiety among health care professionals. *Health and Community Psychiatry, 40,*507–510.

Watson, J. B. (1924). *Behaviorism.* New York: People's Institute.

Weber, J. (1993). *Patterns of intergroup attributional bias and intergroup conflict.* Unpublished doctoral dissertation, University of California, Los Angeles.

Weber, M. (1930). *The Protestant ethic and the spirit of capitalism.* New York: Scribner's Sons. (Original work published 1904)

Weiner, B. (1980a). A cognitive (attribution)–emotion–action model of motivated behavior: An analysis of judgments of help giving. *Journal of Personality and Social Psychology, 39,* 186–200.

Weiner, B. (1980b). May I borrow your class notes? An attributional analysis of judgments of help giving in an achievement-related context. *Journal of Educational Psychology, 72,* 676–681.

Weiner, B. (1985). An attributional theory of achievement-related emotion and motivation. *Psychological Review, 29,* 548–573.

Weiner, B. (1986). *An attributional theory of motivation and emotion.* New York: Springer-Verlag.

Weiner, B. (1988). An attributional analysis of changing reactions to persons with AIDS. In R. A. Berk (Ed.), *The social impact of AIDS in the U.S.* (pp. 123–132). Cambridge, MA: Abt Books.

Weiner, B. (1991a). Metaphors in motivation and attribution. *American Psychologist, 46,* 921–930.

Weiner, B. (1991b). On perceiving the other person as responsible. In R. A. Dienstbier (Ed.), *Nebraska symposium of motivation* (Vol. 38, pp. 165–198). Lincoln: University of Nebraska Press.

Weiner, B. (1992). Excuses in everyday interaction. In M. L. McLaughlin, M. J. Cody, & S. R. Reed (Eds.), *Explaining one's self to others* (pp. 131–146). Hillsdale, NJ: Erlbaum.

Weiner, B. (1993a). AIDS from an attributional perspective. In J. B. Pryor & G. D. Reeder (Eds.), *The social psychology of HIV infection* (pp. 287–304). Hillsdale, NJ: Erlbaum.

Weiner, B. (1993b). On sin versus sickness: A theory of perceived responsibility and social motivation. *American Psychologist, 48,* 957–965.

Weiner, B., Amirkhan, J., Folkes, V. S., & Verette, J. A. (1987). An attributional analysis of excuse giving: Studies of a naive theory of emotion. *Journal of Personality and Social Psychology, 52,* 316–324.

Weiner, B., & Brown, J. (1984). All's well that ends. *Journal of Educational Psychology, 76,* 169–171.

Weiner, B., Figueroa-Munoz, A., & Kakihara, C. (1991). The goals of excuses and communication strategies related to causal perceptions. *Personality and Social Psychology Bulletin, 17,* 4–13.

Weiner, B., & Graham, S. (1989). Understanding the motivational role of affect: Life-span research from an attributional perspective. *Cognition and Emotion, 3,* 401–419.

Weiner, B., Graham, S., & Chandler, C. C. (1982). Pity, Anger, and guilt: An attributional analysis. *Personality and Social Psychology Bulletin, 8,* 226–232.

Weiner, B., Graham, S., Peter, O., & Zmuidinas, M. (1991). Public confession and forgiveness. *Journal of Personality, 59,* 281–312.

Weiner, B., & Handel, S. J. (1985). A cognition–emotion–action sequence: Anticipated emotional consequences of causal attributions and reported communication strategy. *Developmental Psychology, 21,* 102–107.

Weiner, B., & Kukla, A. (1970). An attributional analysis of achievement motivation. *Journal of Personality and Social Psychology, 15,* 1–20.

Weiner, B., Perry, R. P., & Magnusson, J. (1988). An attributional analysis of reactions to stigmas. *Journal of Personality and Social Psychology, 55*, 738–748.

Weisman, A., Lopez, S. R., Karno, M., & Jenkins, J. (1993). Mexican American families with schizophrenia. *Journal of Abnormal Psychology, 102*(4), 601–606.

Whitley, B. E., Jr. (1990). The relationship of heterosexuals' attributions for the causes of homosexuality to attitudes toward lesbians and gay men. *Personality and Social Psychology Bulletin, 16*, 369–377.

Williams, S. (1984). Left–right ideological differences in blaming victims. *Political Psychology, 5*, 573–581.

Winer, D. L., Bonner, T. O., Jr., Blaney, P. H., & Murray, E. J. (1981). Depression and social attraction. *Motivation and Emotion, 5*, 153–166.

Wispé, L. (1991). *The psychology of sympathy.* New York: Plenum Press.

Wright, B. A. (1983). *Physical disability: A psychological approach* (2nd ed.). New York: Harper & Row.

Young, L. M., & Powell, B. (1985). The effects of obesity on the clinical judgments of mental health professionals. *Journal of Health and Social Behavior, 26*(3), 233–246.

Zucker, G. S., & Weiner, B. (1993). Conservatism and perception of poverty: An attributional analysis. *Journal of Applied Social Psychology, 23*, 925–943.

# Author Index

# Subject Index

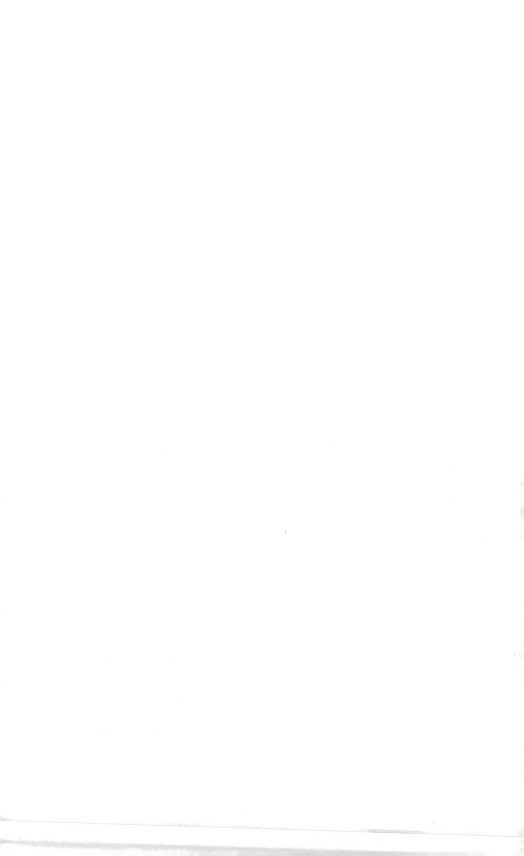